HEALTH MAINTENANCE FOR WOMEN: PERIODIC SCREENING GUIDELINES

Data	5-14	15-19	20-29	30-34	35-39	40	50	60	70
Interval physical exam and history:			q 3 yrs			q 2 yrs		q 1-2 yrs	
Professional breast exam			q 1-3 yrs						
Pelvic exam			q 1-3 yrs			q 1-2 yrs	q 1 yr		
Pap smear		q 1-3 yrs after 2 neg tests				q 1 yr			
Breast self-exam			Monthly			q 2 yrs		q 1 yr	
Blood pressure	At every visit					q 6 months-1 yr		q 6 months	
Laboratory/screening tests:									
HCT or Hgb		q 5 yrs unless otherwise indicated							
Total cholesterol		q 5 yrs if normal				q 3 yrs		q 1 yr	
Fasting blood sugar			q 3-5 yrs if within normal limits						
U/A and x-ray	When indicated								
Electrocardiogram						Baseline test, then q 5 yrs		q 3 yrs	
STD/TB screen	High risk only								
Other exams:									
Eyes including vision	Before starting school					q 3-5 yrs	q 1 yr		
Rectal exam/occult blood				q 5 yrs		q 1 yr			
Thyroid assessment						Baseline test	q 2 yrs		
Proctosigmoidoscopy							q 3-5 yrs		
Mammography: baseline at age 35					Baseline test	q 1 yr			
Endometrial sample in high-risk women at menopause							One baseline test; then as indicated		

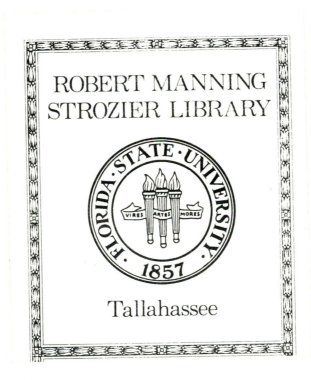

WOMEN'S HEALTH CARE

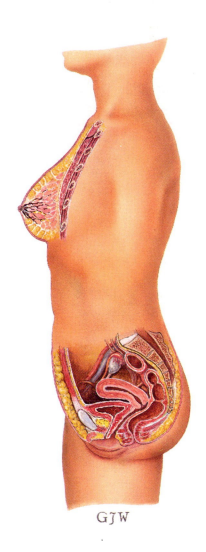

GJW

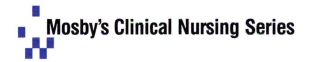

Mosby's Clinical Nursing Series

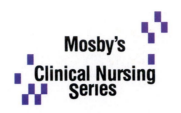

Mosby's
Clinical Nursing
Series

Cardiovascular Disorders
by Mary Canobbio

Respiratory Disorders
by Susan Wilson and June Thompson

Infectious Diseases
by Deanna Grimes

Orthopedic Disorders
by Leona Mourad

Renal Disorders
by Dorothy Brundage

Neurologic Disorders
by Esther Chipps, Norma Clanin, and Victor Campbell

Cancer Nursing
by Anne Belcher

Genitourinary Disorders
by Mikel Gray

Immunologic Disorders
by Christine Mudge-Grout

Gastrointestinal Disorders
by Dorothy Doughty and Debra Broadwell Jackson

Blood Disorders
by Anne Belcher

Ear, Nose, and Throat Disorders
by Barbara Sigler and Linda Schuring

Women's Health Care
by Valerie Edge and Mindi Miller

AIDS and HIV Infection
by Deanna Grimes and Richard Grimes

Skin Disorders
by Marcia Hill

WOMEN'S HEALTH CARE

VALERIE EDGE, RN, EdD

Nursing Faculty
North Harris College
Department of Human Performance and Health Sciences
Rice University
Houston, Texas

MINDI MILLER, RN, PhD

Department of Human Performance and Health Sciences
Rice University
Houston, Texas
M.L.A. Consultants
Conroe, Texas

Original illustrations by

GEORGE J. WASSILCHENKO
Tulsa, Oklahoma
and

DONALD P. O'CONNOR
St. Peters, Missouri

Original photography by

Patrick Watson
St. Louis, Missouri

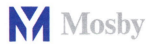

St. Louis Baltimore Boston Chicago London Philadelphia Sydney Toronto

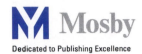

Publisher: *Alison Miller*
Editor: *Sally Schrefer*
Developmental Editor: *Penny Rudolph*
Project Manager: *Mark Spann*
Production Editor: *Melissa Martin*
Layout: *Celeste Clingan*

Composition by The Clarinda Company
Printed by Von Hoffmann Press

Printed in the United States of America

Mosby—Year Book, Inc.
11830 Westline Industrial Drive
St. Louis, Missouri 63146

Library of Congress Cataloging–in–Publication Data

Edge, Valerie.
    Women's health care / Valerie Edge, Mindi Miller.
      p.   cm.— (Mosby's clinical nursing series)
    Includes bibliographical references and index.
    ISBN 0–8016–8013–1
    1. Gynecologic nursing. 2. Gynecology. 3. Women—Diseases.
I. Miller, Mindi. II. Title. III. Series.
    [DNLM: 1. Genital Diseases, Female. 2. Women's Health. WP 140
E23w 1993]
RG105.E34 1993
618.1—dc20
DNLM/DLC
for Library of Congress   93–32614

93 94 95 96 97 CL/CD/VH 9 8 7 6 5 4 3 2 1   CIP

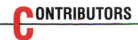

CONTRIBUTORS

Andrew W. Campbell, MD
Medical Director
Center for Immune, Environmental, and Toxic Disorders
Houston, Texas

Rae W. Langford, RN, EdD
Rehabilitation Nurse Consultant
Houston, Texas

Harriett Linenberger, RNC, MSN
Administrative Director
Hospital Education
Hermann Hospital
Houston, Texas

Mona Rae Merryman, RN, BSN, BA, CCRN
Critical Care Clinician
Long Beach, California
Adjunct Faculty
Mt. San Antonio College
Walnut, California

Christine L. Mudge-Grout, RN, MS, PNP, CNN
Clinical Nurse Specialist
Assistant Clinical Professor
University of California—San Francisco
San Francisco, California

Carol A. Norman, RN, MEd, MSN
Nursing Faculty
North Harris College
Houston, Texas

Helen M. Starkweather, RN, MSN
Nursing Faculty
North Harris College
Houston, Texas

Katherine Stefos, PhD, RPh
Division of Pharmacy
The University of Texas
M. D. Anderson Cancer Center
Houston, Texas

CONSULTANTS

Meryl Cohen, MEd
Director of Education and Training
Planned Parenthood of Houston
and Southeast Texas, Inc.
Houston, Texas

Vicki M. Dodson and Carole J. Leggett
Cancer Survivors and Cofounders of VIP Answering
Service and Franchise
Conroe, Texas

Joseph R. Feste, MD
Clinical Associate Professor
Department of Obstetrics and Gynecology
Baylor College of Medicine and
University of Texas School of Medicine
Houston, Texas

Phyllis Randolph Frye, Attorney
Executive Director
International Conference on Transgender Law and
Employment Policy, Inc.
Houston, Texas

M. Kay Garcia, RN, DrPH
Director
Occupational Health for Nurses
Southwest Center for Occupational and Environmental
Health
The University of Texas School of Public Health
Houston, Texas

Harriett Linenberger, RNC, MSN
Administrative Director
Hospital Education
Hermann Hospital
Houston, Texas

Frances Moncure, RN, PhD
Retired Professor of Nursing
AIDS Care Team Volunteer
Christ the King Lutheran Church
Houston, Texas

Martine Aliana Rothblatt, Attorney
Director for Health Law Project
International Conference on Transgender Law and
Employment Policy, Inc.
Houston, Texas

June M. Thompson, RN, MS, DrPH(C), CEN
Nursing Research
Children's Hospital
Columbus, Ohio

Marilyn Tompkins, RNC, FNP, MSN
Assistant Director
Lifecheq
The University of Texas
M. D. Anderson Cancer Prevention Program
Houston, Texas

Pam Wilson, RNC, FNP, MSN
Administrative Director
LifeCheq
The University of Texas
M. D. Anderson Cancer Prevention Program
Houston, Texas

Preface

Women's Health Care is the thirteenth volume in Mosby's Clinical Nursing Series, a new kind of resource for practicing nurses. The series is the result of the most extensive market research ever undertaken by Mosby. First we surveyed hundreds of practicing nurses to determine what kinds of resources they want to meet their advanced information needs. Next we asked clinical specialists, authors, and recognized experts to develop a format that would meet these needs. We presented their results to nine focus groups composed of working nurses and used their comments and suggestions to refine the format's organization and style. In the final stages we published a 32-page, full-color sample so that detailed changes could be made to improve physical layout and appearance, section by section and page by page. The result is a new genre of professional books for nursing professionals.

The goal of *Women's Health Care* is to present an overview of disorders that occur mainly in women, accompanied by guidelines for disease prevention and health promotion. The content focuses on the adult, nonpregnant female, although health issues throughout a woman's life span are discussed. The book primarily addresses conditions with high incident rates, although rare disorders are sometimes summarized to complete a discussion or to present information for comparison. The five-step nursing process is used to outline nursing care for both specific and general female disorders and health risks.

Chapter 1 begins with a colorful atlas of the female reproductive system. Illustrations of normal adult female anatomy and physiology are included so that abnormalities and pathophysiology can be contrasted in subsequent chapters.

Chapter 2 describes assessment data relevant to the health history of women. The physical examination of breast and gynecologic structures is depicted in a colorful, step-by-step pictorial guide.

Chapter 3 gives a full-color representation of diagnostic procedures used in women's health care, including MRI, CT, ultrasonography, and the latest endoscopic procedures, biopsy techniques, and laboratory tests. An easy-to-follow, consistent format allows quick referencing.

Chapter 4 centers on the symptomology that often occurs with female disorders. Pain, bleeding, and monthly variations are delineated.

Chapters 5 and 7 present information on structural and cellular variations of the breast and gynecologic organs. Illustrations include anatomic and histologic slides.

Chapters 6 and 8 describe breast and gynecologic cancers and discuss cancer detection and treatment choices.

Chapter 9 provides a summary of sexually transmitted diseases and other inflammatory processes. Illustrations show causative organisms, as well as physical symptoms, such as skin lesions.

Chapter 10 highlights systemic disorders that frequently afflict women and presents specific interventions for major disease processes.

Chapter 11 provides information relevant to fertility, infertility, and contraception, procreative choices are pertinent to all women during their reproductive years.

Chapter 12 describes some of the therapeutic and elective procedures and surgeries available to women. A few cosmetic options are presented, as well as traditional breast and gynecologic therapies.

Chapter 13 outlines breast, gynecologic, and systemic events that may occur during growth and development stages. Normal life-cycle parameters are contrasted with potential disorders.

Chapter 14 presents data for detecting and preventing health risks and addresses health promotion for daily living.

Chapter 15 is a collection of patient teaching guides for use during assessment and education sessions with female patients and their families. These guides are particularly useful for teaching self-examination techniques to women.

Chapter 16 presents pharmacologic guidelines for the treatment of some female disorders. The drug outlines help to identify areas where additional drug information may be needed.

Contents

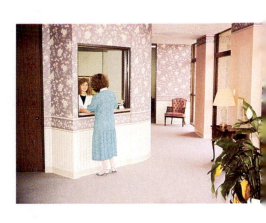

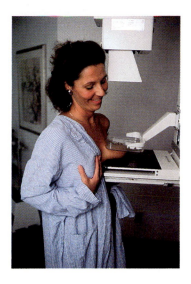

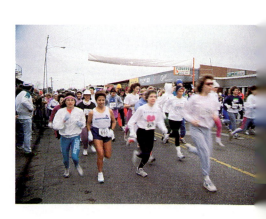

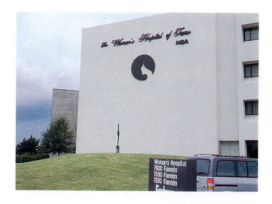

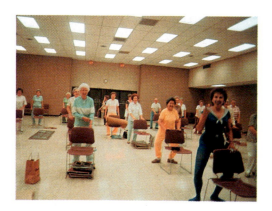

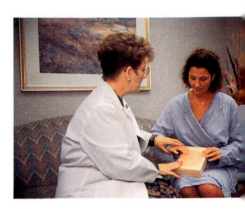

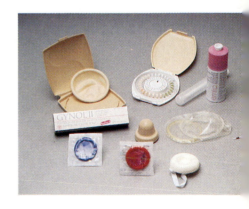

Color Plates

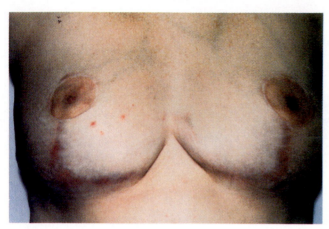

PLATE 1
Implant leakage resulting in prominent incision lines and flat breasts.

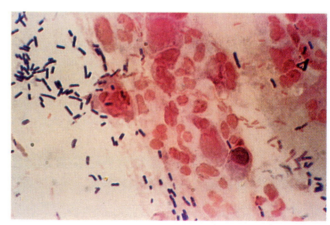

PLATE 2
Implant leakage resulting in breast asymmetry in size and shape and in differences in nipple directions.

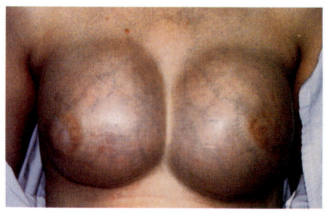

PLATE 3
Irritation and edema of breasts from implant material resulting in tight, grossly enlarged, shiny breasts.

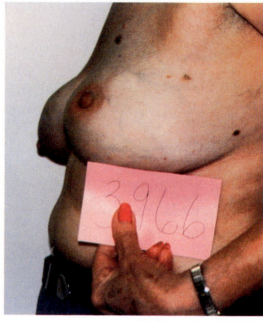

PLATE 4
Gram stain of normal vaginal flora with lactobacilli and gram-negative rods.

Color plates 4 through 16 courtesy The Centers for Disease Control, Atlanta, Ga.

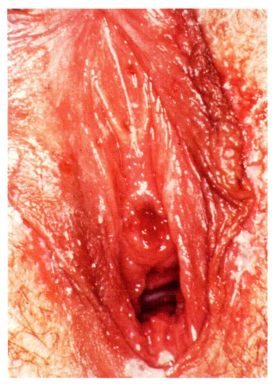

PLATE 5
Herpes infection of the labia.

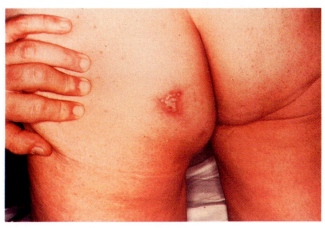

PLATE 6
Herpes infection of the buttocks.

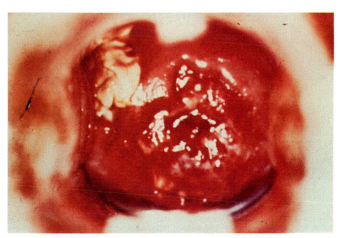

PLATE 7
Herpes infection of the cervix.

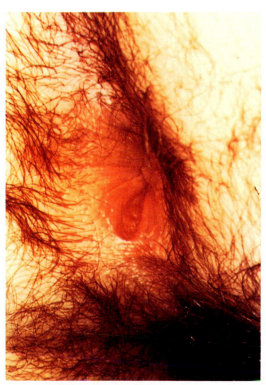

PLATE 8
Primary syphilis near the anus.

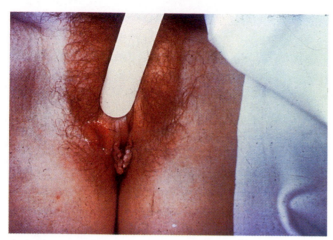

PLATE 9
Primary syphilis of the vulva with condyloma at bottom of labia near rectum.

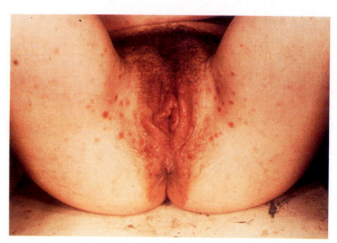

PLATE 10
Rash of secondary syphilis over vulva and thighs.

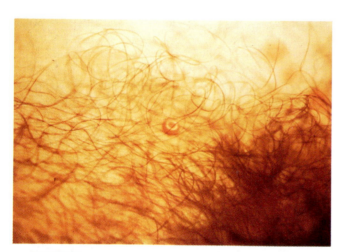

PLATE 11
Papule caused by molluscum contagiosum virus (MCV).

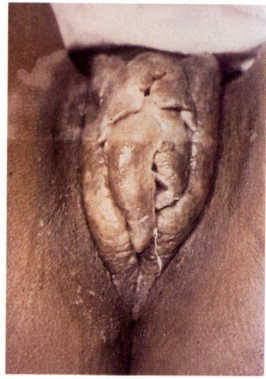

PLATE 12
Chronic lymphogranuloma venereum (LGV) causing genital elephantiasis.

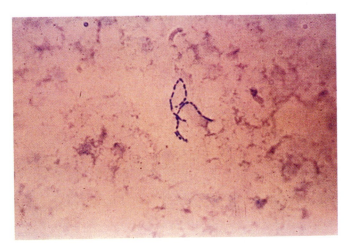

PLATE 13
Gram stain of H. ducreyi, which causes chancroid formation.

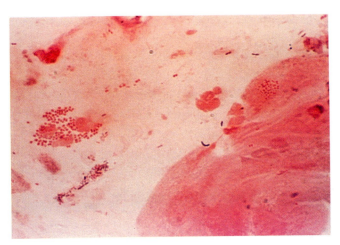

PLATE 14
Gram stain showing cervical gonorrhea.

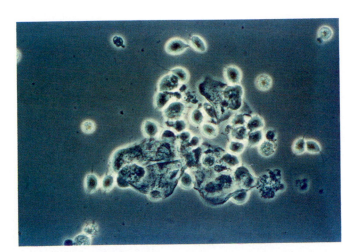

PLATE 15
Wet mount showing vaginal trichomoniasis.

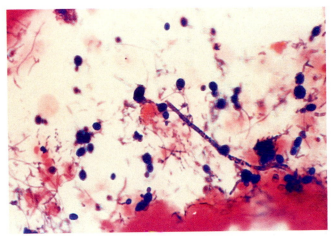

PLATE 16
Gram stain showing vaginal candida.

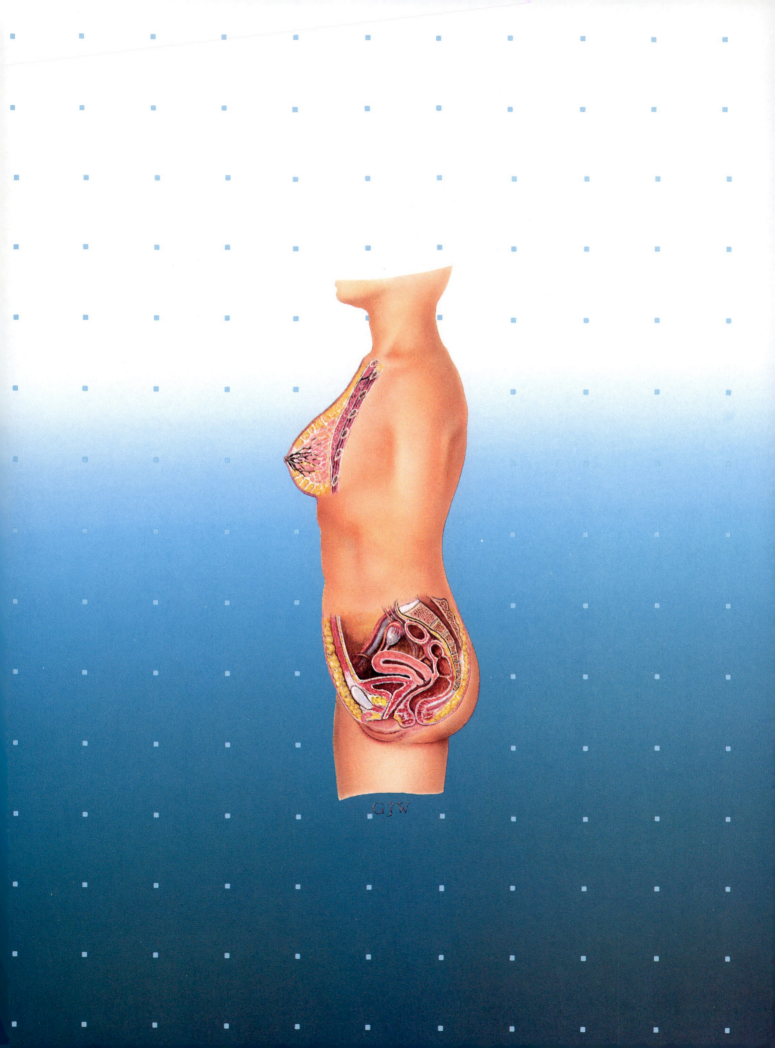

CHAPTER 1

Color Atlas of Female Anatomy and Physiology

Female anatomy and related physiology typically differ from those of males in the following areas: mammary glands; external genitalia; internal reproductive organs; and pelvic bone structure. Adult female mammary glands, or breasts, usually are larger than those of adult males, and female breasts produce milk during lactation. The female external genitalia, including the mons pubis, labia, and vestibule, provide support for copulation. Most of the female external genitalia cannot be seen if the outer fleshy folds of the labia majora are closed. Internal female organs, consisting of the ovaries, uterine tubes (oviducts or fallopian tubes), uterus, cervix, and vagina, are vital to procreation. Pelvic bone measurements are slightly different between the sexes; a woman's pelvis is wider than a man's to facilitate childbirth.

■Throughout the text, the terms *Fallopian* and *uterine* are used interchangeably.

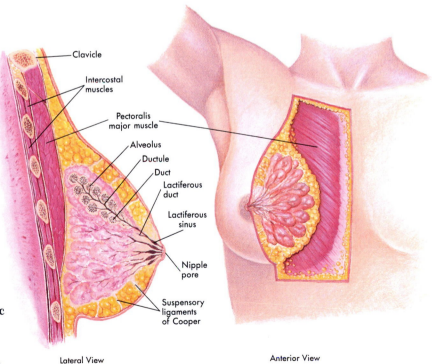

Clavicle
Intercostal muscles
Pectoralis major muscle
Alveolus
Ductule
Duct
Lactiferous duct
Lactiferous sinus
Nipple pore
Suspensory ligaments of Cooper

Lateral View

Anterior View

FIGURE 1-1
Major anatomic structures of the breast. (From Seidel.[96])

BREASTS

Mammary glands are similar to large sebaceous (sweat) glands. They consist of glandular lobes and adipose (fat) tissue. Female breasts are located between the parasternal and the anterior axillary lines, although breast tissue extends into the axilla and epigastrium. Breasts usually extend between the second and seventh ribs. Breast skin is smooth and contains hair follicles and sweat and sebaceous glands. Cooper's ligaments (connective tissue) support the breasts and attach them to the pectoral muscles.

The breasts are composed of lobes, lobules, and alveoli (Figures 1-1 and 1-2). Fifteen to 20 separate lobes (divisions) subdivide into several lobules, which further divide into 10 to 100 grapelike acini, or alveoli, which secrete milk during lactation. The lobes pass to the nipple via small lactiferous ducts. Each duct connects to only one triangular or pyramid-shaped lobe. Several ducts connect to the nipple, where they terminate in lactiferous sinuses (ampullae), giving the internal bud a spokelike, wheel appearance. The areola, a flat, darker area surrounding the nipple, contains the duct openings of Montgomery's glands, which form Morgagni's tubercles near the areolar periphery. Cooper's ligaments (connective tissue or thick fascial bands) support the breasts and attach them to the pectoral and serratus anterior muscles. These breast structures are surrounded by a fat layer. The amount of fat is determined by diet, estrogen, and heredity.

The epithelium of the breast reacts to hormonal fluctuations as does endometrial tissue. Water retention, vascular engorgement, enlarged ductal lumina, and increased secretory activity usually occur premenstrually. The cellular activity of the ducts increases during the follicular phase. During the luteal phase, the ductal system of the breast dilates, and alveolar cells become secretory cells. Areolar tissue responds to estrogen and progesterone stimulation.

During menstruation, the cellular activity of the alveoli (acini) decreases and breast ducts become smaller. However, during lactation, milk forms in the secretory cells of the alveoli, and the collecting ducts of the lobules transport milk from the alveoli to the excretory ducts of each lobe.

Breast tissue develops during adolescence. The amount of glandular tissue in the breast is about the same in all women. Differences in breast size result from the fat, or adipose tissue, deposits between the mammary gland and the connective tissue. Breast shape changes during the life span.

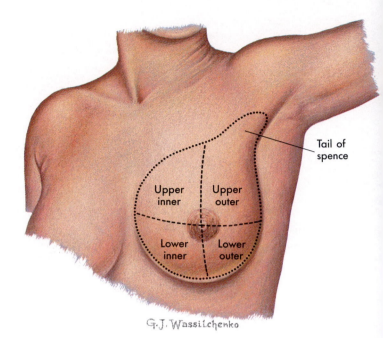

G.J. Wassilchenko

FIGURE 1-2
Quadrants of the left breast and axillary tail of Spence.

STRUCTURAL SUPPORT

The mammary glands (breasts) are located bilaterally on the anterior chest wall between the level of the second and seventh ribs. The upper two-thirds region is attached to the *pectoralis major muscle*, and the lower one-third region is attached to the *serratus anterior muscle* (Figure 1-3). The serratus anterior muscle supports or stabilizes the scapula on the chest wall. The largest muscle, the latissimus dorsi, spirals around the *teres major muscle*. Muscular tissue and the connective tissue of Cooper's ligaments support neural and blood structures.

BLOOD SUPPLY

The mammary gland (breast) receives a rich blood supply (see Figure 1-3). Most of the blood is supplied by the perforating branches of the *internal mammary (internal thoracic) artery*, which is a branch of the *subclavian artery* that descends vertically close to the sternum, sending out small branches that reach into the intercostal spaces. The *lateral cutaneous branches* of the anterior rami of the third, fourth, and fifth intercostal arterial branches provide the lateral breast area with a rich blood supply. Branches of the *axillary artery* supply the mammary and lower muscles: The *superior thoracic branch* supplies the pectoralis major muscle; the *pectoral branch of the acromiothoracic artery* supplies the pectoral muscle and overlying

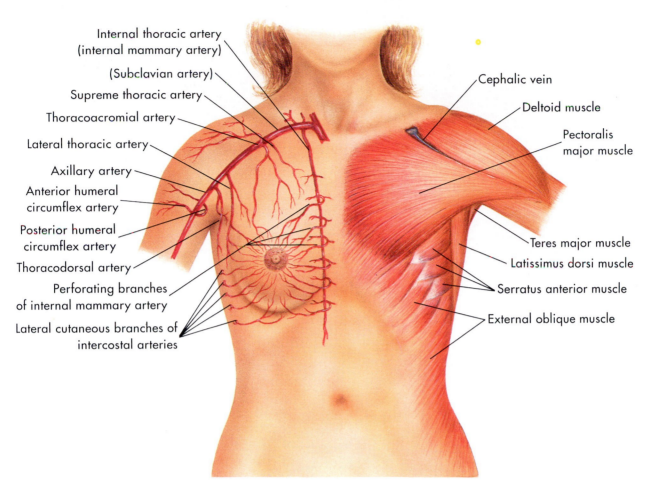

Internal thoracic artery
(internal mammary artery)

(Subclavian artery)

Supreme thoracic artery

Thoracoacromial artery

Lateral thoracic artery

Axillary artery

Anterior humeral
circumflex artery

Posterior humeral
circumflex artery

Thoracodorsal artery

Perforating branches
of internal mammary artery

Lateral cutaneous branches of
intercostal arteries

Cephalic vein

Deltoid muscle

Pectoralis
major muscle

Teres major muscle

Latissimus dorsi muscle

Serratus anterior muscle

External oblique muscle

FIGURE 1-3
Musculature and blood supply of the breast.

breast tissue; the *lateral thoracic*, or *external mammary artery*, extends downward along the lateral thorax to supply the lateral breast through branching, and the *subscapular branch* supplies the subscapular muscle and lateral breast. Additionally, a series of *anastomotic branches* between the lateral thoracic and mammary arteries ensure an abundant blood supply to the mammary gland. These branches also ensure an abundant blood supply to the nipple and surrounding area by forming a *circular plexus* around the areola. The mammary venous pattern follows the same pattern as the arterial supply. The circular venous plexus around the areola is referred to as the *circulus venosus*.

LYMPHATICS

The breast has an abundant network of lymph vessels (lymphatics) that drain breast tissue (Figure 1-4). The main lymphatic pathways travel upward and laterally, passing through lymph nodes along the way. Most breast lymphatics empty into 20 to 30 *central axillary lymph nodes*, which follow the course of the axillary

vein and empty into *subclavian lymph nodes*. The lymphatics that drain the central breast area pass through four to six *anterior pectoral nodes*, which are laterally located along the thoracic artery near the lateral pectoral region. These lymphatics empty into the central axillary nodes. The lymphatics that drain the medial breast area pass through the paramammary *route of Gerota* to the liver and *subdiaphragmatic nodes*. Additional deep fascial breast lymphatics drain through the *thoracoacromial vessels* to the subclavian lymph nodes *(Grozzman's pathway)*. Superficial mammary lymphatics drain to the opposite axillary lymphatics via the *cross-mammary pathway*. The lymphatics, particularly the central axillary lymphatics, are the main route of metastases for breast carcinoma and usually are removed during surgery.

INNERVATION

Sensory innervation of the breast is supplied by *cutaneous branching* of the *cervical* and *thoracic spinal nerves*. Cutaneous branches of the third and fourth

A

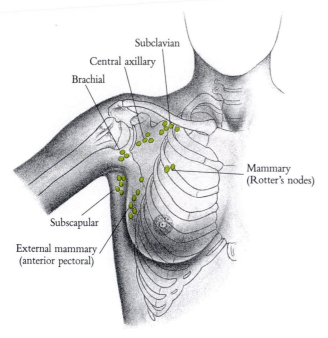

B

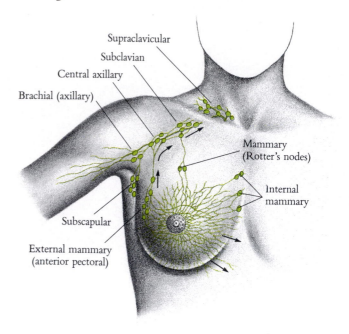

FIGURE 1-4
A, Lymph nodes of the axilla. **B,** Lymphatic drainage of the breast. (From Seidel.[96])

nerves of the cervical plexus pass downward to the anterior thorax, ending at the level of the second rib. These branches supply sensation to the upper breast area. The *thoracic spinal nerves,* T_3-T_6, form intercostal nerves and emerge near the sternum as branching cutaneous nerves. The *anterior cutaneous branches* emerge from the pectoralis major muscle near the sternum to supply sensation to the medial breast area, and the *lateral cutaneous branches* emerge from serrati muscles to supply sensation to the lateral breast area. The branching of T_2 enters the upper limb as the *intercostobrachial nerve* and supplies sensation to the axilla. Innervation of the areola and nipple is supplied by the *long thoracic nerve,* which has multibranched, bulbous endings.

EXTERNAL GENITALIA

Several terms are used in referring to the external female genitals, such as pudenda, perineum, and vulva. The *pudenda* generally refers to all visible external structures from the symphysis pubis to the perineum (Figure 1-5). The *perineum* is the area below the vaginal introitus (entrance or opening), which extends to the anus and contains the fourchette. The *vulva* refers to the labial folds and the enclosed structures within these folds. Typically the vulva includes the *mons pubis (mons veneris), labia majora* and *minora, clitoris,*

urethral opening, hymen (if present), and *vestibule* (entryway). The genitals may differ in appearance among women as a result of differences in size, shape, coloring, childbearing history, age, race, heredity, and hormonal influence. External structures are best observed when a woman assumes a semireclined position with the thighs apart.

The *mons pubis (mons veneris)* is a fat deposit below the umbilical area, over the pubic bone near the groin (junction of the thighs), and superior to the labia majora. Hair grows over the mons at puberty. This soft, fatty area may function to cushion the symphysis pubis during sexual intercourse, or coitus. *Mons veneris* means "mountain of Venus" (the Roman goddess of love) in Latin.

The *labia majora* (large lips) protect the underlying labia minora, urinary meatus, and vaginal introitus. The labia majora, which are thick and more pigmented (darker) than the surrounding structures, have a slight distribution of hair on the external surface. The inner, lateral surfaces are moist and smooth and contain sweat and sebaceous glands. The labia majora are sensitive, because they contain many nerve and vascular networks. When closed, the labia majora usually cover the labia minora.

The *labia minora* are additional folds located between the labia majora. They are moist, pink folds similar in texture to vaginal mucosa. The labia minora are very sensitive, since they are highly innervated and vascular. The connective tissue of the labia minora contains sebaceous glands that drain lubricating, bactericidal secretions onto this delicate tissue.

The *vestibule* is the space between the labia minora that is formed by the labia minora, clitoris, and

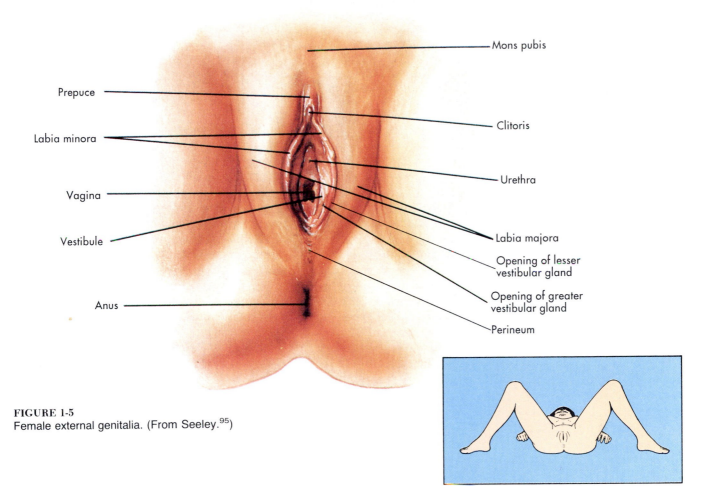

FIGURE 1-5
Female external genitalia. (From Seeley.[95])

Vagina Few nerve endings; anterior vaginal wall under the urethra analogous to the male prostate gland because fluid may be emitted during orgasm; attached to pelvic floor musculature and fascia

Mons pubis (mons veneris) Triangular escutcheon (coarse hair); cushionlike elevation over symphysis pubis; soft subcutaneous fatty (adipose) tissue; loose connective tissue; sebaceous (oil) glands

Clitoris Homologue of male penis, 0.5 cm, innervated, sensitive glans (tip); corpus (body) and two crura (elongation attached to inferior rami of pubis); vascular plexus (erectile tissue), sebaceous glands, nerves, and blood vessels; short, cylindric structure, about 6 x 6, 1.5 to 2 cm long; minora form prepuce above frenulum below clitoris

Vestibule Ovoid (boat shaped), enclosed by labia minora; houses urinary orifice (urethral meatus, hymen, and vaginal introitus)

Skene's glands (paraurethral or lesser vestibular glands) Inside urethral meatus

Bartholin's glands (vulvovaginal or greater vestibular glands) Paired structures, 1.5 cm long

Labia majora (pair) Labium majus (single fold); outermost rounded folds with hair; composed of adipose and connective tissue; sebaceous follicles on inner surfaces; extends from mons pubis to perinum, encircling vestibule

Labia minora (pair) Labium minus (single fold); hairless skin between majora; composed of connective tissue and nerves; extends from anterior frenulum (fold) of clitoris to posterior frenulum (merged folds) of labia

Perineum Muscular area with elastic fibers, fibrous tissue, and connective tissue; triangular area dorsal to pubic arch and superior to coccyx tip; lateral to pubic and ischial rami (hip bones); extends from fourchette (fold below vagina) to anus; supports distal sections of urogenital and gastrointestinal tracts

fourchette. The labia minora form the prepuce, which covers the clitoris. The anterior vestibule surrounds or houses other genital structures. Six openings are found within the vestibule: the vaginal introitus (orifice), hymen (if present), urethra (urinary orifice and meatus), and the paired ducts of Bartholin's and Skene's glands.

Clitoris is a Greek word that means "key," referring to the central part of female sexuality. The clitoris lies under the arch of the pubis. The tip, or glans, of the clitoris is very sensitive. The sebaceous glands of the tip secrete smegma, a cheeselike substance that may contain an erotic odor. Two corpora cavernosa (spongy erectile tissue) are located within the clitoris. These cylindric blood sinuses become engorged with blood and expand during sexual excitement.

The *prepuce* is a hoodlike covering in the lateral portion of the clitoris. It may look like a meatus or opening, but it is a closed structure. The *frenulum* of the clitoris is formed by the inner parts of the labia minora below the surface of the glans; the merged folded areas of the labia minora form this frenulum. The *fourchette* is a transverse skin fold found below the vaginal orifice, where the labia majora and labia minora meet. If the hymen remains intact, the depression between the hymen and the fourchette is known

as the *fossa navicularis.*

The *vaginal orifice* (introitus) is located in the lower end of the vestibule and may vary in size. Although the hymen may be completely or partly ruptured, remnants may be seen. Separation of the vaginal introitus and gaping of the labia are common after childbirth. The *urethral orifice* is a small, pink, vertical, puckered opening in the midline of the vestibule, anterior to the vaginal introitus, about 2.5 cm below the clitoris.

Skene's glands, also called the lesser vestibular glands or paraurethral glands, are located inside the urethral meatus. These glands produce a lubricating mucus. *Bartholin's glands*, also called the greater vestibular glands or vulvovaginal glands, are located in the posterior lateral aspect of the vaginal vestibule. Bartholin's glands produce an alkaline mucus during coitus that may promote sperm survival.

■NTERNAL REPRODUCTIVE ORGANS

The internal organs of the female reproductive system include the structures of the vagina, cervix, uterus,

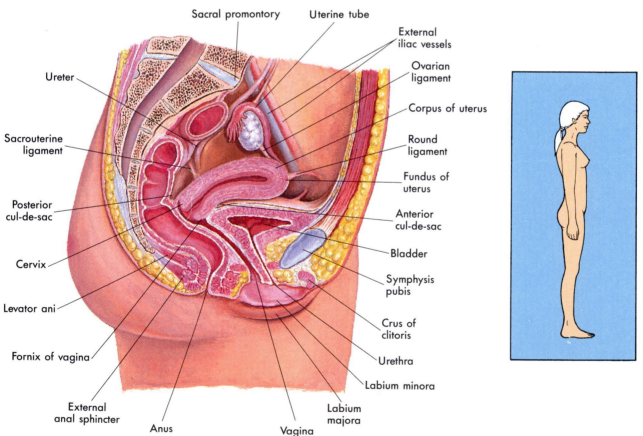

FIGURE 1-6
Midsagittal view of female pelvic organs. (From Seidel.[96])

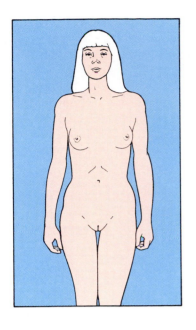

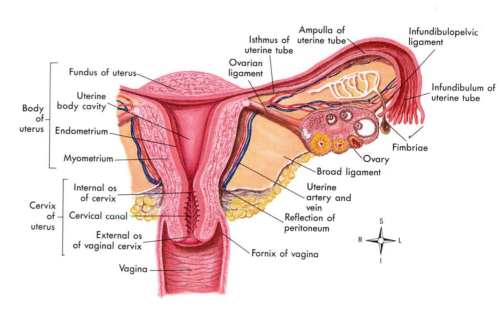

FIGURE 1-7
Cross-sectional view of internal female genitalia and pelvic contents. (From Seidel.[96])

uterine tubes (fallopian tubes or oviducts), and ovaries (female gonads). These organs are located within the somewhat protective bony pelvis in the lower pelvic cavity (Figures 1-6 and 1-7).

The *vagina* (birth canal) connects the vestibule of the external genitalia with the cervix of the uterus in the midpelvic area. The vagina lies between the bladder and the rectum and has a vestibular opening covered by a membranous tissue, called the hymen. The vagina is a thin-walled, collapsible, tubelike canal. It is 10 to 15 cm long and is made up of a smooth mucosal inner lining of moist, stratified squamous epithelium and a layer of smooth muscle covered with a glandular mucous membrane. The anterior wall (7 to 8 cm) is shorter than the posterior wall (9 to 10 cm), where the cervix is located. The vagina consists of four layers: the inner epithelial layer, which contains mucus-producing cells; the middle layer, which contains vessels, lymphatics, and nerves; the next layer, which contains smooth muscle; and the vascular outer layer, made up of connective tissue.

The *fornices* of the vagina are recessed areas that surround the cervix. The posterior fornix (the area nearest the rectum) is the deepest recess. The vagina has longitudinal folds and transverse ridges, or rugae, which allow it to stretch during coitus and childbirth. It also has a continual flow of vaginal secretions, which promotes self-cleansing. Removal of mucosal cells occurs mainly during menstruation and pregnancy. An acidic pH of 4 or 5 in the vagina protects against some

infections; pH is lower at midcycle and higher before menstruation. The vaginal mucosa responds to estrogen and progesterone stimulation. The vagina serves as the organ for sexual intercourse, as a duct for excreting menstrual flow, and as a birth canal.

The *cervix*, which connects the external os (opening) of the vagina with the internal os of the uterus, has a diameter and length of about 2.5 cm. It is composed of fibrotic connective tissue, elastic smooth muscle, and some muscle fibers. The cervix has few nerve endings, although women may experience sensations of pressure and stretching during childbirth. Mucus production by the cervix changes during the menstrual cycle and pregnancy in response to hormonal stimulation. The endocervical lining turns from pink to blue during pregnancy. The cervical os can stretch to 10 cm in diameter during labor.

The *uterus* (womb) is located in front of the rectum and behind the symphysis pubis and urinary bladder. It usually tilts anteriorly (forward) and is slightly anteflexed. When the bladder is full, the uterus moves backward toward the rectum; when the rectum is full, the uterus moves forward against the bladder. The uterus is an inverted (upside down), pear-shaped, hollow, flat, muscular, thick-walled organ. Its average dimensions are 7.5 × 3.5 × 2 cm, and it weighs about 56 g (2 ounces). The upper two thirds of the uterus is the corpus (the body or central section). The corpus is attached to the fundus (the upper rounded section), which contains the cornua (the portion where the fallopian tubes enter). The lower uterus contains the isthmus (uterine canal), which leads into the cervical and vaginal canals. The uterus can stretch from fist size to spaces capable of holding a full-term infant or several neonates.

The *uterine (fallopian) tubes* are held by the mesosalpinx. The infundibulum is the ovarian end of the expanded uterine tube. The ostium, the opening of the infundibulum, is surrounded by fimbriae, which direct the ova into the oviduct. The infundibulum leads to the ampulla, which narrows and becomes the isthmus. It attaches to the uterine tube that connects to the uterus. The uterine tube is made up of an inner mucosa with simple, ciliated columnar epithelium, a middle muscular layer, and an outer serosal layer.

STRUCTURAL SUPPORT

The uterus is supported by the broad, round, uterosacral and cardinal ligaments (transverse and Mackenrodt's ligaments) and by the anterior (pubocervical) ligament and the posterior (rectovaginal) liga-

ment. The posterior ligament forms a pocket called the cul-de-sac, or pouch of Douglas. The fundus (upper), corpus (body), and cervix (lower) uterus consist of expandable smooth muscle fibers. The uterus consists of three layers: the perimetrium, or outer layer, made up of serous membrane; the myometrium, or middle layer, made up of smooth muscle; and the endometrium, the inner mucous membrane that forms the interior wall of the uterus. The endometrial lining is shed during menstruation. A serous abdominal sac, the peritoneum, covers the uterus.

The ovaries are supported by the mesovarium, the broad ligament, and the suspensory and ovarian ligaments. The ovarian epithelium of the peritoneum and the tunica albuginea cover the ovaries.

The paired *ovaries* are divided into a medulla, which contains nerves, blood, lymph vessels, and a cortex, which contains follicles. Each healthy, productive ovary undergoes a monthly cell division (meiosis) to mature an ovum and release it from an ovarian follicle. This process is called ovulation. After ovulation, the follicle degenerates into a corpus luteum, which secretes progesterone, a hormone necessary for maintaining a rich, vascular endometrium, which is needed for implantation of a fertilized ovum.

Perineal support is provided by the *urogenital diaphragm* and the *levator ani, transverse perineal, bulbocavernosus,* and *ischiocavernosus* muscles (Figure 1-8). Four ligaments on each side support and position the uterus: the *round* (upper anterior), the *uterosacral* (lower posterior), the *cardinal or Mackenrodt's* (lateral), and the *broad* (dividing the pelvis into anterior and pos-

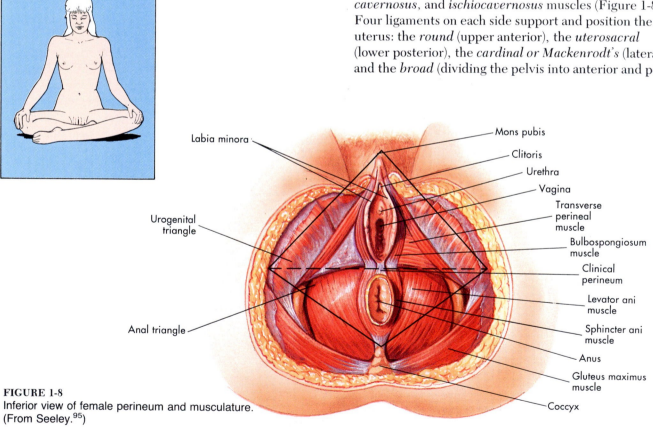

FIGURE 1-8
Inferior view of female perineum and musculature. (From Seeley.[95])

Labia minora

Urogenital triangle

Anal triangle

Mons pubis

Clitoris

Urethra

Vagina

Transverse perineal muscle

Bulbospongiosum muscle

Clinical perineum

Levator ani muscle

Sphincter ani muscle

Anus

Gluteus maximus muscle

Coccyx

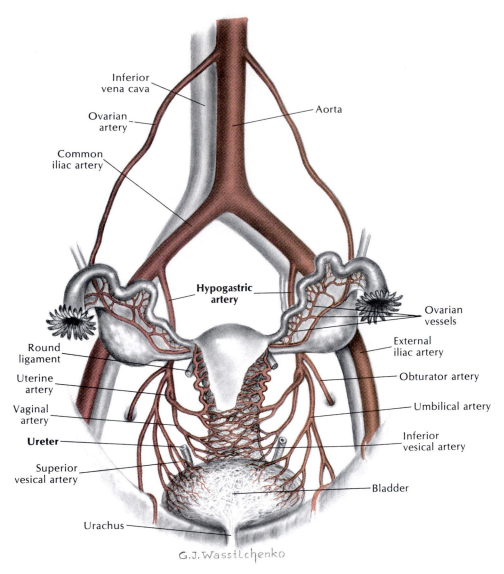

Inferior
vena cava

Ovarian
artery

Common
iliac artery

Aorta

**Hypogastric
artery**

Ovarian
vessels

Round
ligament

External
iliac artery

Uterine
artery

Obturator artery

Vaginal
artery

Umbilical artery

Ureter

Inferior
vesical artery

Superior
vesical artery

Bladder

Urachus

G.J. Wassilchenko

FIGURE 1-9
Pelvic blood supply. (From Bobak.[13])

terior regions). Two single ligaments, the *anterior pu-bosacral* ligament and the *posterior rectovaginal* ligament, support the lower uterine region. The ovaries and oviducts lie embedded between sheaths of the broad ligament. Both the ovaries and oviducts are somewhat supported by the broad ligament but the oviducts receive support from the *mesovarian* ligament, and the ovaries also receive support from the *suspensory* and *ovarian* ligaments. The vagina is supported by the pelvic floor musculature. The bony *pelvis* surrounds and protects the internal structures. It consists of the two *innominate* bones, the *sacrum* and the *coccyx*, which are held together by ligaments that stretch during childbirth.

BLOOD SUPPLY

The reproductive organs have an abundant blood supply (Figure 1-9). Bifurcation of the *common iliac artery* gives rise to the *anterior hypogastric (internal iliac) artery*, from which the *uterine artery* arises to supply the uterus. On each side, the *ascending branch* of the uterine artery passes through the broad ligament, forming *anterior* and *posterior branches* that supply the uterine body (corpus) and cervix. The corresponding *descending branch* divides into several branches along the uterine body and further branches into the myometrium and endometrium, ensuring a rich blood supply. Additionally, the uterine artery's descending branch joins the *vaginal artery*, giving the vagina a rich blood supply.

The *internal iliac artery* continues though the pelvis as the *internal pudendal artery, the artery of the clitoris,* and the *perineal arteries,* supplying the vagina and external genitalia. The *external iliac artery* and extensions of the *femoral artery* supply the labia. The *ovarian artery* travels downward through the broad ligament to the ovary, where it sends several branches to supply the ovary. The main artery continues inward to the uterus to join with the *uterine artery,* giving the uterus a rich dual blood supply. Venous blood returns through the *uterovaginal plexus* and the *pudendal* and *vaginal veins* to the *uterine veins,* which travel the same course as the uterine arteries. The right uterine vein empties into the inferior vena cava, whereas the left uterine vein must first empty into the left *renal vein.*

LYMPHATICS

Several chains of lymph nodes follow the major arterial systems, including the *femoral, internal, external common iliac, superficial* and *deep inguinal, lumbar,* and *paraaortic nodes* (Figure 1-10). The uterus contains three lymphatic networks near the endometrium, myometrium, and peritoneal areas. The lymphatics of the *uterine corpus (body)* occur as four or five pathways. These pathways are located below the oviducts and travel upward along the ovarian blood vessels that commute with ovarian lymphatics to empty into *internal* and *external iliac nodes* and the *superficial inguinal nodes.* The lymphatics of the *lower uterine* segment join *cervical* lymphatics, which empty into the *obturator* and *iliac lymph nodes.* The lymphatics that drain the *upper uterus (fundus), oviducts,* and *ovaries* follow the ovarian veins to empty into *lumbar (paraaortic) lymph nodes.* The lymphatics of the external genitalia empty into the *superficial inguinal lymph nodes.*

INNERVATION

The reproductive organs are supplied by nerves from the *lumbosacral plexus* (L_1-L_4), whose principal branches innervate the external genitalia via the *ilioinguinal branch* and the *genitofemoral branch.* The *sacral plexus* ($L_{4,5}$ and $S_{1,2,3}$) also innervates the reproductive organs via the *pudendal plexus.* The main nerve of the pudendal plexus, the *pudendal nerve,* branches at $S_{2,3,4}$ to form the *interior hemorrhoidal branch,* which supplies the labia majora, and the *dorsal nerve of the clitoris,* which supplies the dorsal and distal external genitalia. Afferent and efferent fibers function independently of the autonomic nervous sys-

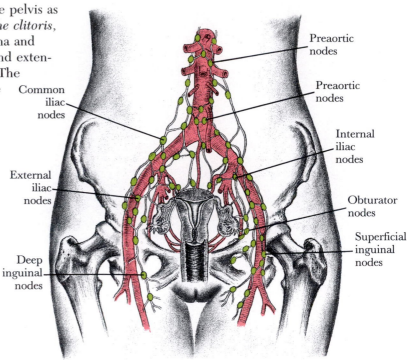

FIGURE 1-10
Lymphatic drainage of the female genital tract. (From Seidel.[96])

tem. Efferent fibers pass from the dorsal ganglia of the eleventh and twelfth thoracic spinal roots downward through the *aortic, hypogastric,* and *pelvic (uterovaginal) plexuses* to innervate uterine smooth muscle at the base of the uterosacral ligament. Afferent fibers travel upward through the same plexus pathway to the dorsal roots of the eleventh and twelfth thoracic spinal roots, where they continue to the thalamus. The ovaries are innervated through the *aortic-ovarian plexus,* and the relatively insensitive vagina receives minimal innervation via the *pudendal plexus.*

MENSTRUAL CYCLE

The hypothalamus and pituitary in the brain and the ovaries in the pelvis are the main sites of regulation of the menstrual cycle (Figure 1-11). The complex sequence of events that produces menses is thought to be controlled by the hormones produced within the very follicle destined to ovulate.

The hypothalamus directs the pulsatile secretion of gonadotropin-releasing hormone (GnRH) in a critical frequency and concentration. This stimulates the pituitary to produce follicle-stimulating hormone (FSH)

THE MENSTRUAL CYCLE

Menstrual phase: Days 1 to 4

Ovary:	Estrogen levels begin to rise, preparing follicle and egg for next cycle.
Uterus:	Progesterone stimulates endometrial prostaglandins that cause vasoconstriction; upper layers of endometrium shed.
Breast:	Cellular activity in the alveoli decreases; breast ducts shrink.
Central nervous system (CNS) hormones:	FSH and LH levels decrease.
Symptom:	Menstrual bleeding may vary, depending on hormones and prostaglandins.

Postmenstrual, preovulatory phase: Days 5 to 12

Ovary:	Ovary and maturing follicle produce estrogen. *Follicular phase* —egg develops within follicle.
Uterus:	*Proliferative phase* —uterine lining thickens.
Breast:	Parenchymal proliferation (increased cellular activity) of breast ducts occurs.
CNS hormone:	FSH stimulates ovarian follicular growth.

Ovulation: Day 13 or 14

Ovary:	Egg is expelled from follicle into abdominal cavity and is drawn into the uterine (fallopian) tube by fimbriae and cilia; follicle closes and begins to form corpus luteum. Fertilization of egg may occur in outer one third of tube if sperm are unimpeded.
Uterus:	End of proliferative phase; progesterone causes further thickening of the uterine wall.
CNS hormones:	LH and estrogen levels increase rapidly; LH surge stimulates release of egg.
Symptom:	Mittelschmerz may occur with ovulation; cervical mucus is increased and is stringy and elastic (spinnbarkeit).

Secretory phase: Days 15 to 20

Ovary:	Egg (ovum) is moved by cilia into the uterus.
Uterus:	After the egg is released, the follicle becomes a corpus luteum; secretion of progesterone increases and predominates.
CNS hormones:	LH and FSH decrease.

Premenstrual, luteal phase: Days 21 to 28

Ovary:	If implantation does not occur, the corpus luteum degenerates. Progesterone production decreases, and estrogen production drops and then begins to rise as a new follicle develops.
Uterus:	Menstruation starts around day 28, which begins *day 1* of the menstrual cycle.
Breast:	Alveolar breast cells differentiate into secretory cells.
CNS hormones:	Increased levels of GnRH cause increased secretion of FSH.
Symptoms:	Vascular engorgement and water retention may occur.

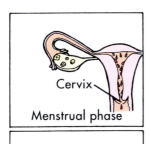

Cervix

Menstrual phase

Lining of uterus

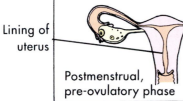

Postmenstrual, pre-ovulatory phase

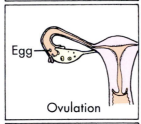

Egg

Ovulation

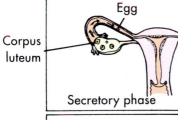

Egg

Corpus luteum

Secretory phase

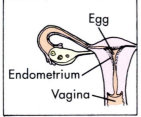

Egg

Endometrium

Vagina

Premenstrual, luteal phase

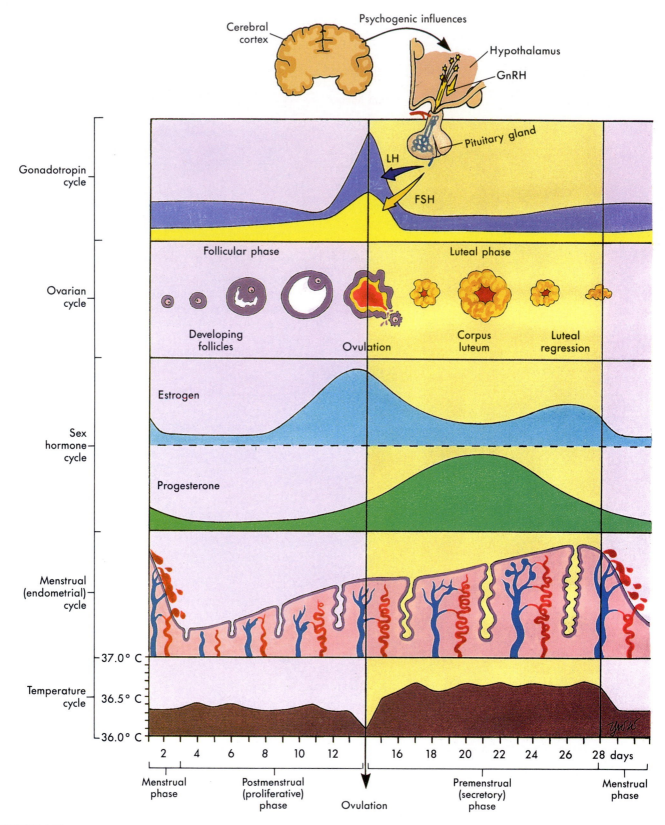

FIGURE 1-11
Female menstrual cycle. The diagram shows the interrelationship of the cerebral, hypothalamic, pituitary, ovarian, and uterine functions throughout a standard 28-day menstrual cycle. The variations in basal body temperature are also shown. (From Thibodeau.[103])

MAJOR HORMONES AFFECTING THE FEMALE REPRODUCTIVE ORGANS

Central nervous system hormones

Luteinizing hormone (LH)—Acts in conjunction with follicle-stimulating hormone to cause maturation of the follicle and ovum, release of estrogen, and ovulation.

Follicle-stimulating hormone (FSH)—Stimulates the ovarian follicles to mature and secrete estrogen.

Gonadotropin-releasing hormone (GnRH)—Stimulates LH and FSH.

Ovarian hormones

Estrogen and progesterone—Steroids that stimulate development of secondary sexual characteristics; these hormones also decrease GnRH levels after ovulation.

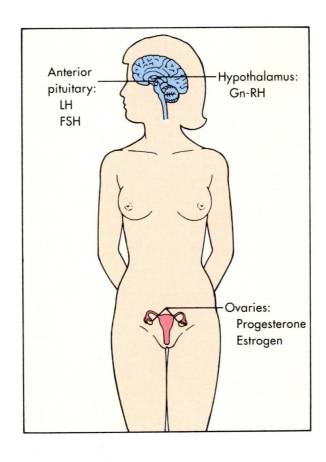

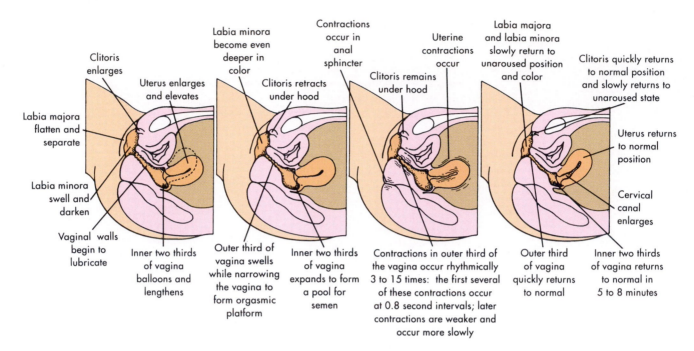

FIGURE 1-12
Female sexual response.

and luteinizing hormone (LH). The follicles in the ovaries respond to the increased levels of FSH by producing increasing amounts of estrogen. Likewise, LH increases steadily to a surgelike burst at midcycle that is essential for ovulation.

After ovulation, LH promotes the development of the corpus luteum from the follicle that produced the egg. The corpus luteum produces all three classes of sex steroidal hormones: androgens, estrogens, and progestins. Normally the progesterone level rises sharply after ovulation, reaching a peak 8 days after the LH surge, and then declines rapidly, resulting in menses.

FEMALE SEXUAL RESPONSE

The female sex drive is stimulated by steroids from the ovaries and androgens from the adrenal gland (Figure 1-12). Parasympathetic responses activate the erectile tissue of the clitoris and produce engorgement of blood in the bulb of the vestibule. The vaginal introitus tightens and simultaneously begins to secrete mucus from glands beneath the labia minora and in the vagina. The resulting vaginal lubrication facilitates entry of the penis during intercourse. A controversial "erotic" zone, called the "G-spot," has been described near the anterior vaginal wall below the urethra. Some professionals consider the G-spot to be analogous to the male prostate gland. These professionals say the G-spot may be aroused to orgasm and ejaculation of prostatic-like fluid into the urethra during sexual stimulation. However, the existence of the G-spot is regarded with considerable skepticism, because the data supporting it are inconsistent.

CHAPTER 2

Assessment

An evaluation specific to women begins with a detailed history, followed by systematic physical examination of the breasts, genitalia, and pelvic organs. These findings are supplemented with relevant diagnostic and laboratory tests. Nonverbal and verbal behavior should also be assessed. Breast and gynecologic examinations are parts of the total health assessment that should be included in routine or yearly physical evaluations.

HISTORY

Obtaining the patient's health history serves two purposes. First, it gives the woman time to become comfortable with the examiner. Second, the data obtained provide direction for a more thorough examination of possible health problems. Risk factors associated with breast, endometrial, cervical, and ovarian cancer can be assessed, and additional diagnostic procedures performed as indicated by the history. Although breast and gynecologic health histories concentrate on factors specific to women, a broad range of data is collected to identify interrelated risks or disorders. For example, the endocrine system directly affects cyclic events, such as menstruation. The breast and gynecologic histories often are taken together. Therefore information may be collected once and used for both the gynecologic and the breast assessments.

BREAST ASSESSMENT

The physical examination of the breasts is done after the breast and gynecologic histories have been taken.

PATIENT CONSIDERATIONS

Because the history and physical examination can be embarrassing for a woman, the nurse should be sure to provide a private, comfortable environment. All procedures should be adequately explained, and the patient should be encouraged to ask questions. Women often are knowledgeable about their health needs or risk factors, and their self-examinations and opinions should not be discounted or discredited.

Provide a warm room and adequate lighting. The patient may be more comfortable if she begins by demonstrating how she performs breast self-examination. Use a sheet or gown to cover areas that do not need to be exposed.

Hand washing before any examination is imperative to control infection. Before beginning the examination, assemble all equipment that may be needed: gloves, glass slide, and cytologic fixative (if nipple discharge is present); small pillow or folded towel; flashlight for transillumination; and ruler (if lump is present).

To examine the breasts and axillae thoroughly, the

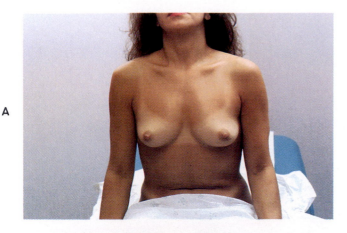

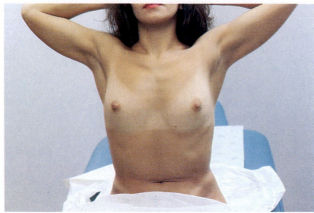

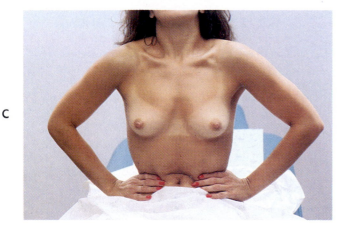

FIGURE 2-1
Patient positions for inspection of breasts. **A,** Patient sits with arms loosely at sides. **B,** Patient extends arms over head. **C,** Patient presses hands on hips. **D,** Patient clasps hands together in front of chest.

nurse uses inspection and palpation techniques. A four-quadrant breast diagram may be used to document findings (see Figure 1-2). The patient must assume a variety of positions to allow adequate inspection of the mammary, axillary, and supraclavicular regions. Contraction of the pectoral muscles and pulling of the suspensory ligaments may help exaggerate abnormalities. Retractions are more readily observed when the hands are placed against the hips or raised above the head. Changes in the lower skinfold (inframammary fold) are more pronounced when the arms are raised. Dusting a light coating of talc on the examiner's fingers may reduce friction and aid in palpating deep breast tissue.

Explain each part of the examination as it is being performed. Besides being courteous, this helps to teach or review the steps of breast self-examination (BSE).

INSPECTION

Inspect the breasts as the woman assumes the following positions (Figure 2-1):

Sits or stands with arms held loosely at her sides
Extends arms over her head
Presses hands on hips or pushes hands together in front of chest
Sits and leans over
Assumes a supine position with hands behind (not above) her head

Inspect both breasts, areolae, and nipples, and compare them for:

Size, symmetry, and position
Contour or bulging
Skin color or presence of erythema
Skin texture or smoothness
Venous patterns
Lesions or rashes
Nipple inversion, eversion, retraction, or dimpling
Bleeding, discharge, ulcerations, or edema
Supernumerary nipples

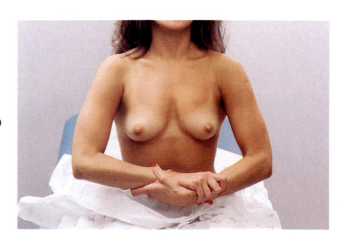

BREAST HEALTH HISTORY

General considerations

These general considerations pertain to an adult woman. Menopausal data would be addressed if appropriate for the patient's age. From the outset any complaint of breast, chest, and axillary pain or unusual breast symptoms should be noted. The dates and results of the last breast examination, mammogram, or other diagnostic studies should be listed.

Patient's age

Any changes in breast characteristics: pain, tenderness, lumps, discharge, skin changes, changes in size or shape

Changes in the breast that occur with the menstrual cycle: tenderness, swelling, pain, enlarged nodes

Date of first day of last menstrual period

Menopause: onset, course, associated problems, residual problems

Breast support used with strenuous exercise or sports activities

Skin irritation under pendulous breasts from tissue-to-tissue contact or from rubbing of bra

Medications, particularly oral contraceptives or other hormones: name, dosage, length of time used

Caffeine intake

Breast self-examination: frequency; when done in the menstrual cycle (have patient describe her procedure)

Risk factors for benign breast disease

Risk factors for breast cancer

Past medical history

Previous breast disease or conditions: cancer, stage, neoplasms, histologic type, fibrocystic changes, infections, trauma, lesions, epithelial proliferative lesions, unilateral/bilateral descriptions

Surgery: breast biopsies, aspirations, implants, reduction plasties, oophorectomy; if previous bilateral augmentation mammoplasty (BAM) has been done, note type of implant material (silicone gel–filled implants require further evaluation, such as autoimmune risks)

Menstrual history: age of menarche or menopause; cycle length and regularity; duration and amount of flow; associated breast symptoms (nipple discharge, pain or discomfort)

Pregnancy: age at each pregnancy, length of each pregnancy, date of delivery or termination

Lactation: number of children breast-fed; duration of time for breast-feeding; date of termination of last breast-feeding; medications used to suppress lactation

Past use of endogenous or exogenous hormones: name and dosage, reason for use (contraception, menstrual control, relief of menopausal symptoms), length of time hormones were used, date of termination

Exposure to diethylstilbestrol (DES) or other potential toxins

Previous medical records may need to be obtained concerning the patient and the women in her family

Family history

Breast cancer: which relative was affected (particularly mother or sister); type of cancer; age at time of occurrence; treatment and results

Other breast disease in female or male relatives: type of disease; age at time of occurrence; treatment and results

Current problem (if applicable)

Breast discomfort
- Temporal sequence: gradual or sudden onset; length of time symptom has been present; does symptom come and go, or is it always present
- Relationship to menses: timing, severity
- Character: stinging, pulling, burning, drawing, stabbing, aching, throbbing; unilateral or bilateral; localization; radiation
- Associated symptoms: lump or mass, discharge from nipple
- Contributory factors: skin irritation under breasts from irritants; strenuous activity; recent injury

Breast mass or lump
- Temporal sequence: length of time since lump was first noted; does lump come and go, or is it always present; relationship to menses
- Symptoms: tenderness or pain, dimpling or change in contour
- Changes in lump: size, character, relationship to menses (timing or severity)
- Associated symptoms: nipple discharge or retraction, tender lymph nodes

Nipple discharge
- Character: gradual or sudden onset, duration, color, consistency, odor, amount
- Associated symptoms: nipple retraction; breast lump or discomfort
- Associated factors: relationship to menses or other activity; medications (contraceptives, phenothiazines, digitalis, diuretics, steroids); recent injury to breast

HEALTH HISTORY—cont'd

GYNECOLOGIC HEALTH HISTORY
General considerations

These general considerations are pertinent to an adult woman of childbearing age. Obstetric data may not be pertinent to an adolescent patient. Parts of the menstrual history would not be relevant to a premenopausal woman who has had a hysterectomy or to a woman after menopause. Any current problem or abnormality should be noted from the start and correlations assessed throughout the history. Previous medical records should be obtained for the patient and her family as needed. The date and findings of the last gynecologic examination, including the results of a Papanicolaou (Pap) smear, should be recorded.

Menstrual history
- Age of menarche
- Date of last menstrual period: first day of last cycle
- Number of days in cycle and regularity of cycle
- Character of flow: amount (type of pads, mini or maxi, number of pads or tampons used in 24 hours), duration, presence and size of clots
- Dysmenorrhea: characteristics, duration, frequency (occur with each cycle?), relief measures
- Intermenstrual bleeding or spotting: amount, duration, frequency, timing in relation to phase of cycle
- Intermenstrual pain: severity, duration, timing; association with ovulation
- Premenstrual symptoms: headaches, weight gain, edema, breast tenderness, irritability or mood changes, frequency (occur with every period?), interference with activities of daily living, relief measures
- Menopausal symptoms: menstrual changes, signs of hormonal shifts

Obstetric history
- Gravity (number of pregnancies)
- Parity (number of births); term, preterm
- Number of abortions; spontaneous or induced
- Number of living children
- Complications of pregnancy, delivery, postpartum, or with fetus/newborn (including prematurity, congenital defects)

Douching history
- Frequency: length of time since last douche; number of years douching
- Method
- Solution used
- Reason for douching

Cleansing routines: use of sprays, powders, perfume, antiseptic soap, deodorants, or ointments

Contraceptive history
- Current method or combination of methods, if used: length of time used, effectiveness, consistency of use, side effects, satisfaction with method
- Previous methods: duration of use for each, side effects, reasons for discontinuing each

Infertility
- Length of time attempting pregnancy, sexual activity pattern, knowledge of fertile period in menstrual cycle
- Abnormalities of vagina, cervix, uterus, fallopian tubes, ovaries
- Contributing factors: stress, nutrition, chemical substances
- Partner factors
- Diagnostic evaluation to date

Other systems
- Head to toe review
- Genitourinary and gastrointestinal health is pertinent to assessment of a woman's genital and reproductive organs
- Neuromuscular disorders, endocrine function, and systemic diseases such as diabetes and autoimmune disorders influence a woman's health
- Psychiatric evaluation may be needed to assess physical or sexual abuse

Sexuality
- Difficulties, concerns, problems
- Satisfaction with current practices, habits, and sexual relationships
- Number of partners
- Sexual preference

Exposure risks
- Medications: prescription, over-the-counter (OTC) drugs; allergies
- Tobacco, alcohol, illegal drug use
- Toxins, radiation, occupational hazards

HEALTH HISTORY—cont'd

Past medical history

Recent pregnancies, abortions, or gynecologic procedures
Past gynecologic procedures or surgery (tubal ligation, hysterectomy, oophorectomy, laparoscopy, cryosurgery, conization)
Sexually transmitted diseases
Pelvic inflammatory disease
Vaginal infections
Previous illnesses and disorders
Cancer of reproductive organs

Family history

Diabetes
Cancer of reproductive organs
Mother received DES while pregnant with patient
Multiple pregnancies
Congenital anomalies

Current problem (if any)

Abnormal bleeding
- Character: shortened interval between periods (<19-21 days), lengthened interval between periods (>37 days), prolonged menses (>7 days), bleeding between periods
- Change in flow: nature of change, number of pads or tampons used in 24 hours (tampons/pads soaked?), presence of clots
- Temporal sequence: onset, duration, precipitating factors, course since onset
- Associated symptoms: pain, cramping, abdominal distention, pelvic fullness, change in bowel habits, weight loss or gain

Menstrual dysfunction or amenorrhea
- Exercise history
- Medications or systemic disorders that may cause disorder
- Factors from menstrual history indicating changes or worsening condition

Pain or pruritus
- Temporal sequence: date and time of onset, sudden or gradual onset, course since onset, duration, recurrence
- Character: specific location, type and intensity of pain
- Associated symptoms: vaginal discharge or bleeding, gastrointestinal symptoms, abdominal distention or tenderness, pelvic fullness, itching
- Association with menstrual cycle: timing, location, duration, changes
- Relationship to bodily functions and activities: voiding, eating, defecation, flatus, exercise, walking up stairs, bending, stretching, sexual activity
- Aggravating or relieving factors
- Previous medical care for this problem
- Effectiveness of treatment or medications (prescription or over the counter)

Vaginal discharge
- Character: amount, color, odor, consistency, changes in characteristics
- Occurrence: acute or chronic
- Medications: birth control pills, antibiotics
- Douching habits
- Clothing habits: use of cotton or ventilated underwear and pantyhose, tight pants or jeans
- Discharge or symptoms in sexual partner
- Associated symptoms: itching; tender, inflamed, or bleeding external tissues; dyspareunia; dysuria or burning on urination; abdominal pain or cramping; pelvic fullness

Urinary symptoms (dysuria, burning on urination, frequency, urgency)
- Character: acute or chronic; frequency of occurrence; past episodes; onset; course since onset; does patient feel as if bladder is empty or not after voiding; pain at start, throughout, or at cessation of urination
- Description of urine: color, presence of blood or particles, clear or cloudy
- Associated symptoms: vaginal discharge or bleeding, abdominal pain or cramping, abdominal distention, pelvic fullness, flank pain

Postmenopausal problems: bleeding, itching, urinary symptoms, dyspareunia, change in sexual desire

PALPATION

Ask the woman to assume a supine position with her hands behind (not above) her head.

Press lightly, or palpate, by using a back-and-forth method or a systematic circular or rotating movement, to ensure that all tissue is felt (Figure 2-2). Repeat the palpation with deeper pressure.

With all variations of palpation, use firm pressure but do not compress tissue against the rib cage. Do not lift the finger pads from the breast during palpation. If the breasts are large, perform bimanual palpation (Figure 2-3). Figure 2-4 shows how to palpate a breast lesion.

Stand on the side that is being examined, and palpate the tail of Spence as it enters the axilla (Figure 2-5). Use the fingertips (flat or pad area) to palpate all four breast quadrants and over the areola for lumps or nodules. After completely examining one side, repeat the procedure on the other side. Different positions and body elevations help distribute breast tissue; having the least tissue possible between the skin and chest wall when palpating yields the most accurate results.

Palpate the nipples between the index finger and thumb, using compression rather than pinching movements (Figure 2-6). Note the position of the nipple on each side in relation to the intercostal space. While compressing the nipple, check for any discharge. If a discharge is noted, a Pap smear may be indicated.

To palpate for axillary, supraclavicular, and infraclavicular lymph nodes, have the woman in a seated posi-

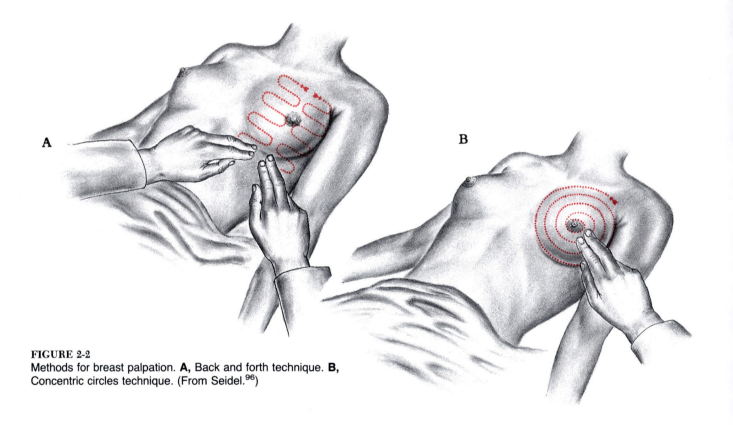

FIGURE 2-2
Methods for breast palpation. **A,** Back and forth technique. **B,** Concentric circles technique. (From Seidel.[96])

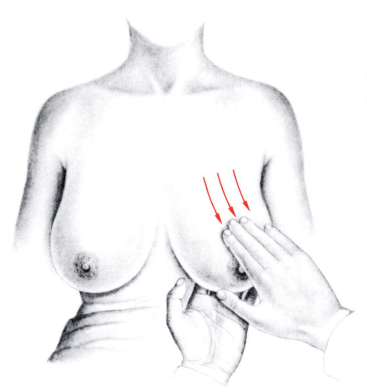

FIGURE 2-3
Bimanual palpation of large breasts. (From Seidel.[96])

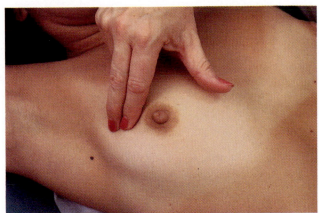

A

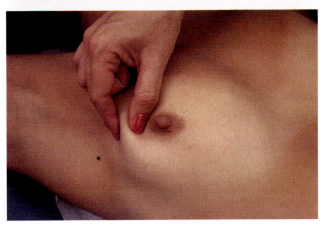

B

FIGURE 2-4
A, Palpating for consistency of breast lesion. **B,** Palpating for delineation of borders and mobility of breast mass.

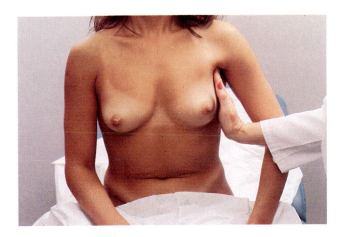

FIGURE 2-5
Palpating the tail of Spence.

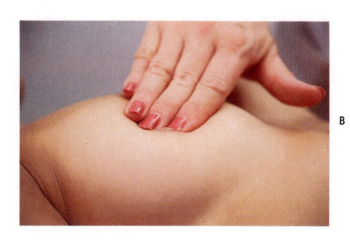

FIGURE 2-6
A, Palpation of the nipple. **B,** Palpation of the areolar area.

tion with arms flexed at the elbow (Figure 2-7). While one hand palpates, the other should support the woman's arm, allowing her chest wall muscles to relax. Palpate the apex (anterior or pectoral), medial (central), and lateral (posterior) aspects near the rib cage. Also palpate along the upper arm surface, pectoral muscles, and border of scapula.

Use the palmar finger surfaces (cupped hand) to palpate into the axillary hollow. Gently roll tissues against the muscles and chest wall of the axilla, since lesions may be hidden under fatty or muscle tissue. Palpate the supraclavicular area for lymph nodes by rotating the fingers over the clavicle.

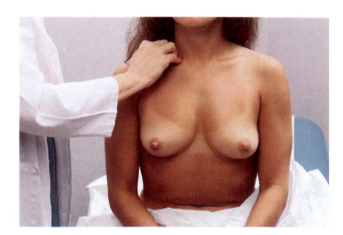

FIGURE 2-7
Palpation of supraclavicular lymph nodes.

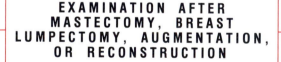

EXAMINATION AFTER MASTECTOMY, BREAST LUMPECTOMY, AUGMENTATION, OR RECONSTRUCTION

Assess the unaffected breast. Then palpate the scar area with two fingers. Use circular motions to detect any edema or tenderness. Examine the mastectomy site for signs of lumps or nodules, lesions, edema, thickening, inflammation or redness, other color changes, rash, scar irritation, or irregularities.

Using three or four finger pads, palpate the chest wall with smooth, sweeping movements. Note any edema, lumps or nodules, and thickening or tenderness. Assess the axillary and supraclavicular areas for any lymph nodes, edema, or muscle loss.

If the patient has had reconstruction, lumpectomy, or augmentation, use the usual thorough procedure to assess the breasts. Note any new tissue or scar formation.

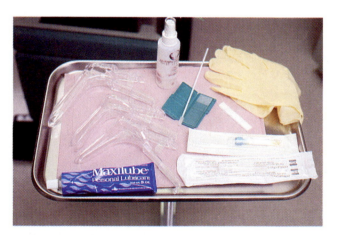

FIGURE 2-8
Equipment for pelvic examination.

GYNECOLOGIC ASSESSMENT

A pelvic examination usually follows the breast examination in routine screening. Any woman who is sexually active or has reached 18 years of age should have a pelvic examination at least yearly, including a Pap smear. The following equipment should be assembled before beginning this assessment (Figure 2-8):

Clean, disposable gloves; vaginal speculums (Graves' for multiparas, Pedersen's for nulliparas [other types of speculums are Sims', bivalve, large Graves', and pediatric]); water-soluble lubricant; flexible lamp; nitrazine pH paper; sterile cotton swabs moistened with saline; glass slides; culture plates and test tubes; plastic spatula or cervical brush devices (cytobrush); cytologic fixative; chlamydial enzyme immunoassay kit.

Wash hands before all examinations. Double gloves may be worn if the patient is bleeding, infection is suspected, or the examiner or patient has any cuts or lesions on hands.

Have the woman empty her bladder (unless incontinence is being assessed). Drape her to preserve as much modesty as possible. The patient usually assumes a lithotomy (dorsosacral) position with her feet in the stirrups and the buttocks near the edge of the table (Figure 2-9). A side-lying position (Sims' or left lateral prone position with the top knee raised toward the chest) may be used. A standing position is used to assess prolapse and incontinence.

INSPECTION

Wearing gloves, begin by inspecting the external genitalia. Inspect hair distribution, texture, and appearance, including symmetry and cleanliness of mons pubis and labia majora. Before touching the patient, inserting a speculum, palpating, or performing any cultures or tests, explain each step to the woman. Let her know when to expect pressure or other sensations.

PALPATION

Gently place a hand on the woman's thigh (remember to explain each procedure first). Separate the labia majora with the fingers, and inspect the labia minora for symmetry and characteristics (Figure 2-10). Palpate the

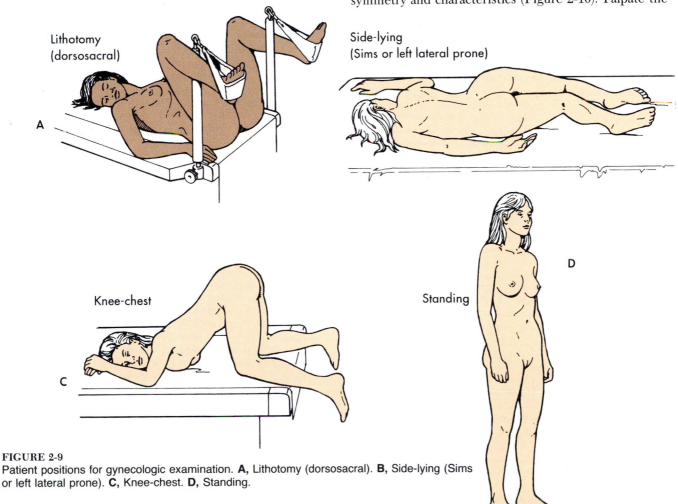

Lithotomy (dorsosacral)

A

Side-lying (Sims or left lateral prone)

B

Knee-chest

C

Standing

D

FIGURE 2-9
Patient positions for gynecologic examination. **A,** Lithotomy (dorsosacral). **B,** Side-lying (Sims or left lateral prone). **C,** Knee-chest. **D,** Standing.

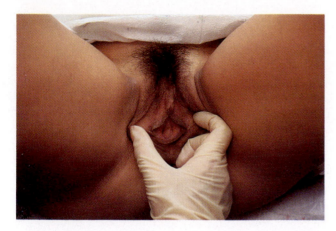

FIGURE 2-10
Palpation of the labia.

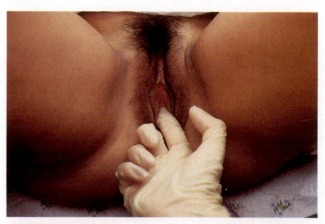

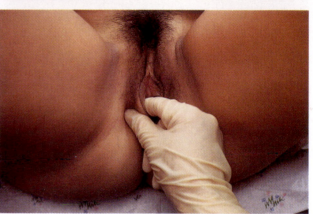

FIGURE 2-11
A, Palpation of Skene's glands. **B,** Palpation of Bartholin's glands.

inguinal nodes. Palpate the labia minora between thumb and finger. Inspect the clitoris, urethral orifice, vaginal introitus, and perineum. Note the appearance of the vestibule and the characteristics of structures.

Place the index finger into the vagina. With the index finger, gently exert upward pressure on the anterior of the vagina, and examine and milk Skene's glands. Palpate Bartholin's glands between the thumb and index finger (Figure 2-11). Inspect and palpate the perineum. Place the index and middle fingers into the vagina and have the client bear down on your finger to check pelvic support. Some slight bulging is normal. Then have the client tighten her vaginal muscles around your two fingers to check muscle tone.

SPECULUM EXAMINATION

Begin the examination of the internal genitalia by wetting the correctly sized speculum (smallest size possible while maintaining visualization) with warm water (do not use a lubricant, because it interferes with cultures and Pap smear results). Separate the labia majora and minora, and gently insert two fingers of the nondominant hand into the vagina (Figure 2-12, *A*). The pelvic muscles

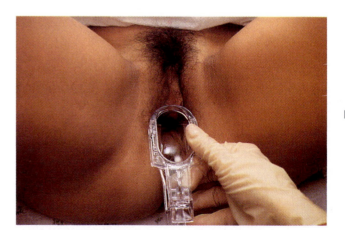

FIGURE 2-12
Examination of the internal genitalia with a speculum. **A,** Gently insert the closed speculum blades into the vagina. **B,** Insert the speculum further, rotating the speculum downward toward the rectal wall.

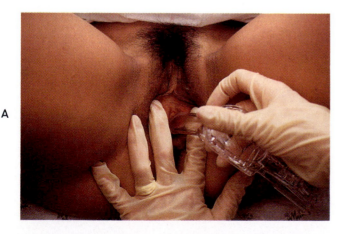

may relax if the woman breathes slowly through her mouth.

Press posteriorly on the fourchette to retract the vaginal wall. Avoid pressure on the urethral meatus. Gently insert the closed speculum blades next to the fingers; the speculum's handle should be pointing sideways. Insert the speculum partway, rotating it downward toward the rectal wall (Figure 2-12, *B*). The handle is now pointing down. After the speculum has been advanced, open the blades slowly to avoid pinching, and inspect the vagina.

Open the blades to expose the cervix, and lock the speculum into place. Inspect the cervix. Obtain smears and cultures as needed. Cultures and smears should be obtained in the following order: (1) Pap smear, (2) gonococcal specimen, (3) chlamydial specimen, (4) wet prep. Close the blades and carefully remove the speculum while inspecting the vagina. Ask the woman to cough to evaluate muscle tone and to check for evidence of urinary stress incontinence.

BIMANUAL PELVIC EXAMINATION

Explain how a bimanual examination is performed. Then insert the lubricated index and middle fingers of one hand into the vagina, and place the other hand on the midline of the abdomen (Figure 2-13). With slight pressure, palpate the vaginal walls. Locate the cervix. Note the size, shape, length, position, and mobility of the cervix and the patency of the os. Gently grasp the cervix and move it from side to side.

Palpate the fornices, the pouch of Douglas, and the uterosacral ligaments for masses. Palpate the uterus to determine its location, position, size, shape, contour, consistency, and mobility. The ovaries and tubes are located by placing two fingers of one hand to the side of the cervix and pushing back and up while the other hand (on the abdomen) pushes downward near the anterosuperior iliac spine. Note the characteristics of the uterus, cervix, and ovaries. The adnexa (tubes and ovaries) may be difficult to palpate.

RECTOVAGINAL EXAMINATION

Although often deferred, a rectovaginal assessment should be part of every examination. Gloves should be changed after each entry into an orifice. Explain the procedure, and then perform rectovaginal palpation as appropriate. Insert the index finger into the vagina and the middle finger into the anus (Figure 2-14). Assess the sphincter tone. Palpate the rectovaginal septum for thickness and tone. Palpate the posterior aspect of the uterus and the anterior and posterior rectal wall. Note any stool characteristics on glove. Conduct a guaiac test on stool if the woman is over 40 years of age.

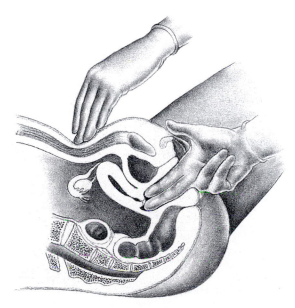

FIGURE 2-13
Bimanual pelvic examination. (From Seidel.[96])

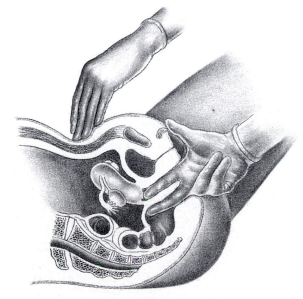

FIGURE 2-14
Rectovaginal examination. (From Seidel.[96])

EXAMINATION AFTER HYSTERECTOMY

Follow the same steps for assessing the woman's genitalia and pelvic organs. Note information from the history concerning the reason for the surgery and whether it was a partial or total hysterectomy. A vaginal cuff (surgical scar) may be present; this scar may appear as a white or pink suture line in the posterior fornix of the vaginal canal.

A Pap smear is performed by using the blunt spatula end to remove cells from the suture line (this specimen should be labeled as vaginal cells). Gonococcal and chlamydial specimens may be taken from the vestibule.

Assess for age-related changes in the vaginal rugae and secretions, especially if a total hysterectomy was performed without hormone replacement therapy being given. The cervix will be absent. Also examine for signs of rectocele, cystocele, and stress incontinence.

A bimanual examination is performed to assess for lumps or masses, adhesions, irregularities, and tenderness. The uterus cannot be palpated, but the ovaries and tubes must be assessed if the patient has had a partial hysterectomy. The bladder and bowel areas may be more easily palpated after a hysterectomy.

BREAST AND GYNECOLOGIC EXAMINATION: NORMAL FINDINGS AND CLINICALLY SIGNIFICANT DEVIATIONS

Normal findings	Clinically significant deviations
Breasts	**Breasts**
Size varies, usually slight asymmetry in size	Tenderness unrelated to menstrual cycle
Will hang bilaterally equal	Inflammation
Smooth texture, feels lobular	Irregular contour
Even color (same as body surfaces)	Increase in unilateral size
Elastic, movable, dense, firm	Obvious asymmetry
Sagging with age, multiparity, poor support	Skin retraction, dimpling, or bulging
May have visible bilateral venous patterns and striae	Fixation (shortening or nonmobile appearance)
Four quadrants and tail of Spence have equal tissue when palpated	Change in convex pattern
Bilaterally smooth, diffuse, granular, usually nontender; fine and granular in older women	Erythema or hyperpigmentation
	Roughness or thickened tissue
	Tissue heat
	Lesions
May have premenstrual engorgement, fibrocystic changes of bilateral thick nodular consistency	Sudden engorgement unrelated to menstrual cycle
Inframammary ridge bilaterally firm at 4 to 8 o'clock position	Edema (peau d'orange, texture similar to orange peel)
Young adult breasts are located between third and sixth rib, nipples near fourth intercostal space	Sudden unilateral vascular pattern
	Hard, fixed, irregular, nontender nodes
	Nodular, fibrocystic patterns
	New, tender, or changing moles
Areolae	**Areolae**
Bilateral, equal, round or oval, 2 to 12 cm in diameter	Asymmetry
Pink or darker than body surfaces; color changes with puberty and pregnancy	Change in shape or pigmentation
Smooth Montgomery tubercles	Masses, lesions, excoriation, inflammation

BREAST AND GYNECOLOGIC EXAMINATION: NORMAL FINDINGS AND CLINICALLY SIGNIFICANT DEVIATIONS—cont'd

Normal findings	Clinically significant deviations
Nipples Bilateral, equal, pointing in same direction Location may drop with obesity, age, or after lactation Smooth, slightly wrinkled Touching causes puckering and nipple erection Homogeneous color May have supernumerary nipples May have nipple inversion, bilateral or unilateral Bilaterally smooth, equal, and nontender when palpated	**Nipples** Asymmetry (distorted nipple) Recent retraction or inversion, bilateral or unilateral Edema, inflammation, or redness Change in shape, direction, or pigmentation unrelated to puberty or pregnancy Ulceration, erosion, scaling or crusting, dryness Discharge (serous, bloody, or odorous)
Lymph nodes Not usually palpable	**Lymph nodes** Palpable nodes
External genital structures **Mons pubis/veneris** Triangular escutcheon, inverse shape, coarse hair Hairline may extend to umbilicus Cushionlike elevation over symphysis pubis Smooth, soft, subcutaneous fatty (adipose) tissue Loose connective tissue Sebaceous (oil glands)	***External genital structures*** **Mons pubis/veneris** Diamond hair pattern (male distribution) Hair absent or patchy Parasites, nits, lice Scars, lesions, masses, rashes, excoriation, lacerations, discoloration, edema, or inguinal swelling Unilateral appearance or symptoms
Labia majora (pair) Labium majus (single fold) outermost rounded fold with hair, darker pigmentation May gap or close over labia minora (more gapping with multiparas, may obstruct view of urethral orifice) May be moist or dry Dark pink pigmentation Adipose and connective tissue Sebaceous follicles on inner surfaces Extend from mons to perineum, encircling vestibule Homologous to male scrotum	**Labia majora** Pronounced irregularity or asymmetry Inflammation, irritation, lesions, masses, nodules, ulcerations, excoriation, lacerations, discharge, hernias, or swelling Leukoplakia (white patches) Edema (may indicate carcinoma or vulvar varicosities)
Labia minora (pair) Labium minus (single fold) hairless skin between labia majora Usually thinner than labia majora with slight asymmetry Sexual activity and childbirth produce natural gapping of labia minora More prominent after childbirth	**Labia minora** Lesions, excoriation, inflammation, leukoplakia, uneven color, or pronounced asymmetry

Continued.

BREAST AND GYNECOLOGIC EXAMINATION: NORMAL FINDINGS AND CLINICALLY SIGNIFICANT DEVIATIONS—cont'd

Normal findings	Clinically significant deviations
Connective tissue and nerves extend from anterior frenulum (fold) of clitoris to posterior frenulum (merged folds) of labia minora Generally moist, soft, darker pink than labia majora Homologous to bottom side of penis	
Fourchette (connects labia minora to posterior vulva) Symmetric fold Smooth texture; even, pinkish color	**Fourchette** Tenderness, irritation Irregular shape Nodules
Vestibule Ovoid (boat shaped), enclosed by labia minora Houses urinary orifice (urethral meatus), hymen, and vaginal introitus (orifice)	**Vestibule** Lesions, inflammation, ulceration, discharge (smegma), fistulas, polyps, masses, sebaceous cysts, ulcerations, edema Caruncles (outpouching of urethral mucous membrane) Venereal lesions Urinary incontinence
Clitoris Cylindric Size varies (should not exceed 3 cm) Innervated, sensitive glans (tip) Corpus (body) and two crura (elongations attached to inferior rami of pubis) Vascular plexus (erectile tissue), sebaceous glands, nerves and blood vessels Labia minora form prepuce above and frenulum below clitoris (medial aspect covered by prepuce) Glans of clitoris homologous to glans of penis Shaft of clitoris homologous to male corpus cavernosum	**Clitoris** Size abnormality (atrophy, enlargement) Adhesions, lesions Inflammation Drainage
Vaginal introitus May be thin vertical slit or large orifice Moist, pink tissue May have no hymen or hymenal caruncles (irregular edges); many varieties of normal hymen shape Tight squeeze or tone in nullipara Less tone in multipara	**Vaginal introitus** Profuse discharge Inflammation, edema, lesions Unable to constrict vaginal orifice Cystocele, rectocele, enterocele (hernial bulge or sac), uterine prolapse
Vulva **Lesser vestibular area:** Contains paired tubular Skene's (paraurethral) glands inside urethral meatus	**Vulva** Irregularity Nodules Tenderness

BREAST AND GYNECOLOGIC EXAMINATION: NORMAL FINDINGS AND CLINICALLY SIGNIFICANT DEVIATIONS—cont'd

Normal findings	Clinically significant deviations
Greater vestibular area: Contains paired 1.5 cm long Bartholin's (vulvovaginal or greater vestibular) glands; glands not palpable; bulb of vestibule homologous to male bulbourethral glands	Discharge Palpable glands
Perineum Triangular area dorsal to pubic arch and superior to tip of coccyx; lateral to pubic and ischial rami (hip bone); extends from fourchette (fold below vagina) to anus Supports distal sections of urogenital and gastrointestinal tracts Muscular area with elastic fibers, fibrous tissue, and connective tissue Smooth tissue; may have episiotomy scar Thick in nullipara; thinner, more rigid in multipara	**Perineum** Marked scarring, fistulas, lesions, masses, discharge, inflammation, excoriation Weak muscle tone Tenderness Thinness
Internal genital structures **Vagina** Moist, smooth, pink, firm, homogeneous tissue Rugae (folds that diminish in multipara) Thin, odorless, clear or cloudy, minimum or moderate discharge	*Internal genital structures* **Vagina** Tenderness Nodules, red lesions, pale tissue (possible anemia) Leukoplakia (patches) Lesions, cracks, dry areas, bleeding (without menses), edema, nodules, cysts, or masses Yellow, gray, green, thick, white frothy, curdy, profuse, or odorous discharge that adheres to vaginal wall Bulging of posterior vaginal wall at orifice indicates rectocele Bulging of anterior wall indicates cystocele Other protrusions may indicate urethrocele, enterocele, or uterine prolapse
Cervix Smooth, moist, pink Feels like moist, round button with recessed center May feel like tip of a nose Evenly pink, symmetric, midline position, may point anterior or posterior 2.5 cm to 4 cm in diameter May lie 1 to 3 cm into vagina Usually 1 to 3 cm fornices (folds in vagina around cervix) Erythema (redness) near os Small, round os in nullipara Slit, star, or irregularly shaped os in multipara	**Cervix** Pale (possible anemia, menopause) Blue (possible pregnancy) Diameter >4 cm Lateral cervical position Position into vagina more than 3 cm Patchy erythema, irregular borders, asymmetric os, granular os, inflammation Lesions, red or white patches, strawberry spots Bleeding unrelated to menses Nodules or lacerations Odor or yellow, gray, or green discharge Enlarged or irregular Very soft or hard

Continued.

Normal findings	Clinically significant deviations
Pliable os; may insert fingertip about 0.5 cm	Stenosed os
May have mucous plug in os	Pain on palpation
Cyclic changes in discharge	"Stretch tenderness" when moved may indicate ectopic pregnancy
Smooth, ovoid	
May have nabothian cysts (small, yellow, raised, round, smooth areas)	
Cervix in horizontal position indicates midpositioned uterus	
May have odorless discharge	
Flexible; moves 1 to 2 cm without tenderness	
Uterus	**Uterus**
Pear-shaped, 5.5 to 8 cm long (enlarges slightly with parity)	Tenderness
Flexible and not tender	Enlarged (>5 cm)
Usually in anteroposterior plane and anteverted position	Fundus above pubis
Fundus (top) at pubis level (not always palpable)	Irregular, soft
Round, firm, smooth fundus	Masses or nodules
Cervix points along vaginal canal axis if midpositioned, retroflexed and anteflexed	Fixed, nonmobile
Cervix points anteriorly if retroverted	
Adnexa (ovaries and tubes)	**Adnexa (ovaries and tubes)**
May not be palpable	Markedly tender ovary
Walnut size (about 4 cm) ovary; firm, smooth, ovoid shape	Enlarged ovary
About 3 cm × 2 cm × 1 cm	Immobile masses or nodules in ovaries or tubes
Flexible, slightly tender ovaries when palpated	Pulsations
Fallopian tubes may be sensitive to pressure	Palpable tubes
Homologous to testes	
Rectovaginal area	**Rectovaginal area**
Anal surface darker pink and coarser	Anal area skin tags, scars, lesions, inflammation, fissures, excoriation, lumps, polyps, modules, masses, induration
Rectal wall thin, smooth, soft, pliable	
External anal sphincter contracts when touched	Thick or nodular septum
Fundus usually palpable through rectovaginal pouch	Tenderness
Smooth surface	Relaxed sphincter
Tight anal sphincter	Fecal incontinence
Stool brown without blood	Black or bloody stool
Deep perineal pouch	**Deep perineal pouch**
Same structure as in men but without bulbourethral glands; contains dorsal nerve of clitoris and vaginal parts	Evidence of stress incontinence
Contains sphincter urethrae muscle, perineal nerve branches to sphincter urethrae, and internal pudendal vessels	Relaxed muscle tone

CHAPTER 3

Diagnostic and Laboratory Procedures

ULTRASONOGRAPHY

Ultrasonography is a procedure that uses a harmless, high-frequency sound wave to obtain an image of an organ. The patient lies on an examining table in the supine position. A greasy paste is liberally applied to the skin to enhance transmission and reception of the sound waves. The transducer is moved along the skin in a vertical and then a horizontal line. A pictorial image is produced, and a realistic Polaroid picture of the organ is obtained. The image produced allows a three-dimensional view of the organ. Ultrasonography requires no contrast medium and has no associated radiation, which makes it especially valuable in evaluating women in their reproductive years who might be pregnant. The procedure is inexpensive, noninvasive, and highly accurate in distinguishing between cystic and solid masses.

INDICATIONS

Ultrasonography is used to distinguish between cystic and solid masses, especially in the pelvis, breasts, abdomen, heart, and pregnant uterus (Figure 3-1). It does not distinguish between benign and malignant solid tumors.

CONTRAINDICATIONS

None

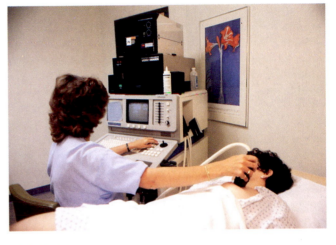

FIGURE 3-1
Ultrasonography of the breast. (From Belcher.[9a])

NURSING CARE

Patient preparation varies according to the organ being scanned.

Breasts: No special preparation needed.

Pelvis: The patient must have a full bladder to enhance visualization of the uterus and adnexa. The procedure is painless and does not require anesthesia. Enemas may be needed if an outline of the intestine is desired. If the gallbladder is being studied, the patient must be kept NPO after midnight on the day of the test. No diet or medication alterations are required. Informed consent must be obtained. No postprocedural care is required.

PATIENT TEACHING

In addition to explaining the procedure, inform the patient that she will not be exposed to radiation. Tell her that the procedure is painless and has no known risks. The only discomfort she may feel will be from lying still on a hard surface with a full bladder. Physicians specially trained in ultrasonography supervise the procedure and interpret the findings. No care is required after the procedure, and the patient can drive without assistance. Since the patient usually can see the monitor during the examination, she may observe negative or abnormal findings. Provide emotional support.

COMPUTED TOMOGRAPHY

Computed tomography (CT) is a method of body section roentgenography. It is a noninvasive, diagnostic scanning technique that incorporates detectors, a scanner, and a computer to produce three-dimensional cross-sectional images (Figure 3-2). With the patient lying supine on a narrow bed, several x-ray beams are passed through the body at different angles. A television monitor displays the image produced and records it by means of a Polaroid-type camera. Computed tomography is highly accurate in distinguishing between benign and malignant lesions. The study can be conducted with or without a contrast agent and may be used in conjunction with ultrasonography or magnetic resonance imaging (MRI). When an intravenous contrast material is used, vascular structures can be identified. A CT study is routinely used to guide fine-needle biopsies.

INDICATIONS

To diagnose:
   Breast disorders
   Kidney tumors
   Liver, pancreatic, or splenic tumors
   Adenomas
   Uterine or ovarian tumors
   Lymphadenopathy tumors
   Primary or metastatic chest wall tumors
   Disorders of the pelvic organs
   Mediastinal tumors
   Hematomas
   Biliary or gallbladder tumors
   Meningiomas
   Pulmonary tumors
   Esophageal tumors

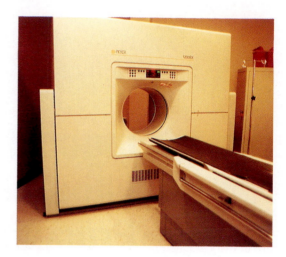

FIGURE 3-2
Clinical setting for computed tomography (CT). (From Belcher.[9a])

   Granulomas
   Pheochromocytomas
   Intracranial tumors
   Carcinomas
   Retroperitoneal tumors

CONTRAINDICATIONS

Pregnancy
Obesity (>300 pounds)
Allergy to iodinated dye or shellfish
Unstable vital signs
Unstable conditions requiring continuous life support
Implanted metal objects or fragments (e.g., intrauterine device [IUD], pacemaker, metallic orthopedic device, metal aneurysm clips)

NURSING CARE

No activity, food, or fluid restrictions or alterations in medication are required unless contrast medium is to be used. The patient should be kept NPO for at least 4 hours before the oral contrast medium is given. Assess the patient for the contraindications listed. Have the patient remove all metal objects and empty her bladder before the test. Obtain informed consent if required. After the examination no special care is needed unless contrast medium was used. If a contrast dye was used, encourage the patient to drink fluids to prevent renal complications and to promote excretion of the dye.

PATIENT TEACHING

In addition to explaining the procedure, inform the patient that there is no more exposure to radiation than would be involved in a series of regular x-rays, and that the procedure has no known risks. Tell the patient that she will hear a clicking sound during the procedure, but she will not feel the scanning machine rotate. A major concern of patients is being confined in the close quarters of the CT equipment. Antianxiety drugs may help those with mild claustrophobia. The patient's compliance (i.e., remaining still) is required during the entire procedure. Explain to the patient that she must remain motionless during the procedure (any movement can cause artifacts on the scan). The only discomfort the patient may feel may be from lying still on a hard surface for a prolonged period. If contrast dye is used, she may feel a warm flush of the face or body. Occasionally nausea occurs when the dye is injected. If possible, use a picture of the CT machine to encourage the patient to talk about any anxieties she may have. Tell the patient that the procedure is performed by a radiologic technologist and takes 30 to 45 minutes. If contrast dye is used, add 30 to 45 minutes to the procedural time. The technician observes the patient from an adjoining room and can communicate with her by intercom. No postprocedural care is required, and the patient can resume all activities.

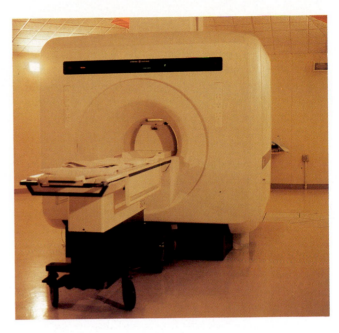

FIGURE 3-3
Magnetic resonance imaging (MRI) equipment. (From Mourad.[81a])

MAGNETIC RESONANCE IMAGING

Magnetic resonance imaging (MRI) is a noninvasive, diagnostic scanning technique that provides valuable information about the body's biochemistry. It provides multiplane, cross-sectional imaging based on the magnetism inherent in certain nuclei in the human body and the interaction of that magnetism with radio waves. A huge electromagnet is used to detect hidden tumors by mapping the vibrations of the various atoms in the body on a computer screen. The patient lies supine on a narrow bed, which is slid into the desired position inside the MRI scanner (Figure 3-3). She must remain motionless during the scan, since any movement can cause artifacts. The MRI scanner uses a powerful magnetic field and radiofrequency energy to produce images. The MRI computer monitors the images and then processes and displays them on a video monitor for interpretation or photographing for later interpretation.

MRI has several advantages over computed tomography scanning: MRI involves no exposure to radiation; cross-sectional views can be obtained in any plane, not just axially; MRI "sees" through bone; MRI provides better contrast between normal tissue and pathologic tissue; and several types of pathologic tissue can be recognized.

INDICATIONS

To detect primary and metastatic tumors in the following areas:
 Head, face, and surrounding structures
 Spine and surrounding structures
 Heart and great vessels
 Kidneys
 Bones and joints
 Extremities and soft tissue
 Neck
 Mediastinum
 Liver
 Breasts
 Pelvis

CONTRAINDICATIONS

Obesity (>300 pounds)
Claustrophobia
Implanted metal objects or fragments (e.g., intrauterine device [IUD], pacemaker, metallic orthopedic device, metal aneurysm clips)
Pregnancy
Confusion, agitation
Unstable conditions requiring continuous life support

NURSING CARE

No activity, food, or fluid restrictions or alterations in medication are required. Have the patient remove all metal objects and empty her bladder before the test. Explain the procedure, and obtain informed consent if required. No special postprocedural care is needed. Assess the patient for the contraindications listed.

PATIENT TEACHING

Explain the procedure. A major concern of patients is being confined in the close quarters of the MRI equipment. Antianxiety drugs may help those with mild claustrophobia. The patient's compliance (i.e., remaining still) is required during the entire procedure. Explain to the patient that she must remain motionless during the procedure (any movement can cause artifacts on the scan). Inform the patient that there is no exposure to radiation with MRI and that the procedure has no known risks. Tell the patient that the MRI equipment makes a thumping sound during the procedure. The only discomfort she may feel may be from lying still on a hard surface, or possibly from a tingling in metal teeth fillings. If possible, use a picture of the scanning machine to encourage the patient to talk about any anxieties she may have. Tell the patient that the procedure is performed by a radiologic technologist and takes 30 to 90 minutes. Physicians specially trained in magnetic resonance imaging interpret the findings. No postprocedural care is required, and the patient can drive without assistance.

MAMMOGRAPHY

Film mammography and xeromammography are x-ray examinations of the breast. These procedures produce image contrasts that are sensitive and specific enough to detect small invasive and even noninvasive breast tumors. Radiation exposure with these techniques has been reduced, and overall image quality and diagnostic value have significantly improved. A mammogram may detect cancer 1 to 2 years before it becomes clinically palpable, especially in women with pendulous breasts. It provides a reliable means for following women at high risk for developing breast cancer. The patient may sit on a chair or stand during the procedure. One breast is rested on a table above an x-ray cassette, and the technician places a compressor on the breast (Figure 3-4). X-rays are taken from two angles (frontal and lateral), and the procedure is repeated on the other breast. The patient is asked to wait a few minutes until the films are developed to check their quality.

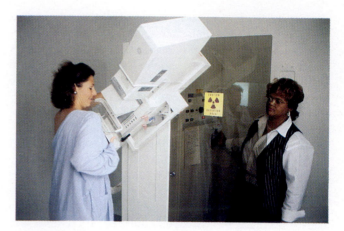

FIGURE 3-4
Patient undergoing mammography.

INDICATIONS

To diagnose:
  Breast cancer
  Benign tumors
  Fibrocystic changes
  Gross cysts
  Breast abscesses
  Suppurative mastitis
  Intraglandular lymphoma nodes
  Mammography is also used to evaluate symptoms of breast disease and to differentiate between noncancerous breast disease and breast cancer.

CONTRAINDICATIONS

Pregnancy

NURSING CARE

The patient should not wear any body powder, creams, or deodorant on the torso the day of the procedure, because they may interfere with the x-rays. No food or fluid restrictions or alterations in medication are required. Have the patient remove all jewelry, metal objects, and clothing above the waist and put on a gown that opens in the front. Obtain informed consent if required. No postprocedural care is needed. The patient may resume normal activity after the procedure.

Assess the patient for the contraindication given, i.e., pregnancy. She may feel discomfort when her breast is compressed, but the compression is brief. A minimal dose of radiation is involved.

PATIENT TEACHING

Explain the procedure, discussing recent advances in mammography and the minimal risks associated with mammograms. Allow the patient to express her feelings about this examination, since some women are embarrassed by the procedure. Provide emotional support. Tell the patient when to expect a report. Take this time to instruct the patient in the techniques for monthly breast self-examination. Explain the American Cancer Society's recommendations for clinical breast examinations and mammography. The results of diagnostic tests must be considered with the physician's clinical findings to be meaningful. Test results alone rarely are enough to determine a precise diagnosis.

BREAST BIOPSY AND ASPIRATION

A breast biopsy (often performed by needle aspiration) usually is done in an outpatient setting, as a diagnostic procedure after discovery of a breast lump and after a mammogram has been performed. The test is conducted to determine whether the lump is benign or malignant. A local anesthetic is administered, and the specimen is aspirated through a needle inserted into the breast (Figure 3-5). A small amount of tissue is incised, or the entire lesion and some surrounding tissue are removed. Either method takes only a few minutes. If an incision is made, it is closed and a dressing is applied. The specimen can be examined immediately by the pathologist (frozen section) for confirmation of malignancy as well as for more detailed staging and grading to determine further treatment and prognosis. Approximately 80% of breast lumps biopsied are benign.

INDICATIONS

To confirm suggestive clinical and/or mammography findings.

CONTRAINDICATIONS

Surgical risk increases with obesity, stress, smoking, poor nutrition, and recent or chronic illness.

NURSING CARE

The patient is kept NPO after midnight on the day of the biopsy. No activity restrictions or alterations in medication are required. Assess the patient for the contraindications listed, and obtain informed consent if required. Postprocedural care includes checking vital signs until they are stable and providing pain medication if needed. An ice bag may be used on the site. Provide support for the patient.

PATIENT TEACHING

Explain the procedure, and reassure the patient that it usually causes only momentary discomfort. If sutures

were required, they must be removed at a later date. Encourage the patient to wear a supportive bra for 24 hours a day until the site has completely healed. Advise the patient to avoid vigorous exercise for 2 weeks after surgery but to resume normal activity as soon as possible. At home a heating pad will relieve pain in the surgical area. The patient should report pain, swelling, redness, bleeding, or any other signs of infection to her physician immediately. Tell her that her nipple may be numb for a few weeks. Additionally, make sure that the patient understands the need to perform monthly breast self-examination, and teach her the proper technique.

If a malignancy is identified, the patient and her family will need emotional support as well as referral for appropriate treatment and follow-up. Treatment alternatives should be discussed with the physician before the biopsy.

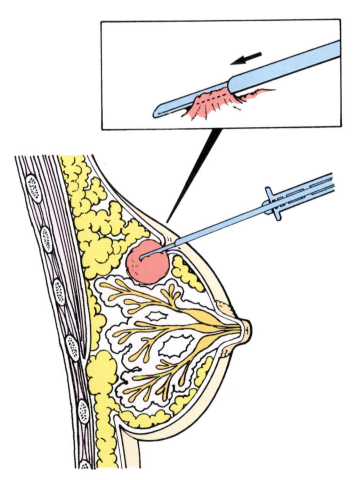

FIGURE 3-5
Breast biopsy and aspiration.

STEREOTACTIC BREAST BIOPSY SYSTEM

The stereotactic needle biopsy system provides an alternative method of performing breast biopsy. The system combines mammography with a computer guided system and an aspiration needle or biopsy gun needle. The film digitizer (computer system) provides precise guidance for the needle for pinpoint accuracy. A rotating table or platform works with gravity, providing better visualization and access to the breast, chest wall, and axillary breast tissue.

The patient is positioned on the rotating table on her abdomen with the breast pendulus through an aperture. The breast is compressed with the questionable lesion centered in the biopsy window. Stereotactic images are taken. The mammography film is placed on the digitizer; coordinates are determined and displayed. The coordinates guide the needle to the desired location and depth of the questionable lesion, and the aspirate is drawn, or a sample is obtained for biopsy.

This system allows the physician to quickly perform a very accurate fine-needle aspiration and needle core biopsy with minimal discomfort and no disfigurement for the patient. Because the procedure requires only local anesthetic, it can be performed in an outpatient or ambulatory setting. No postprocedural care is necessary.

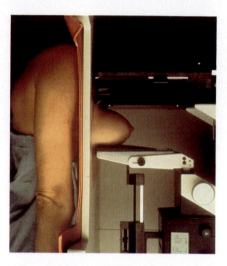

The patient is positioned on the table with the breast pendulus through the aperture. The breast is compressed with the target lesion centered in the biopsy window.

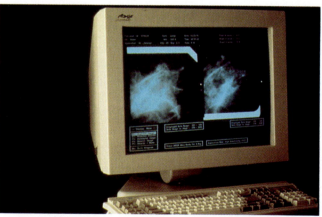

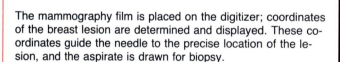

The mammography film is placed on the digitizer; coordinates of the breast lesion are determined and displayed. These coordinates guide the needle to the precise location of the lesion, and the aspirate is drawn for biopsy.

PAPANICOLAOU SMEAR

The Papanicolaou (Pap) smear is recommended as a routine part of the pelvic examination for women over 18 years of age. It is used to detect neoplastic cell secretions from the cervix and vagina. This test can detect early cellular changes in premalignant or existing malignant conditions. It has been found to be 95% accurate in detecting cervical carcinoma and 40% accurate in detecting endometrial carcinoma. If a Pap smear is found to be abnormal, one method used to determine the appropriate treatment is shown in Figure 3-6.

During the procedure, the patient lies in the lithotomy position on an examining table with stirrups.

After a speculum has been positioned in the vagina and the cervix has been visualized, a swab or spatula is introduced through the speculum and cells are collected for examination (Figure 3-7). The patient feels no discomfort during the procedure except during insertion of the speculum. The cells collected are applied to a clean slide, fixed before drying, and sent to the laboratory for analysis. A notation of the patient's name, age, parity, last menstrual period, and medication history, as well as the reason for the test, should be sent with the sample to the laboratory.

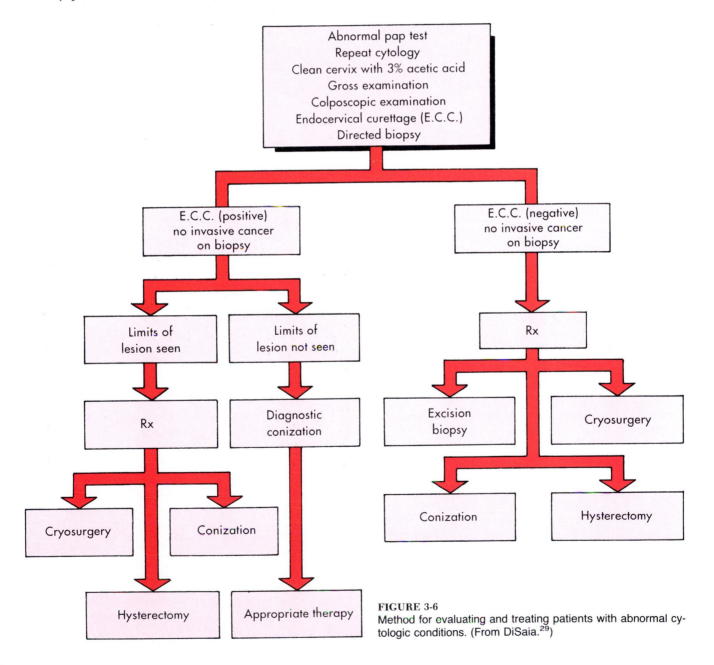

FIGURE 3-6
Method for evaluating and treating patients with abnormal cytologic conditions. (From DiSaia.[29])

INDICATIONS

To detect:
Cervical and vaginal cancer cells
Cervical intraepithelial neoplasia
Endometrial cancer
Premalignant conditions

CONTRAINDICATIONS

Menses

NURSING CARE

No food or fluid restrictions or alterations in medication are required. The patient should not be menstruating, nor should she douche or take a tub bath for 24 hours before the Pap smear. Have the patient empty her bladder before the procedure, and assess her for the contraindications listed. Help the patient onto the examination table, and drape her for privacy. Collect the specimen or assist another practitioner, and appropriately label the specimen. No follow-up care is required.

PATIENT TEACHING

Explain the procedure, and instruct the patient not to douche or take a tub bath for 24 hours before the test. Abstinence from sexual intercourse for 24 to 48 hours before the smear may be requested. Explain to the patient that she should feel no discomfort, except when the speculum is inserted.

DILATION AND CURETTAGE

Dilation and curettage (D & C) is a procedure in which the cervix is dilated and the uterine endometrium is surgically scraped or curetted. The procedure is performed for both diagnostic and therapeutic reasons; it is one of the most common gynecologic procedures performed. A D & C is done with the patient in the lithotomy position. A routine bimanual pelvic examination is performed, and the cervix is visualized through a speculum inserted into the vagina. The cervical os is dilated, and a curette is inserted into the uterus to scrape out the endometrium. Tissue is sent to the laboratory for analysis.

INDICATIONS

To diagnose:
To detect uterine malignancy
To evaluate fertility
To evaluate dysfunctional uterine bleeding
Therapeutic uses
To treat heavy bleeding
Dysmenorrhea
Incomplete abortion

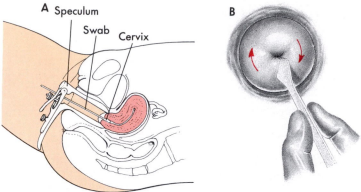

FIGURE 3-7
Papanicolaou (Pap) smear. **A,** Cross-section view of the process of obtaining a cervical specimen. (From Grimes.) **B,** Cervix is scraped with bifid end of a spatula to obtain Pap smear. (From Seidel.[96])

To remove polyps
Therapeutic abortion

CONTRAINDICATIONS

None

NURSING CARE

No activity restrictions are required. Food and fluid are restricted for 12 hours before the procedure. Have the patient put on a surgical gown and empty her bladder before the procedure. Obtain informed consent if required. After the procedure, check the patient's vital signs until they are stable. Provide pain medication if needed. Monitor the patient for infection, lacerations, or uterine perforations.

PATIENT TEACHING

Explain the procedure, and discuss any anxieties the patient has. After the procedure, the patient can expect some vaginal bleeding. Instruct her to monitor her temperature and the bleeding, and to notify her physician immediately if any symptoms of infection (e.g., elevated temperature and chills or an offensive odor of discharge), laceration, or uterine perforation develop. Tell her not to use tampons or douches and to refrain from sexual intercourse for at least 2 weeks. A mild analgesic may be taken for pain, and a heating pad probably will relieve abdominal cramping.

ENDOSCOPY

Endoscopic procedures allow direct visualization of hollow organs or body cavities by means of a lighted flexible instrument. Different endoscopes have been developed specifically for each area to be visualized (e.g., the **culdoscope** for the female pelvic organs, the **laparoscope** for the abdominal cavity, the **colposcope** for the vagina and cervix, and the **hysteroscope** for the uterus and fallopian tubes).

LAPAROSCOPY

Laparoscopy is used to visualize the female abdominal organs. This procedure can be used for diagnosis as well as surgery. With the patient in modified lithotomy or Trendelenburg's position, a needle is inserted through a small incision in the peritoneal cavity and the peritoneal cavity is filled with 3 to 4 liters of CO_2 to enhance visualization of abdominal organs. Another small incision is made and the laparoscope is inserted into the peritoneal cavity (Figure 3-8). If minor surgery (such as a tubal ligation) is planned, a second tube will be inserted through an additional incision, through which surgical instruments can be inserted. Following the procedure, gas is released, tubes are removed, and incisions are closed. The entire procedure usually takes about 40 minutes.

INDICATIONS

To diagnose:
   Pelvic adhesions
   Tubal and uterine causes of infertility
   Ectopic pregnancy
   Salpingitis
   Ovarian tumors and cysts
   Endometriosis
   Ruptured ovarian cyst
   Stage of carcinoma
Therapeutic uses:
   Lysis of adhesions
   Tubal ligation
   Cholecystectomy
   Retrieval of ova for in vitro fertilization (IVF) or gamete intrafallopian transfer (GIFT)
   Removal of IUD
   Removal of biopsy specimen
   Appendectomy

CONTRAINDICATIONS

Local peritonitis
Suspected intraabdominal hemorrhage
History of multiple surgeries

NURSING CARE

Keep the patient NPO after midnight before the procedure. Enemas may be ordered. Follow general anes-

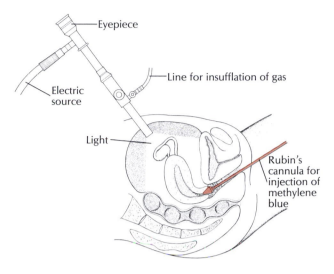

FIGURE 3-8
Laparoscopy. (From Bobak.[13])

thesia precautions, if appropriate. Have the patient empty her bladder before the procedure. Intravenous fluids may be started. Obtain informed consent. After the procedure, monitor the patient's vital signs, level of pain, and urinary output until they are stable. Protect the patient from injury until she has recovered from the anesthetic. Have the patient refrain from drinking carbonated beverages for 48 hours, since these can react with the carbon dioxide used for insufflation and cause vomiting. The length and type of immediate recovery care depend on the anesthetic used.

PATIENT TEACHING

Explain the procedure, and obtain informed consent. Assess the patient for the contraindications listed. Inform the patient that she may feel some pain in the shoulder and abdomen after the procedure; reassure her that this pain usually resolves within 24 hours.

COLPOSCOPY

Colposcopy is the visualization of the vagina and cervix with a binocular microscope. The examination is used to rule out invasive cancer of the cervix. Colposcopy is also used to monitor precancerous abnormalities and recurrent abnormalities and women whose mothers received diethylstilbestrol (DES) during pregnancy. Colposcopy is effective in identifying a suspicious lesion, especially for biopsy, and may eliminate the need for cervical conization.

The procedure is performed with the patient in the lithotomy position. The vagina and cervix are exposed with a speculum and then swabbed with 3% acetic acid to remove mucus and improve visibility. Suspicious lesions are diagramed, and photographs are taken using the light and magnification of the colposcope.

INDICATIONS

Dysplasia
Condylomas
Abnormal Pap smear
Invasive carcinoma
Atrophic changes (usually from aging)

CONTRAINDICATIONS

None

NURSING CARE

Provide emotional support, and encourage the patient to express her concerns. No activity restrictions are required. Antibiotic vaginal creams should be discontinued 1 month before the examination. Have the patient put on a surgical gown and empty her bladder before the procedure. Obtain informed consent if required.

PATIENT TEACHING

In addition to explaining the procedure, inform the patient that the procedure usually causes only momentary discomfort. The results must be considered with the clinical findings of her physician to be meaningful.

CULDOSCOPY

Culdoscopy is the visualization of the pelvic organs. The patient usually is sedated; a general anesthetic is not used. The culdoscope is introduced into the peritoneal cavity through a small incision made in the posterior vaginal fornix and into the perineal space between the rectum and the uterus. Laparoscopy has largely replaced culdoscopy because it gives superior visualization with carbon dioxide insufflation. The culdoscope may be inadequate because of pelvic adhesions. Also, the infection rate is lower with the abdominal approach used in laparoscopy. Culdoscopy may still be used for tubal sterilization in very obese women because of the danger in using general anesthetic in obese patients.

INDICATIONS

Investigation of infertility
Congenital abnormalities
Tubal sterilization in very obese women

CONTRAINDICATIONS

None

NURSING CARE

No activity, food, or fluid restrictions or alterations in medication are required. Obtain informed consent if required. Observe the patient for bleeding and infection after the procedure.

PATIENT TEACHING

Explain the procedure, and inform the patient that she probably will have some shoulder pain if carbon dioxide was introduced into the pelvic cavity during the procedure. Reassure her that the pain usually resolves within 24 hours.

HYSTEROSCOPY

Hysteroscopy is the visualization of the uterine cavity with an endoscope to evaluate infertility, abnormal uterine bleeding, possible malignancies, and fallopian tube competency. After administration of an anesthetic, a rigid endoscope is inserted into the uterine cavity, which is distended with carbon dioxide to allow visualization.

INDICATIONS

Investigation of infertility
To remove a foreign body
Investigation of suspected endometrial cancer
Diagnosis of uterine bleeding

CONTRAINDICATIONS

Pregnancy

NURSING CARE

No activity, food, or fluid restrictions or alterations in medication are required. Obtain informed consent if required. Observe the patient for bleeding and infection after the procedure.

PATIENT TEACHING

Explain the procedure, and inform the patient that she probably will have some shoulder pain if carbon dioxide was introduced into the pelvic cavity during the procedure. Reassure her that the pain usually resolves within 24 hours.

HYSTEROGRAPHY

Hysterography involves instillation of a radiopaque contrast dye through the cervix to define the size, position, and shape of the uterus. Instilling contrast media into the rectum and bladder will enhance the hysterogram, especially when malposition is related to pelvic tumors.

INDICATIONS

Malposition of the uterus

CONTRAINDICATIONS

Pregnancy

NURSING CARE

No activity, food or fluid restrictions, or alterations in medication are required. Obtain informed consent if required. Observe the patient for bleeding and infection after the procedure. After the procedure, monitor the patient's vital signs until they are stable.

PATIENT TEACHING

After the procedure, a vaginal packing or tampon probably will be left in place for several hours. Some spotting is expected, but any unusual bleeding or severe pain should be reported immediately. Tell the patient to avoid strenuous exercise and sexual intercourse for 24 hours after the procedure.

HYSTEROSALPINGOGRAPHY

Hysterosalpingography is a fluoroscopic x-ray study of the uterus and fallopian tubes performed to evaluate fertility in women, to confirm tubal ligation, to evaluate uterine competency, and to detect uterine anomalies. It is best to perform the procedure 4 to 5 days after the end of menstruation because debris from menstruation can temporarily occlude the fallopian tubes. The risk of unknown pregnancy is also reduced with this timing.

The patient lies in the lithotomy position on an examining table with stirrups. After a speculum is positioned in the vagina and a tenaculum, attached to the speculum, holds the cervix in place, a dye is injected through a cannula into the uterine cavity and the fallopian tubes (Figure 3-9). X-rays are taken as the dye fills the uterus and fallopian tubes. The patient may be repositioned for several films and may be asked to wait until the films are developed.

INDICATIONS

To confirm:

 Fallopian tube abnormalities, adhesions, or obstructions (indicated by repeated miscarriage, failure to attain pregnancy, and painful menstruation)

 Uterine abnormalities (e.g., foreign objects or injuries)

 Fistulas or adhesions close to the fallopian tubes

CONTRAINDICATIONS

Pregnancy

Menstruation

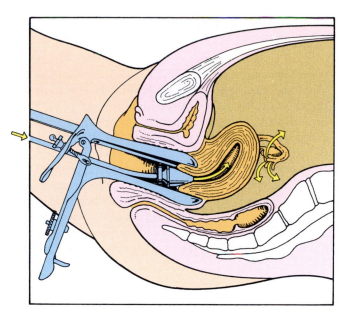

FIGURE 3-9
Hysterosalpingography. (Adapted from Bobak.[13])

Allergy to x-ray contrast material

Undiagnosed vaginal bleeding or pelvic inflammatory disease (PID)

NURSING CARE

No activity, food, or fluid restrictions or alterations in medication are required. Have the patient remove her clothes and change into a surgical gown. Have her empty her bladder before the procedure. Obtain informed consent. Sedatives or antispasmodics may be ordered to reduce fallopian tube spasm. After the procedure, observe the patient for any allergic reactions, cramps, nausea, and dizziness. Although these are uncommon, reassure the patient that they usually are temporary. Shoulder pain, caused by irritation of nerves from the dye, is more common.

PATIENT TEACHING

Explain the procedure, and obtain informed consent if required. Assess the patient for the contraindications listed. Tell the patient that pain may result from tubal spasm and uterine cramping. Inform her that she may have a vaginal discharge (sometimes bloody) for 1 to 2 days after the procedure, and she may need to wear a perineal pad. Instruct the patient to report any signs of infection (e.g., fever, foul odor from discharge) to her physician. Provide emotional support and encourage the patient to discuss her concerns. Explain the postprocedural care, and tell the patient that the results of diagnostic tests must be analyzed in conjunction with clinical findings.

CERVICAL BIOPSY

A cervical biopsy is performed with the patient in the lithotomy position. Local anesthesia is not required, because the cervix is not sensitive to cutting or burning. After a routine bimanual pelvic examination is completed and the cervix has been visualized through a colposcope, atypical areas on the cervix are identified. A biopsy forceps is inserted through the speculum, and a direct punch biopsy is performed. The tissue is sent to the laboratory for analysis. Any bleeding that occurs is stopped with pressure or chemicals. A cervical biopsy should be performed 1 week after menses begins to minimize the possibility that the patient is pregnant.

INDICATIONS

To confirm cancer diagnosis after a questionable or abnormal Pap smear
Abnormal cervical secretions
Exposure to diethylstilbestrol (DES) in utero

CONTRAINDICATIONS

Pregnancy

NURSING CARE

Assess the patient for the contraindication listed. No activity restrictions are required. Restrict food or fluid intake for 12 hours before the procedure. The patient should not have sexual intercourse or douche for 48 hours before the procedure. Use of antibiotic vaginal creams should be discontinued 1 month before the procedure, and the examiner should be informed of any other medications being taken, especially birth control pills. Have the patient put on a surgical gown and empty her bladder before the procedure. Obtain informed consent if required. After the procedure, monitor the patient's vital signs until they are stable. A vaginal packing or tampon probably will be left in place for several hours. Some spotting is expected, but any unusual bleeding or severe pain should be reported immediately.

PATIENT TEACHING

In addition to explaining the procedure, inform the patient that the procedure usually causes only momentary discomfort. Provide emotional support, and encourage the patient to discuss her concerns. A biopsy should be performed 1 week after the menses begins. Encourage the patient to adhere to the recommended 24 hours of bed rest. Tell the patient to avoid strenuous exercise for 8 to 24 hours after the biopsy. Tell her she also must abstain from sexual intercourse and refrain from inserting anything into the vagina (except a tampon) until the biopsy site has healed (usually about 72 hours). Remind her to report excessive bleeding (more than one pad per hour) to her physician. A biopsy report usually is available within 72 hours. However, the results must be considered with the clinical findings of her physician to be meaningful.

CERVICAL CONIZATION (CONE BIOPSY)

Cervical conization is the removal of a cone-shaped portion of the cervix for diagnostic purposes (Figure 3-10).

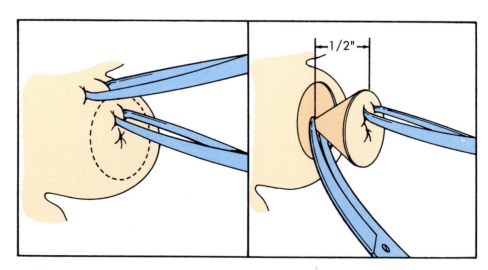

FIGURE 3-10
Conization of the cervix.

This procedure has been replaced by colposcopy in many cases. Schiller's test often is performed in conjunction with but before cervical conization to stain cervical lesions to be biopsied. An aqueous iodine solution is applied to the cervix. Normal tissue turns a deep brown; abnormal tissue does not stain. The patient is placed in the lithotomy position, and a vaginal speculum is inserted to allow visualization of the cervix. A cold knife or laser is used to cut a circular incision around the external os. A cone-shaped piece of tissue is removed for biopsy; the cervix is sutured if needed, and a D & C is performed (see D & C).

INDICATIONS

Positive result on endocervical curettage (ECC)
Discrepancy between Pap smear and cervical biopsy

NURSING CARE

No activity, food, or fluid restrictions or alterations in medication are required. Obtain informed consent if required. Observe the patient for bleeding and infection.

PATIENT TEACHING

Explain the procedure to the patient. Tell the patient that menstrual bleeding should be normal after conization but may be heavier with a brownish premenstrual discharge. Complications after conization may include infertility or incompetent cervix during pregnancy.

ENDOMETRIAL BIOPSY

An endometrial biopsy is used to monitor precancerous abnormalities, ovulatory abnormalities, and women whose mothers took diethylstilbestrol (DES) during pregnancy. This procedure usually is conducted to obtain a sample of tissue for pathologic examination. The procedure is performed on a nonfasting, unsedated patient in the lithotomy position. No anesthesia is required, but a local anesthetic and/or medication such as ibuprofen may be given. After a routine bimanual pelvic examination is done to determine the position of the uterus, the cervix is exposed and cleaned. A tenaculum is placed on the cervix to stabilize it, and a metal sound is introduced into the uterus to measure it. A curette is introduced into the uterus, and biopsy samples are collected from the endometrium. The samples are sent to the laboratory for histologic examination (Figure 3-11).

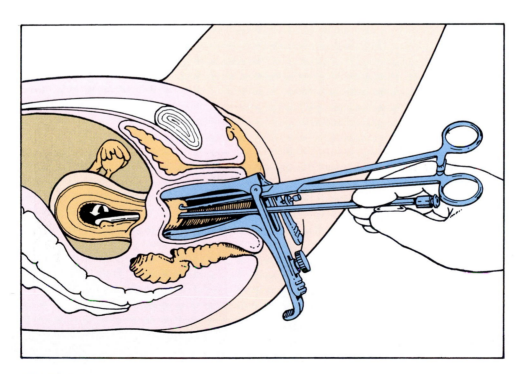

FIGURE 3-11
Endometrial biopsy.

This procedure is a bit more uncomfortable than a cervical biopsy. The pain is sharp, but only momentary as the instruments are introduced into the cervix and uterus. Because some bleeding is expected, vaginal packing or a tampon probably will be put in place.

INDICATIONS

To diagnose:
>   Endometrial cancer
>   Tuberculosis
>   Polyps
>   Inflammatory condition

Endometrial biopsy is also used to determine whether ovulation is occurring and/or the effects of estrogen on the endometrium.

CONTRAINDICATIONS

Patients in whom the cervix cannot be visualized (due to abnormal position or previous surgery)
Infection
Pregnancy

NURSING CARE

No activity restrictions are required. Assess the patient for the contraindications listed. Provide emotional support, and encourage the patient to express her concerns. Restrict food or fluid intake for 12 hours before the procedure. A biopsy should be performed 1 week *after* the menses begins to minimize the possibility that the patient is pregnant. To determine whether ovulation has occurred, the procedure should be conducted 3 to 5 days *before* the normal menses. The patient should not have sexual intercourse or douche for 48 hours before the procedure. Use of antibiotic vaginal creams should be discontinued 1 month before the procedure, and the examiner should be informed of any other medications being taken, especially birth control pills. Have the patient put on a surgical gown and empty her bladder before the biopsy. Obtain informed consent if required. After the biopsy, monitor the patient's vital signs until they are stable. Vaginal packing or a tampon probably will be left in place for several hours. Some spotting is expected, but any unusual bleeding or severe pain should be reported immediately.

PATIENT TEACHING

In addition to explaining the procedure, inform the patient that a biopsy usually causes only momentary discomfort. Encourage her to adhere to the recommendation for bed rest for 24 hours after the procedure; strenuous exercise and heavy lifting should be avoided. Douching and intercourse are not permitted for at least 72 hours after the biopsy. Inform her that she must abstain from sexual intercourse and refrain from inserting anything into the vagina (except a tampon) until the bi-

opsy site has healed (usually about 72 hours). Remind the patient to report excessive bleeding (more than one pad per hour) to her physician. A biopsy report usually is available within 72 hours, but the results must be considered with the clinical findings of her physician to be meaningful.

BONE DENSITOMETRY

Bone densitometry is used to determine bone mineral content, especially in the diagnosis and evaluation of osteoporosis in postmenopausal women (Figure 3-12). Dual-photon absorptiometry or a quantitative CT scan of the metabolically active trabecular bone in the spine is the procedure of choice. Dual-energy x-ray absorptiometry, another method being tested, has shown promising results. All measure bone density to determine the loss of mineral content of bone.

CONTRAINDICATIONS

None

NURSING CARE

No activity, food, or fluid restrictions or alterations in medication are required. Have the patient remove all metal objects and empty her bladder before the test. Obtain informed consent if required. No postprocedural care is required.

PATIENT TEACHING

Explain the procedure, especially noting that the patient must lie motionless on an examination table during the procedure, because any movement can cause artifacts on the scan. Provide encouragement and support for the patient.

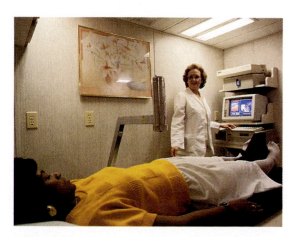

FIGURE 3-12
Bone densitometry.

BONE SCAN

A bone scan is used to identify areas of increased osteolytic and osteoblastic activity. Bone scanning involves several steps. First, a radioactive material is injected into a vein in the arm. The patient then is encouraged to drink water over the next 1 to 3 hours to aid renal clearance of any radioisotope not picked up by the bone. After voiding, the patient is positioned on an examination table and must remain motionless during the scan (Figure 3-13). Any movement by the patient can cause artifacts on the scan. A scintillation camera scans the entire body, identifying areas that absorb the radionuclide given and outlining areas of osteoblastic and osteolytic processes in the bones, such as malignant tumors or osteoporosis. Areas of concentrated nucleotide uptake may represent a tumor or other abnormality. These areas of concentration can be detected days or weeks before an ordinary x-ray can reveal a lesion. The findings are analyzed by a specialist in nuclear medicine imaging.

INDICATIONS

Metastatic tumors of the bone, breasts, kidneys, lungs, thyroid, and urinary bladder
Hidden bone trauma and fracture
Degenerative bone disorders

CONTRAINDICATIONS

Pregnancy (due to risk of fetal damage)
Lactation (due to risk of contaminating the infant)

NURSING CARE

No activity, food, or fluid restrictions or alterations in medication are required. Have the patient remove all metal objects, change into a surgical gown, and empty her bladder. Obtain informed consent if required. Assess the need for pain medication or a sedative to help the patient lie still for the prolonged scanning period. Assess the patient for the contraindications listed. Voiding before the scan clears the pelvic region of the tracer. Encourage the patient to drink fluids to clear the radionuclide. Observe the venipuncture site for discoloration, discomfort, and swelling. Applying warm

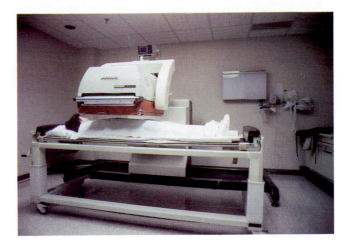

FIGURE 3-13
Patient positioned for bone scan. (From Mourad.[81a])

compresses every 2 to 4 hours should relieve any discomfort.

PATIENT TEACHING

An explanation of the procedure should reassure the patient that the scanning process does not cause radiation effects. The radiation dose is less than that received from regular diagnostic x-rays. No fasting or sedation is needed. Minor localized discomfort at the injection site occurs when the dose of radiation is injected. Lying on the hard table during the procedure can also be uncomfortable. The radioactive substance will not affect other people and usually is excreted in the urine within 6 to 24 hours. The scanning machine detects radiation from the patient, but does not *emit* radiation. Inform the patient that the machine makes a clicking sound during scanning.

After the intravenous injection, the waiting period before scanning is approximately 1 to 3 hours. Tell the patient exactly when the scanning will be conducted, and encourage her to drink several glasses of water to aid renal clearance. A nuclear medicine technician conducts the scan, which takes 30 to 60 minutes. The venipuncture may become discolored, sore, or swollen. Instruct the patient to apply warm compresses to the site every 2 to 4 hours to relieve any discomfort.

DIAGNOSTIC EXAMINATIONS FOR SPECIFIC FEMALE CONDITIONS AND DISEASES

Condition/disease	Name of diagnostic test ordered	To determine	Differential diagnosis
Addison's disease	▪ Serum cortisol response to ACTH	▪ Low value indicates Addison's disease	
Amenorrhea "secondary" amenorrhea (prior normal menses)	▪ Pregnancy test ▪ Thyroid-stimulating hormone (TSH) ▪ Prolactin ▪ Progestin challenge ▪ If above tests are negative, check follicle-stimulating hormone (FSH) and luteinizing hormone (LH) levels	▪ Pregnancy ▪ Rule out (R/O) hypothyroidism ▪ R/O hyperprolactinemia ▪ Assess level of estrogen and competence of uterus ▪ Assess pituitary function	▪ Pregnancy ▪ Hypothyroidism ▪ Hyperthyroidism ▪ Complete Asherman's syndrome ▪ Hypothalamic amenorrhea ▪ Ovarian failure
Anovulation	▪ History of abnormal or absent menstrual function ▪ Thyroid function test ▪ FSH/LH levels ▪ Serum testosterone/ dehydroepiandrosterone sulfate (DHEAS) if indicated	▪ R/O hypothyroidism or hyperthyroidism ▪ R/O perimenopause or intermittent ovarian failure	▪ Thyroid disease ▪ Obesity ▪ Polycystic ovary disease (PCO) ▪ Premature ovarian function ▪ Hypogonadotropic hypogonadism ▪ Congenital adrenal hyperplasia
Cushing's syndrome	▪ Dexamethasone suppression test ▪ 24-hour urinary free cortisol measurements	▪ Adrenal function	
Dysmenorrhea	▪ Good history/clinical examination ▪ If clinically indicated, pelvic ultrasound ▪ If indicated, laparoscopy and/or hysteroscopy	▪ R/O secondary disease or disorder	▪ Primary dysmenorrhea ▪ Fibroids ▪ Endometriosis ▪ Adenomyosis
Endometriosis	▪ History ▪ Physical examination ▪ Laparoscopy ▪ If indicated, surgery		▪ Ovarian cysts ▪ Fibroids ▪ Pelvic adhesions ▪ Irritable bowel
Genital bleeding ▪ Dysfunctional bleeding ▪ Premenarcheal or postmenopausal bleeding	▪ Thorough physical examination ▪ Pap smear ▪ Endometrial biopsy ▪ Depending on history, pelvic ultrasound or hysteroscopy	▪ R/O cervical lesion ▪ Endometrial pathologic condition ▪ R/O polyp or fibrosis	▪ Anovulation ▪ Hormonal replacement therapy (dosage changes) ▪ Endometrial polyp or hyperplasia ▪ Cervical lesion or laceration ▪ Fibroids ▪ Adenomyosis/endometriosis
Infertility	▪ Semen analysis ▪ Basal body temperature chart ▪ Hysterosalpingography or hysteroscopy ▪ Endometrial biopsy ▪ Postcoital test ▪ Folliculography	▪ Ovarian function ▪ Recurrent abortion ▪ Genital tract abnormalities ▪ Immunologic causes	▪ Male factor ▪ Thyroid disease ▪ Anovulation ▪ Uterine pathologic condition or anomaly ▪ Luteal phase defect ▪ Sperm antibodies
Systemic lupus erythematosus (SLE)	▪ Physical examination ▪ Urinalysis ▪ CBC, sedimentation rate (Sed) ▪ Lupus erythematosus test (LE cell prep) ▪ Anti-nuclear antibody (ANA) ▪ Complement assay	▪ Renal function ▪ Blood counts ▪ Assess immunologic system ▪ False-positive RPRs are found	▪ Other immunologic disease ▪ Many diseases may mimic several symptoms of SLE, e.g., hepatitis, rheumatoid arthritis

Condition/disease	Name of diagnostic test ordered	To determine	Differential diagnosis
	▪ Antimitochondrial antibody (AMA) and anti–smooth muscle antibody (ASMA) ▪ Immunoelectrophoresis ▪ Rapid plasma reagin (RPR)		
Menopause	▪ History and physical examination ▪ FSH	▪ If increased, suggests menopause in older women	▪ Menopause ▪ *Rare:* Thyrotoxicosis, carcinoid tumor, pheochromocytoma
Multiple sclerosis	▪ Symptoms from history or examination ▪ Spinal tap ▪ CT scan of head	▪ Assess cerebrospinal fluid (CSF) ▪ CT if lesions present in head	▪ Any demyelination disease caused by infections, anoxia, etc.
Osteoporosis	▪ Dual-photon absorptiometry or single-photon absorptiometry ▪ Computed tomography ▪ Fasting urinary calcium/creatine ratio ▪ Serum calcium/phosphate/alkaline phosphates	▪ Assess bone loss ▪ Assess calcium loss ▪ R/O other metabolic diseases	▪ Calcium malabsorption ▪ Estrogen deficiency ▪ Parathyroid dysfunction
Pelvic inflammatory disease	▪ Examination ▪ Endometrial/cervical cultures ▪ Pelvic ultrasound ▪ Blood work: CBC/chemistries	▪ Identify organism ▪ Identify abscesses if present	▪ Ectopic pregnancy ▪ Appendicitis ▪ Bone perforation ▪ Diverticulitis ▪ Other abdominal infections ▪ Ovarian torsion
Polycystic ovary disease	▪ Serum testosterone ▪ DHEAS ▪ LH/FSH ▪ History and examination	▪ Ovarian function ▪ Adrenal function ▪ Pituitary function	▪ Anovulation ▪ Ovarian or adrenal tumor
Precocious puberty	▪ Physical examination: record of growth, Tanner stages, neurologic examination, signs of androgenization ▪ Skull x-ray film/CT scan ▪ FSH/LH ▪ Thyroid function tests ▪ Steroids: DHEAS, testosterone, estradiol, progesterone, 17-OHP ▪ Bone age ▪ Pelvic/adrenal ultrasound	▪ R/O neoplasm, hydrocephalus	▪ Idiopathic/central precocious puberty ▪ CNS lesion ▪ Exposure to exogenous sex steroids ▪ Congenital adrenal hyperplasia ▪ Adrenal tumor ▪ Ovarian cyst ▪ McCune-Albright syndrome ▪ Hypothyroidism
Premenstrual syndrome	▪ Symptom diary	▪ Assess occurrence of symptoms in relation to menstrual cycle	
Toxic shock syndrome	▪ Clinical presentation of fever/rash/hypertension ▪ Culture: blood/throat/CSF ▪ CBC ▪ Serum chemistries	▪ Signs of toxin ▪ Blood, throat, CSF culture are usually negative ▪ Hematologic status	▪ Disseminated infection ▪ Fulminant allergic reaction
Turner's syndrome	▪ Karyotype ▪ Clinical features	▪ Chromosomes	▪ Other genetic conditions: Mosaicism XY gonadal dysgenesis Resistant ovary syndrome

CHAPTER 4

Pelvic Pain, Bleeding, and Menstrual Disorders

Symptoms of gynecologic disorders often appear as pain, changes in the menstrual cycle, or bleeding that is unrelated to menses. Several terms are used to identify such symptoms. *Pelvic pain* may or may not be associated with menses. *Dysmenorrhea* generally refers to pelvic pain during menses. *Bleeding disorders* include a variety of conditions. *Menstrual disorders* include the lack of menstruation, which often is referred to as amenorrhea (missed menses or periods). Abnormal genital tract bleeding unrelated to menses may occur throughout a woman's life cycle and may be caused by many different factors. *Premenstrual syndrome (PMS)* refers to a combination of physiologic and psychologic symptoms that occur prior to menses. Pelvic pain and PMS have been described as "subjective" disorders, since it often is difficult to measure these symptoms objectively.

Pelvic Pain

DYSMENORRHEA

Primary dysmenorrhea (spasmodic, essential, or psychogenic) refers to nonorganic menstrual pain (no known pathologic condition of the pelvis), although an excess of prostaglandins may be the major cause. **Secondary dysmenorrhea** (congestive, acquired, or inflammatory) refers to pain associated with a pathologic condition that is extrauterine (outside the uterus), intrauterine (inside the uterus), or intramural (within the wall of the pelvic cavity).

Primary and secondary definitions of dysmenorrhea mean *without* or *with* objective evidence of pelvic disease.

Approximately 25% to 50% of women experience dysmenorrhea or menstrual cramping. About 10% of women report work or school absences caused by dysmenorrhea. Primary dysmenorrhea begins around age 16 and may subside by age 25. The initial discomfort is noticed anywhere from 6 months to 2 years after menarche. Reports vary as to whether primary dysmenorrhea diminishes after pregnancy. Of women with dysmenorrhea, 90% report nausea and vomiting, 85% report fatigue, 60% have diarrhea, 60% report pain in the lower back, and 45% have headaches. Midcycle pain, called mittelschmerz, usually occurs in women under 30 years of age.

headaches. Midcycle pain, called mittelschmerz, usually occurs in women under 30 years of age.

PATHOPHYSIOLOGY

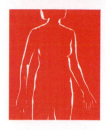

Primary dysmenorrhea is not associated with a pathologic condition. Several theories have been proposed as to the cause of premenstrual and menstrual cramping. Dysmenorrhea is associated with ovulation, and discomfort does not develop until the ovary is mature and secreting progestin. Primary dysmenorrhea does not usually occur until 1 to 2 years after men-

> **Menstrual *molimina* or *dysmenorrhea* refers to the unpleasant pelvic heaviness and discomfort associated with menstruation.**

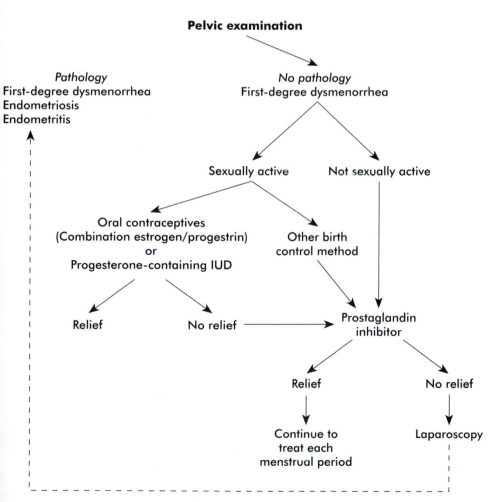

FIGURE 4-1
Evaluation and treatment of dysmenorrhea. (From Frederickson.[35a])

strual function has been established. The endometrium probably produces an excess of prostaglandin $F_{2\alpha}$ ($PGF_{2\alpha}$), which promotes intense uterine contractions, nausea, vomiting, and diarrhea. Increased amounts of vasopressin and leukotrienes and decreased amounts of prostacyclin may also influence contractions. Prostaglandins cause endometrial necrosis and myometrial spasms. Anovular cycles and oral contraceptives reduce prostaglandin, thereby diminishing dysmenorrhea. (Figure 4-1 is an algorithmic representation of the evaluation and treatment of dysmenorrhea.)

Another theory suggests that a thickening of the uterine decidua (membranous dysmenorrhea), caused by excessive activity of the corpus luteum, produces discomfort. Painful uterine contractions may develop in an attempt to expel endometrial fragments or large clots. Also, an imbalance of the uterine autonomic nerve supply may cause muscle spasms. *Mittelschmerz* (midcycle pain) in the area of the iliac fossa may occur from a few minutes to 2 days. This pain probably is caused by the ovulating follicle. Intermenstrual bleeding may occur with mittelschmerz. Midcycle pain has been described as an aspect of both dysmenorrhea and chronic pelvic pain.

Secondary dysmenorrhea by definition refers to identifiable conditions or organic diseases. *Extrauterine* causes include endometriosis, ovarian neoplasms, adhesions, and inflammation. Lower genital tract causes include transverse vaginal septum, congenital absence of the cervix, imperforate hymen, and acquired cervical stenosis. *Intramural* causes include myomas, adenomyosis, and endometrial polyps. A noncommunicating uterine horn may exist. *Intrauterine* causes include intrauterine contraceptive devices (IUDs), pelvic inflammatory disease (PID), adhesions, cervical lesions or stenosis, polyps, and myomas. Secondary dysmenorrhea may occur suddenly after years of asymptomatic menstrual bleeding.

CLINICAL MANIFESTATIONS

The clinical manifestations of dysmenorrhea are numerous and varied: mittelschmerz, infrequently associated with shoulder tip pain or fainting; no fever or muscle guarding; cramping, colicky, spasmodic, or intermittent pain, usually beginning with menses and lasting a few hours to 2 days; a bilateral dull ache in the lower abdomen and back; pain radiating to the medial thighs; bloating; menorrhagia (prolonged and/or profuse menses); dyspareunia (painful sexual intercourse); premen-

strual syndrome (PMS) with breast tenderness, depression, or irritability; gastrointestinal symptoms, including anorexia, nausea, vomiting, and diarrhea; urinary frequency; central nervous system (CNS) symptoms such as headaches, dizziness, fainting, poor concentration, weakness, diaphoresis (sweating), and chills. Findings on examination may include uterine tenderness, uterosacral nodules, enlarged ovaries, fixation of the uterus, and intrauterine pressures similar to or greater than those in active labor.

Table 4-1 shows drugs commonly used to alleviate symptoms of dysmenorrhea.

COMPLICATIONS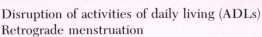

Disruption of activities of daily living (ADLs)
Retrograde menstruation
Infertility
Undetected pregnancy or ruptured ectopic pregnancy, ruptured cysts, uterine perforation from IUD, infection

DIFFERENTIAL DIAGNOSIS

The following conditions may have similar signs and symptoms and should be ruled out:
Adenomyosis/adenomyometritis (invasion of uterine myometrial tissue into the endometrium or of ectopic myometrial tissue into uterine muscle [intrinsic])
Endometriosis (migration of endometrial tissue outside the uterus [extrinsic], often with cysts; endometriosis may replace older adenomyosis terms)
Fibroids (fibroleiomyoma; newer definition, leiomyoma), polyps, ovarian cysts
Cervical stenosis; IUD
Intrauterine adhesions (Asherman's syndrome)
Pelvic inflammatory disease (PID); tuberculosis
Ectopic pregnancy; imperforate hymen; anatomic anomaly
Systemic pain from bowel, urinary, or musculoskeletal disorder
Carcinoma

NURSING CARE

See pages 54 to 57.

Table 4-1

NONSTEROIDAL ANTIINFLAMMATORY DRUGS COMMONLY PRESCRIBED FOR DYSMENORRHEA

Drug	Loading dose	Maintenance dose	Frequency
Ibuprofen	—	200-800 mg	q 4 h
Naproxen	500 mg	250 mg	q 6-8 h
Mefenamic acid	500 mg	250 mg	q 6 h
Aspirin	—	250 mg	q 6 h

From Stenchever.[101]

DIAGNOSTIC STUDIES AND FINDINGS

Diagnostic test	Findings
Pelvic examination and Pap smear; urine and cervical cultures, potassium hydroxide smear (KOH), wet prep; complete blood count (CBC); erythrocyte sedimentation rate (ESR)	To determine the existence of underlying conditions of secondary dysmenorrhea
Ultrasound; endometrial biopsy; laparoscopy; hysteroscopy; dilation and curettage (D & C); hysterosalpingography	To visualize tissue and determine cause

MEDICAL MANAGEMENT

GENERAL MANAGEMENT

Primary dysmenorrhea (management of secondary dysmenorrhea relates to underlying pathologic condition).

Hot baths, heating pad, orgasm, knee-chest position; natural diuretics (e.g., asparagus, parsley); adequate exercise, diet, rest, and hygiene; transdermal electrical nerve stimulation (TENS); acupuncture; biofeedback.

DRUG THERAPY

Nonsteroidal antiinflammatory drugs (Table 4-1): Carboxylates (salicylic, acetic, and propionic acids; fenamates); enolic acids (pyrazolones, oxicams). Prostaglandin inhibitors. Hormonal therapy (e.g., oral steroid contraceptives reduce cramps in 80% of women with dysmenorrhea). Analgesic/antipyretic drugs. Narcotic analgesics.

SURGERY

Cervical dilation (may produce temporary relief).

Presacral sympathectomy (division of the sympathetic superior hypogastric plexus); laparoscopic uterosacral nerve ablation.

Total abdominal hysterectomy and bilateral salpingo-oophorectomy (TAH/BSO) if disorder is secondary dysmenorrhea.

Chronic Pelvic Pain

Noncyclic chronic pelvic pain is constant or intermittent pain that occurs for at least 4 to 6 months. Chronic pelvic pain may be related to an anatomic or physiologic disorder, or the cause may remain unknown.

The incidence of chronic pelvic pain correlates with the underlying pathologic condition. Pain of unknown origin may be related to psychologic factors. Chronic pelvic pain accounts for about 10% of gynecologic consults. An estimated 10% to 35% of laparoscopies and 12% of hysterectomies are performed because of chronic pelvic pain.

PATHOPHYSIOLOGY

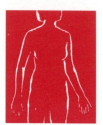 Chronic pelvic pain often is associated with other symptoms such as irregular bowel function, bladder irritability, poor posture, or emotional stressors. Acute conditions may develop into chronically painful ones such as varicosities, anal fissures, and cervical erosion. Structural problems, such as uterine prolapse, can cause persistent, low-grade pain, dyspareunia (painful coitus), and postcoital pain.

The term *chronic pelvic pain* has been used in connection with other etiologic terms such as mittelschmerz and dysmenorrhea. Chronic, *cyclic* pelvic pain has been contrasted with noncyclic, or *acyclic*, causes. Acyclic causes have been further delineated as being *within* or *outside* the reproductive tract, or associated with other anatomic areas. The patient's perception of pain location is usually determined by the affected afferent visceral fiber. Figure 4-2 depicts the dermatome representation of afferent visceral impulses.

Extrauterine causes of pelvic pain include malformations, adhesions, infection, ovarian cysts and tumors, ectopic pregnancy, congestion, pelvic varicosities, and endometriosis. *Uterine* causes may include endometritis, fibroids, polyps, irritation from an intrauterine contraceptive device (IUD), or pelvic relaxation (prolapse). *Urologic* conditions that cause pain include infection, stones, and bladder contractions. *Gastrointestinal* causes of pain may include hernias, elimination problems, obstructions, inflammation, parasites, ulcers, spasms, or dietary intolerance. *Musculoskeletal* causes include herniated discs, pelvic neoplasms, fractures and sprains, fibromyositis (inflammation or hyperplasia), and spondylolysis. *Inflammation, disease, and toxins,* including

herpes zoster, sickle cell disease, diabetes mellitus, and lead poisoning, may cause lower abdominal and pelvic pain. The occurrence of *pelvic vascular congestion syndrome* is debatable. However, vascular congestion may be linked to emotional stress.

Chronic *dyspareunia* may result from several different causes. Painful sexual intercourse may result from vaginismus (spasm), clitoral anomalies, rigid or intact hymen, infections (vulvovaginitis, inflammation of Bartholin's or Skene's glands), vulvar dystrophy, vaginal atrophy, scarring, insufficient lubrication, short vaginal canal, and urinary tract infections (UTIs). Other pathologic conditions of the pelvis that result in dyspareunia include endometriosis, uterine retroversion, and ovarian cysts.

Some theories propose a psychosomatic origin for the pain, especially when the cause of the pain is unknown. Stress may affect the woman's susceptibility to a pain-producing pathologic condition. The regulation of mood by neurotransmitters, such as serotonin and endorphins, and by the limbic system in general is connected with pain perception. In short, depression and stress may deplete the body's ability to cope with pain.

CLINICAL MANIFESTATIONS

The clinical manifestations of chronic pelvic pain are numerous and varied: cyclic or acyclic pelvic pain; chronic pelvic pain associated with underlying pathologic condition; persistent pelvic pain of unknown origin; discomfort out of proportion to cause of pain; dyspareunia and postcoital pain from a malpositioned uterus; signs of depression, abuse, or stress

COMPLICATIONS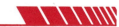

Dependent on underlying cause
Pain that leads to interference with ADLs

DIFFERENTIAL DIAGNOSIS

The following conditions may have similar signs and symptoms and should be ruled out:
Gynecologic disorder
Urinary and bowel pathologic conditions
Gastrointestinal pathologic condition
Musculoskeletal pathologic condition
Orthopedic pathologic condition
Appendicitis
Psychologic disorder

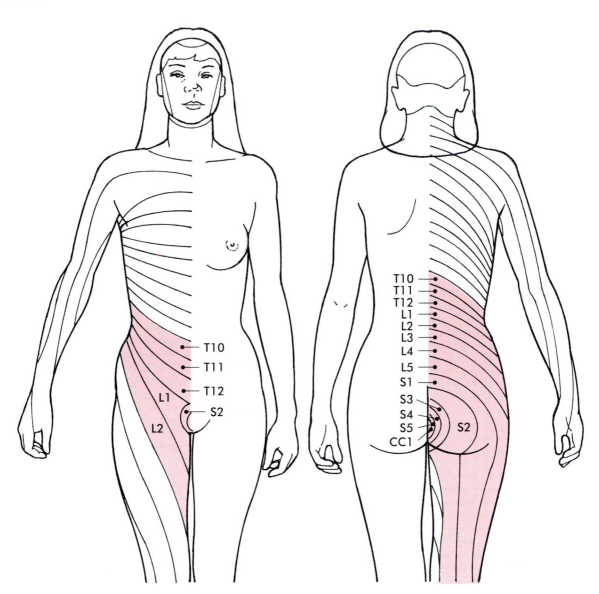

FIGURE 4-2
Dermatome representation of the afferent visceral impulses.

DIAGNOSTIC STUDIES AND FINDINGS

Diagnostic test	Findings
Pelvic examination and Pap smear; complete blood count (CBC)	To identify underlying pathologic condition
Pregnancy test; vaginal, cervical cultures	To identify underlying conditions
Abdominal x-ray, ultrasonography, magnetic resonance imaging (MRI), and computed tomography (CT) scans; laparoscopy	To evaluate possible etiologies
Psychologic tests	To identify factors that may accentuate pain

MEDICAL MANAGEMENT

GENERAL MANAGEMENT

Treatment of underlying pathologic condition; transdermal electrical nerve stimulation (TENS); biofeedback; counseling; pain clinic.

DRUG THERAPY

Analgesics; nonsteroidal antiinflammatory drugs (NSAIDS); gonadotropin-releasing hormone (GnRH) agonists or oral contraceptives to suppress ovulation.

SURGERY

Nerve blocks; laser ablation of uterosacral ligaments; presacral neurectomy; hysterectomy.

1 ASSESS*

ASSESSMENT	OBSERVATIONS	
	DYSMENORRHEA	CHRONIC PAIN
History	Menarche, menses factors (duration, frequency, amount of flow), PMS	Previous medical and surgical treatments and diagnostic tests; pain site and symptoms
	Pain site and symptoms (backache, bloating), chronology and duration, relieving or aggravating factors, medications	Pain chronology, especially onset, intensity, duration (worsening acute conditions; lasting 4 to 6 months)
	Gastrointestinal (GI) and genitourinary (GU) patterns (e.g., nausea, vomiting, diarrhea), CNS symptoms (headache, lethargy, dizziness), sexual and family history (dyspareunia)	Complete systemic history (e.g., GI and GU patterns: dysuria, diarrhea, melena) Sexual and family history (stress, abuse, pain)
Reproductive organs	Examination may reveal uterine tenderness, uterine fixation, pelvic adhesions associated with PID or endometriosis, enlarged uterus from adenomyosis, uterine fibroids or leiomyomas, enlarged ovaries, uterosacral nodules, cervical stenosis	Examination may reveal fissures, pelvic support disorder (prolapse), pelvic adhesions, progressive endometriosis, congestion of pelvic venous system
Psychosocial	Anxiety associated with pelvic pain, knowledge deficit, and/or ineffective coping	

*Nursing care should be well documented in the patient's permanent health care record.

2 DIAGNOSE

NURSING DIAGNOSIS	SUBJECTIVE FINDINGS	OBJECTIVE FINDINGS
Pain or discomfort related to gynecologic disorder	Patient describes location and sensation of pain, aggravating and relieving factors	Tight facial expressions; altered muscle tone; diaphoresis; elevated vital signs; pupillary dilation (findings depend on whether pain is present during examination)
Anxiety related to treatment and prognosis of pelvic pain	Patient expresses anxiety about pelvic pain	Elevated vital signs; diaphoresis; pupillary dilation
Knowledge deficit related to etiology and/or diagnosis and management of pelvic pain	Patient expresses concern about gynecologic symptomatology; requests information on causes of pain and its relief	Active facial expressions and gestures; patient may be talkative and alert or withdrawn
Ineffective individual coping related to stressors that may aggravate pelvic pain	Reports psychologic problems or difficulty managing stressors	Withdrawn or verbally hostile

3 PLAN

Patient goals

1. The patient's pain will be alleviated.
2. The patient's anxiety about her treatment and prognosis will be resolved.
3. The patient will take an active role in selecting treatment options and in pain management.
4. The patient will develop coping strategies and minimize stress.

4 IMPLEMENT

NURSING DIAGNOSIS	NURSING INTERVENTIONS	RATIONALE
Pain or discomfort related to gynecologic disorder	Evaluate character and severity of pain.	To assess pain patterns.
Anxiety related to treatment and prognosis of pelvic pain	Validate patient's fears; identify and correct misconceptions.	To promote patient's self-esteem and help alleviate her anxiety.
	Discuss patient's past coping strategies. Collaborate with health team to present medical and surgical options.	To help reduce patient's fear to enable patient to make an informed choice.

→ › ›

NURSING DIAGNOSIS	NURSING INTERVENTIONS	RATIONALE
Knowledge deficit related to etiology and/or diagnosis and management of pelvic pain	Provide information on pain control (e.g., analgesics, diet, exercise, heat).	To help patient minimize pain.
	Collaborate with physician and health team to ensure effective pain control.	To enhance pain control with team approach.
	Assess patient's feelings about herself and her life.	To clarify patient's feelings.
	Respect patient's need for temporary denial or withdrawal.	To facilitate coping mechanisms.
Ineffective individual coping related to stressors that may aggravate pelvic pain	Explore patient's behavior during dysmenorrhea or chronic pelvic pain.	To identify effects on life-style and coping.
	Encourage problem solving (e.g., counseling), or other resources as needed.	To provide support.

5 EVALUATE

PATIENT OUTCOME	DATA INDICATING THAT OUTCOME IS REACHED
Patient's comfort has increased, or her pain has been relieved.	Patient reports that pain is under control and shows no nonverbal evidence of pain; improvement is documented on pain scale.
The patient understands the etiology and diagnosis of her pelvic pain.	Patient describes the cause, or meaning of unknown etiology, of her pelvic pain.
Patient's anxiety has been minimized.	Patient reports increased psychologic comfort.
Patient selects and implements treatment options and ways to control pain.	Patient and family make informed choice about treatment of condition or control of chronic pain.
Patient realistically minimizes her stressors and identifies her coping resources.	Patient regains self-confidence and accepts her life.

PATIENT TEACHING

Primary dysmenorrhea

1. Discuss the possible causes of pain (behavioral, psychologic, uterine ischemia, and prostaglandin factors), and explore ways to minimize the possible cause.
2. Discuss methods for relieving pain (heat application, effleurage [abdominal massage], orgasm, pelvic tilt exercise, transdermal electrical nerve stimulation [TENS] treatments, acupuncture, biofeedback, laparoscopic uterosacral nerve ablation, cervical digitation).
3. Describe possible pharmacologic treatments.
4. Help the patient identify ways to eat more fruits and vegetables, to minimize bloating and maximize gastrointestinal function.

5. Help the patient identify ways to get adequate rest and exercise and to decrease stress.

Secondary dysmenorrhea and chronic pelvic pain

1. Discuss ways to correct the underlying condition and possible surgical treatment (laparoscopy, dilation and curettage, hysterectomy).
2. Discuss ways to relieve pain (see no. 2 above), and encourage the patient to seek psychologic assistance if needed.
3. Answer the patient's questions as appropriate about pharmacologic options (nonnarcotics, antidepressants).
4. Encourage the patient to discuss her self-perceptions; explore any life-style factors that may be associated with pelvic pain.

Bleeding Disorders

Primary amenorrhea is the failure to menstruate (menarche or first menstruation) by about 16 years of age. **Secondary amenorrhea** is the lack of menstruation for 3 months or longer after menarche. **Premenarcheal (prepubertal) bleeding** is bleeding that occurs before puberty. **Postmenopausal bleeding** is reproductive tract bleeding that occurs 1 year or longer after menopause. **Dysfunctional uterine bleeding (DUB)** refers to abnormal uterine bleeding in the reproductive years.

Primary amenorrhea occurs in fewer than 0.1% of young women. Secondary amenorrhea is a common gynecologic disorder, and menopause and pregnancy are the usual causes. Secondary amenorrhea unrelated to pregnancy or menopause occurs in about 0.7% of women. Dysfunctional uterine bleeding usually is caused by anovulation from neuroendocrinologic factors. Excessive or irregular bleeding from the uterus is one of the most common gynecologic disorders, occurring from puberty through menopause. Twenty percent of cases of dysfunctional uterine bleeding occur during adolescence, 30% during the reproductive years, and

50% in women 40 to 50 years of age. Postmenopausal bleeding is caused by carcinoma in 35% to 50% of women. About 25% of cases involving gynecologic surgery involve abnormal causes of bleeding. Approximately 20% of cases of severe menorrhagia in adolescents involve clotting deficiencies. Oligomenorrhea (markedly infrequent menses) is more common in young women.

PATHOPHYSIOLOGY

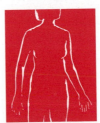

Girls between the ages of 11 and 14 usually have increasingly more estrogenic activity of the ovaries. Ovarian dysgenesis (congenital defects) may result in estrogen deficiency and *primary amenorrhea*. A pituitary pathologic condition, such as pituitary infantilism, is associated with low levels of follicle-stimulating hormone (FSH) and estrogen.

Secondary amenorrhea may result from lack of ovarian production of estrogens. Polycystic ovary syndrome (Stein-Leventhal syndrome) may result in ovarian enlargement and amenorrhea. Premature ovarian failure (premature menopause) may occur if ovarian follicles are absent. Increased prolactin from hypothyroidism, stress, or a tumor may result in amenorrhea. Amenorrhea may also occur with severe diseases such as uncontrolled diabetes, chronic renal disease, and hyperthyroidism. Chronic disease and corticosteroid therapy promote hypothalamic and pituitary suppression. Cushing's syndrome, other adrenal gland tumors, and hyperplasia may result in menstrual cessation.

Anorexia nervosa, bulimia, and starvation produce decreased body fat necessary for hormone production, resulting in hypogonadism and amenorrhea. Heavy athletic activity may also suppress menstruation, especially in thin women with reduced body fat.

When oral contraception is stopped, it may take up to 6 months to reestablish menses. Amenorrhea may also result from prostaglandin inhibitors and exogenous estrogen.

Abnormal bleeding may be caused by benign or malignant tumors of the uterus, cervix, vagina, or vulva. Other causes include hormonal factors, defects of the reproductive tract, foreign bodies, lacerations, lesions, infections, prenatal exposure to diethylstilbestrol (DES), polycystic ovarian disease, systemic diseases (e.g., leukemia, thyroid and liver diseases), blood dyscrasias, and complications of pregnancy. Acquired deficiencies and congenital coagulation defects also lead to bleeding.

Premenarcheal (prepubertal) bleeding is usually the result of hormonal influences or pathologic conditions. Postmenopausal bleeding is reproductive tract bleeding that occurs 1 year or longer after menopause. Causes of postmenopausal bleeding include endometrial hyperplasia, endometrial cancer, or estrogen therapy.

Dysfunctional uterine bleeding (DUB) is painless bleeding associated with anovulation. DUB may vary from spotting to massive hemorrhage and the passage of clots. The condition is *not* associated with one specific etiologic factor. Several different bleeding conditions may occur. *Menometrorrhagia* is painless, heavy, irregular bleeding. *Hypomenorrhea* is inadequate menses; *polymenorrhea* is frequent or repeated menses (occurring less than 21 days apart); and *oligomenorrhea* is infrequent menses (occurring more than 30 days apart). Oligomenorrhea may result from a prolonged proliferative phase of the menstrual cycle. *Menorrhagia or hypermenorrhea* refers to excessive menses (180 ml [5.4 ounces] or more). Menorrhagia may be associated with a high level of prostaglandin, which causes vasodilation and bleeding. *Metrorrhagia* is intermenstrual or irregular bleeding resulting from midcycle fluctuations of estradiol. *Spotting* is the passage of small amounts of pink or dark brown blood. Dysfunctional uterine bleeding may also be classified as mild (irregular, low flow), moderate, or severe (blood loss of 500 ml [15 ounces] or more).

CLINICAL MANIFESTATIONS

The clinical manifestations of bleeding disorders are numerous and varied. If the patient reports that she does not menstruate, primary or secondary amenorrhea may be involved. If she states that her period was delayed, followed by excessive bleeding, anovulation or threatened abortion may be the cause. Infrequent bleeding may indicate DUB, pelvic inflammatory disease, endometriosis, or anovulation. Profuse bleeding may indicate DUB, endometrial polyps, adenomyosis, leiomyomas, or irritation from an intrauterine device (IUD). Irregular or intermenstrual bleeding may be a sign of DUB, endometrial polyps, cervical or uterine cancer, or a problem with oral contraceptives. Weight loss may indicate anorexia and bulimia associated with hypothalamic amenorrhea. The patient also may report menstrual or midcycle pain. Examination findings may include cervical lesions, cervical motion and tenderness, or adnexal tenderness.

COMPLICATIONS

Uncontrolled hemorrhage
Hemodynamic instability
Orthostatic vital signs
Anemia, weight loss
Altered sexual function

DIFFERENTIAL DIAGNOSIS OF ABNORMAL UTERINE BLEEDING

I. Pregnancy related
   A. Intrauterine pregnancy
      1. Threatened abortion
      2. Incomplete abortion
      3. Missed abortion
      4. Septic abortion
   B. Ectopic pregnancy
   C. Gestational trophoblastic neoplasm
      1. Hydatidiform mole
      2. Placental site trophoblastic tumor
      3. Choriocarcinoma
II. Infections/endometritis
   A. Ascending infection and sexually transmitted diseases
   B. Systemic hematogenously derived infections (tuberculosis)
   C. IUD-related infection
   D. Endometritis related to leiomyomas
   E. Postinstrumentation infection
III. Endocrine causes
   A. Anovulation
      1. Hypothalamic
      2. Polycystic ovarian syndrome
      3. Follicle depletion (perimenopausal)
   B. Hypothyroidism and hyperthyroidism
   C. Prolactin-secreting tumors
IV. Neoplasia
   A. Benign polyps
   B. Myomas
   C. Endometrial hyperplasia
   D. Malignancy
      1. Endometrial carcinoma
      2. Cervical or endocervical carcinoma
      3. Ovarian (granulosa cell, metastatic)
      4. Tubal carcinoma
V. Coagulation disorders
   A. Inherited (e.g., von Willebrand's, hemophilia)
   B. Acquired (e.g., idiopathic thrombocytopenic purpura [ITP], leukemia)
   C. Drug induced (coumadin, heparin, aspirin)
VI. Systemic disease
   A. Renal failure
   B. Severe liver disease with secondary coagulopathy
VII. Endometrial atrophy
VIII. Factitious bleeding (not from the uterine cavity)
   A. Gastrointestinal tract origin
   B. Urinary tract origin
   C. Cervical/vaginal bleeding
IX. Unexplained bleeding (dysfunctional uterine bleeding)

From Stenchever.[101]

DIAGNOSTIC STUDIES AND FINDINGS

Diagnostic test	Findings
Amenorrhea	
Developmental studies for puberty	Marshall-Tanner stages
Tests for amenorrhea	(See the box below)
Pregnancy test	To determine underlying conditions

An endometrial biopsy is indicated for chronic anovulation, chronic infection, or persistent bleeding despite hormonal therapy, and in women over 40 years of age.

Bleeding	
Complete blood count; platelets; prothrombin time and partial thromboplastin time (PT/PTT); bleeding time; reticulocytes; stool guaiac; gonococcus and chlamydia cultures; thyroid function tests	To identify anemia, leukocyte levels, and underlying pathologic condition
Ultrasound; dilation and curettage with cervical and endometrial biopsy; hysteroscopy	To assess endometrium for lesions, polyps, or carcinoma
Ovulation tests: basal body temperature, vaginal and cervical cytologic studies, serum and urine progesterone levels	To assess ovulation

---

DIAGNOSTIC TESTS FOR AMENORRHEA

Hypothalamic-pituitary compartment
  Serum hormone levels: LH, FSH, TSH, prolactin, growth hormone, morning and evening cortisol
  Dynamic tests: GnRH, TRH, and CRF challenge tests; insulin tolerance test; water deprivation test
  Imaging: Lateral skull x-ray film, CT scan or MRI of the pituitary and sella
Ovarian compartment
  Serum hormone levels: LH, FSH, estradiol, progesterone
  Diagnostic tests: Progesterone challenge
  Imaging: Pelvic ultrasound, dual-photon absorptiometry or hologic digital radiography, bone age
  Other: Karyotype, ovarian antibody panel, ovarian biopsy, BBT chart
Uterine-vaginal compartment
  Serum hormone levels: hCG
  Dynamic tests: Estrogen plus progestin challenge test
  Imaging: Pelvic ultrasound, hysterosalpingogram, MRI
  Other: Endometrial biopsy
Additional tests of other organ systems
  Serum hormone levels: Testosterone, DHEAS, 3-alpha-androstanediol glucuronide, 17-OH progesterone, thyroxine, T_3 uptake, carotene, insulin, glucose tolerance test
  Dynamic tests: ACTH stimulation test, dexamethasone suppression test, TRH stimulation test
  Imaging: Adrenal CT scan, iodocholesterol scan, thyroid scan
  Other: Selective venous catheterization

ACTH, adrenocorticotropic hormone	hCG, human chorionic gonadotropin
BBT, basal body temperature	LH, luteinizing hormone
CRF, corticotropin releasing factor	T_3, triiodothyronine
DHEAS, dehydroepiandrosterone sulfate	TRH, thyrotropin-releasing hormone
FSH, follicle-stimulating hormone	TSH, thyroid-stimulating hormone
GnRH, gonadotropin-releasing hormone	

From Stenchever.[101]

MEDICAL MANAGEMENT

GENERAL MANAGEMENT

Amenorrhea

Treatment of underlying cause.

DRUG THERAPY

Amenorrhea

Induction of ovulation.

Abnormal uterine bleeding

Nonsteroidal antiinflammatory drugs (NSAIDs); oral contraceptives (estrogens); progesterone or progestin; prostaglandin inhibitors.

SURGERY

Abnormal uterine bleeding

Laser ablation of the endometrium; total abdominal hysterectomy with partial or complete bilateral salpingo-oophorectomy (TAH/BSO); hysteroscopy; hysteroscopic resectoscope for endometrial ablation; dilation and curettage (D & C); polyp excision.

---

1 ASSESS*

ASSESSMENT	OBSERVATIONS	
	AMENORRHEA	**BLEEDING**
History	Age-related factors: onset of menses (primary amenorrhea), breast development and secondary sexual characteristics, menopausal symptoms Cessation of menses (secondary amenorrhea) Diet, stress, exercise Sexual activity Previous D & Cs, postpartum hemorrhage or infection Weight loss or gain Symptoms of systemic disease Genetic abnormalities Use of hormones, antidepressants, alpha-methyldopa, phenothiazines Pregnancy	Characteristics of bleeding (e.g., duration, amount, timing) Last menstrual period (LMP) Diet, stress, exercise Chronic disease or symptoms of disease Pregnancy symptoms Symptoms of infection Weight loss or gain Dental bleeding Dysmenorrhea or midcycle pain Dyspareunia Passing of clots or tissue Use of aspirin, diet pills, or psychotropic drugs

*Nursing care should be well documented in the patient's permanent health care record.

	OBSERVATIONS	
ASSESSMENT	**AMENORRHEA**	**BLEEDING**
Evidence of bleeding	Menstruation not begun at puberty, or cessation of menstruation for at least three cycles	Heavy menstruation Frequent or recurrent menstrual cycle bleeding Infrequent menstruation Bleeding or spotting between menstrual cycles
Psychosocial	Anxiety associated with knowledge deficit about amenorrhea or inappropriate bleeding.	

2   DIAGNOSE

NURSING DIAGNOSIS	SUBJECTIVE FINDINGS	OBJECTIVE FINDINGS
Altered tissue perfusion related to pelvic bleeding	Expresses concern about hemorrhage	Measurable blood expelled
	Describes previous blood loss	Signs of hypovolemia (pallor, tachycardia, tachypnea, hypotension, diaphoresis, oliguria)
Anxiety related to treatment and prognosis of menstrual disorder	Expresses anxiety about amenorrhea or bleeding, its cause, and treatment options	Elevated vital signs, diaphoresis, dilated pupils

3   PLAN

Patient goals

1. The patient will regain and/or maintain adequate perfusion.

2. The patient's fears about the treatment and prognosis for her condition will be resolved.

4   IMPLEMENT

NURSING DIAGNOSIS	NURSING INTERVENTIONS	RATIONALE
Altered tissue perfusion related to pelvic bleeding	Report blood loss, vital signs, signs of hypovolemia; also CBC, hemoglobin (Hgb), hematocrit (Hct), and other pertinent laboratory values.	To provide care and allow emergency treatment, if needed.
	Give fluids and blood products as ordered.	To promote hydration and tissue perfusion.

NURSING DIAGNOSIS	NURSING INTERVENTIONS	RATIONALE
Anxiety related to treatment and prognosis of menstrual disorder	Validate patient's fears about bleeding, and offer encouragement.	To promote self-esteem and self-care.
	Identify and correct misconceptions.	To help patient clarify her fears.
	Discuss patient's past coping mechanisms.	To help reduce patient's fear.
	Collaborate with health team to present medical and surgical options.	To enable patient to make an informed choice of treatment.

5 EVALUATE

PATIENT OUTCOME	DATA INDICATING THAT OUTCOME IS REACHED
Patient's bleeding has been controlled, and perfusion is maintained.	Bleeding is under control, vital signs are stable, and mucosa is pink.
Patient's fears about treatment and prognosis have resolved.	Patient states that she feels less anxiety about the cause of her menstrual disorder and its treatment and prognosis.

PATIENT TEACHING

1. If the patient is hemorrhaging, calmly explain the nursing care involved, including the need to assess vital signs and fluid and blood loss.
2. Encourage the patient to describe bleeding characteristics and to report the symptoms to her physician.
3. Discuss the possible causes of amenorrhea or dysfunctional uterine bleeding as appropriate.
4. Explain the importance of reporting any recurrence of bleeding, including time of occurrence, type of flow, number and type of pads or tampons used, and any precipitating factors such as exercise or coitus, and symptoms that require immediate or emergency treatment.
5. Describe possible treatments, and encourage the patient to explore these options.

Premenstrual Syndrome

Premenstrual syndrome (PMS) is a combination of affective (emotional) and somatic (physical) symptoms that begin around the luteal phase and usually diminish after menstruation begins.

Premenstrual syndrome (PMS) occurs most frequently in women over 30 years of age. It may begin during the late twenties and increase in severity toward menopause. An estimated 50% of women experience PMS sometime in their lives. Currently, 9 million to 12 million women in the United States are affected.

PATHOPHYSIOLOGY

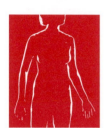

A combination of factors may facilitate the development of PMS. Biologic changes and behavioral symptoms are most pronounced during the late luteal phase of the menstrual cycle. PMS may involve several factors or a combination of factors, such as a rise or fall in estrogen, a decrease in progesterone, vitamin deficiencies, and variations in the levels of aldosterone, renin, angiotensin, melanocyte-stimulating hormone (MSH), and beta-endorphin peptide. Vitamin B_6 is needed for the biosynthesis of serotonin and dopamine, and magnesium aids in the production of neurotransmitters. The mood swings associated with PMS may result from fluctuations of brain neurotransmitters.

Generally, PMS seems to involve a fall in estrogen and progesterone levels, which increases aldosterone production, promoting sodium retention and edema. Fluid retention in turn results from an increase in ovarian steroids and antidiuretic hormone produced by the posterior pituitary gland. Depression may result from decreased brain levels of monoamine oxidase, which stem from the decrease in estrogen. Irritability may result from changing levels of brain catecholamine and monoamine oxidase. Reduced serotonin levels may also influence mood swings.

CLINICAL MANIFESTATIONS

Symptoms begin 5 to 10 days before menstruation and subside 1 to 2 days after the onset of menses. The symptoms of PMS fall into a variety of categories.

General
Lower abdominal and back discomfort; pelvic or abdominal cramping

Hydration (cardiovascular-related)
General feelings of bloating, engorgement, or pelvic edema; peripheral and abdominal edema; weight gain variations of about 1 pound; mastalgia (breast tenderness); oliguria (scanty urinary output); palpitations, diaphoresis (sweating)

Other urologic symptoms
Cystitis, urethritis; enuresis (involuntary urination)

Gastrointestinal
Diarrhea or constipation; nausea, vomiting, compulsive eating, food craving (particularly sweets and salty foods)

Dermatologic
Acne, urticaria (itching), boils, bruising; recurrence of herpes; galactorrhea (milk discharge) if lactating

Ophthalmologic
Recurrent styes, conjunctivitis

Respiratory
Cold and allergy symptoms; recurrent asthma

Neurologic
Headache (including migraine), vertigo (dizziness, lightheadedness), fainting, lability (unsteady when standing); paresthesia (numbness, burning, or pricking sensation) of head and feet, clumsiness

Behavioral
Mood swings, depression, irritability, anxiety, anger, lethargy, fatigue, insomnia or hypersomnia, attention span deficit, loss of motivation or interest, confusion, increased accidents, forgetfulness, crying, guilt, sexual arousal or dysfunction, tension

COMPLICATIONS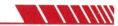

Harmful antisocial behavior
Underlying pathologic or psychologic condition

DIFFERENTIAL DIAGNOSIS

The following conditions may have similar signs and symptoms and should be ruled out:
Endometriosis
Hyperprolactinemia
Nutritional imbalances
Ovarian cysts
Pelvic inflammatory disease (PID)
Psychiatric disorders
Thyroid disease

DIAGNOSTIC STUDIES AND FINDINGS

Diagnostic test	Findings
Medical ovariectomy with gonadotropin-releasing hormone (GnRH) agonist	PMS symptoms vanish if ovulation is suppressed
Complete blood count (CBC); erythrocyte sedimentations rate (ESR): Chem 7 [Na, K, Cl, HCO^3, Glu, BUN (creatinine)]; thyroid panel [T$_3$, T$_4$, TCH, T$_7$ (index computed from T$_3$ and T$_4$)]	To screen for underlying pathologic condition

MEDICAL MANAGEMENT

GENERAL MANAGEMENT

Limit salt intake, caffeine, animal fats, refined sugars, stimulants or mood-altering drugs, and alcohol.

Increase intake of complex carbohydrates, protein, and fiber; increase exercise and stress reduction.

Obtain psychologic support and therapy as needed.

Phototherapy.

DRUG THERAPY

Ovulatory suppression (danazol, GnRH agonists, oral contraceptives); progesterone; antiprostaglandin agents (for cramping and diarrhea); bromocriptine (for breast tenderness); vitamins (B$_6$, E, magnesium); diuretics; mild tranquilizers, anxiolytics, or antidepressants.

SURGERY

Endometrial ablation (removal) if severe pain or underlying pathologic condition warrants it.

1 ASSESS*

ASSESSMENT	OBSERVATIONS
History	Reports history of PMS symptoms (e.g., dysmenorrhea, hydration, and urologic, gastrointestinal, dermatologic, ophthalmologic, neurologic, and/or behavioral symptoms)
Comfort	Describes bloating, pelvic or breast tenderness, or other PMS symptoms
Activity	Describes cyclic-related changes in activities of daily living (e.g., sleep, eating, and work patterns)
Health maintenance	Identifies PMS-related self-care deficits, impaired social interaction, or alterations in perceptual and cognitive abilities

*Nursing care should be well documented in the patient's permanent health care record.

ASSESSMENT	OBSERVATIONS
Self-concept	Reports ineffective self-image associated with PMS psychosomatic factors, which may include relationship and sexual alterations
Psychosocial	Anxiety associated with knowledge deficit about cause, treatment, or prognosis of premenstrual syndrome
Physical examination	Observations made throughout menstrual cycle reveal weight gain, fluid retention, breast engorgement, abdominal bloating (abdominal girth variations), and body system changes, such as increased acne

2 DIAGNOSE

NURSING DIAGNOSIS	SUBJECTIVE FINDINGS	OBJECTIVE FINDINGS
Pain or discomfort related to edema, organ pressure, or hormonal shifts associated with PMS	Describes location, sensation, aggravating and relieving factors (usually lower pelvic pain or breast tenderness)	Grimacing, altered muscle tone, diaphoresis, elevated vital signs, dilated pupils
Activity intolerance related to lethargy, fatigue, and psycho-neuroendocrine dysfunction	Describes PMS symptoms that interfere with usual activities (eating, sleeping, working)	Slow movements, lability, dark circles around eyes, skin breakdown, acne, headaches, change in bowel habits
Altered health maintenance related to cyclic changes associated with PMS	Identifies PMS-associated factors that lead to poor health (systemic disorders, impaired coping)	Recurrence of chronic, intermittent conditions (e.g., herpes, asthma)
Self-esteem disturbance related to PMS	Reports altered sexual attractiveness; expresses low self-esteem due to discomfort or physical dysfunction	Social withdrawal, avoidance of intimacy; lack of eye contact; excessive passivity; work history problems
Anxiety related to treatment and prognosis	Expresses anxiety about consequences of physical and/or behavioral symptoms of PMS	Elevated vital signs; diaphoresis; dilated pupils; irritability, withdrawal, or restlessness; increased muscle tone

__3__ PLAN

Patient goals

1. The patient will obtain relief of PMS symptoms such as fluid retention and breast tenderness.
2. The patient will report a measurable increase or consistency in activities throughout her menstrual cycle, such as adequate sleep and work habits.
3. The patient will achieve optimum health maintenance throughout her menstrual cycle, such as nutritional consistency.
4. The patient will maintain a consistent sense of self-esteem.
5. The patient's anxiety about the treatment and prognosis for her condition will be resolved.

__4__ IMPLEMENT

NURSING DIAGNOSIS	NURSING INTERVENTIONS	RATIONALE
Pain or discomfort related to edema, organ pressure, or hormonal shifts associated with PMS	Evaluate character and severity of PMS symptoms.	To assess patterns of discomfort and dysfunction.
	Provide information on pain control (diet, stress reduction).	To enable patient to minimize pain.
	Document and collaborate with physician and health team to ensure effective pain control.	To enhance pain control with team approach.
Activity intolerance related to lethargy, fatigue, and psychoneuroendocrine dysfunction	Assess patient's usual activity variations, and discuss methods for minimizing cyclic changes.	To encourage patient to maximize own activity level.
Altered health maintenance related to cyclic changes associated with PMS	Help patient identify methods for promoting wellness throughout the menstrual cycle.	To promote self-care.
Self-esteem disturbance related to PMS	Assess patient's feelings about her self-image; encourage problem solving, such as seeking counseling.	To help patient clarify her feelings and to provide external support.
Anxiety related to treatment and prognosis	Validate patient's fears, and identify and correct misconceptions.	To help patient clarify her fears, and to help reduce those fears.
	Discuss patient's past coping strategies.	To promote patient's self-confidence.

→ > >

5 EVALUATE

PATIENT OUTCOME	DATA INDICATING THAT OUTCOME IS REACHED
Patient's pain and PMS symptoms have been relieved.	Patient states that pain is under control, and there is no nonverbal evidence of pain.
Patient's activities of daily living are not interrupted by PMS.	Patient reports consistent well-being throughout her menstrual cycle.
Patient has achieved optimum health maintenance.	Patient describes methods for minimizing adverse symptoms.
Patient has regained a consistent sense of self-esteem.	Patient reports return of self-confidence.
Patient's anxiety has been minimized.	Patient understands the prognosis for PMS.

PATIENT TEACHING

1. Explain that rest, stress reduction, and exercise appear to increase natural endorphins and decrease PMS symptoms, whereas fatigue and stress exaggerate discomfort.
2. Explain that PMS and seasonal affective disorder (SAD) have similar manifestations, and that phototherapy and daylight walks may help improve behavioral symptoms.
3. Help the patient identify foods and vitamins that will help maintain health, such as the natural diuretics (asparagus and parsley).
4. Explain that glucose fluctuations exacerbate PMS symptoms. Small, frequent meals high in protein, complex carbohydrates (grains, rice, potatoes, pasta, cereals), and fruits and vegetables appear to be helpful.
5. Instruct the patient on ways to limit her salt intake from sauces, canned goods, packaged snacks, dairy products, and processed meats, since these foods promote fluid retention and should be avoided.
6. Explain that avoiding coffee, tea, chocolate, cola products, and over-the-counter medications with caffeine may help decrease depression and cyclic breast pain.
7. Explain that a yeast-free diet may eliminate the candidal species that may cause hormonal changes, which increase PMS symptoms.
8. Help the patient explore treatment options (group support, drug therapy, psychotherapy).

CHAPTER 5

Breast Conditions and Benign Variations

A number of breast conditions, such as congenital defects and fibrocystic changes, are not deadly. Nevertheless, congenital defects and developmental anomalies may diminish a woman's self-esteem, and fibrocystic changes, breast masses, inflammation, and trauma may cause physical discomfort and fear about the unknown cause of a lump.

Congenital and Developmental Breast Anomalies

Congenital defects include the absence of nipples *(athelia)*, the absence of breast tissue with or without the presence of nipples *(amastia,* also called amazia), presence of more than two nipples or breasts *(polymastia),* presence of two nipples on one breast *(polythelia),* and inverted nipples (Figure 5-3). **Developmental defects** include small breast size *(micromastia,* also called hypomastia or hypoplasia), excessive breast size *(macromastia,* also called hypermastia, hyperplasia, or gigantism), defective or absent tissue *(aplasia),* and deformities, such as *trunk breasts.* Severe differences in breast size *(anisomastia)* may also occur.

About 80% of all women of childbearing age have minor differences between breasts. Accessory breast tissue occurs in 1% to 2% of the total population and in 2% to 6% of adult women. Polythelia (Figure 5-1) the most common abnormality, may be mistaken as pigmented nevi. Polymastia (Figure 5-2) usually occurs in the axillary region. Polymastia below the thorax is rare, and the absence of nipples or areolae is uncommon.

Approximately 65% of cases of polymastia involve single supernumerary organs, and 30% involve two supernumerary organs; three or more supernumerary

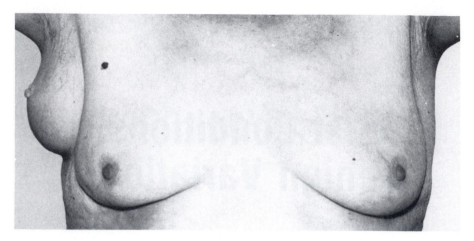

FIGURE 5-1
Unilateral axillary accessory breast (polymastia). (From Isaacs.[63])

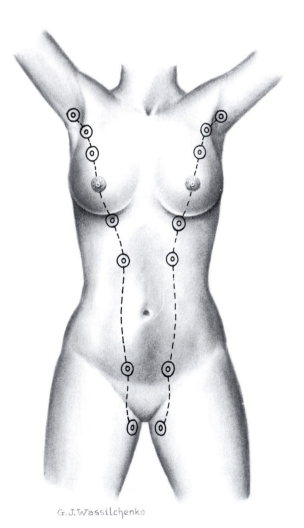

G.J.Wassilchenko

FIGURE 5-2
Common sites for supernumerary nipples. (From Thompson.[104])

breasts occur in a few individuals. The absence of nipples and areolae usually is associated with hypoplasia. It is estimated that 90% of individuals with severe amastia or breast hypoplasia have hypoplasia of the pectoral muscle. However, about 92% of women with pectoral defects have normal breast development. Additional defects occur infrequently, and they usually are associated with such factors as injury and hormonal imbalances.

PATHOPHYSIOLOGY

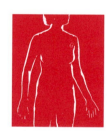

Athelia and *amastia* may occur in males and females from inadequate development of the epithelial primordium from the milk line (mammary ridge) tissue. The mammary duct system cannot bud, branch, or lengthen without an early globular mass. If the epithelial cell line establishes later in fetal life, a nipple may form, but the duct system remains poorly developed. Unilateral or bilateral athelia and amastia may result.

Polymastia (Figure 5-1) occurs in the milk lines of the 5- to 6-week-old embryo. A pair of mammary glands develops in the pectoral region, and the rest of each longitudinal band usually disappears. Occasionally, in both sexes *polythelia* (supernumerary nipples) (Figure 5-2) and extraglandular tissue arise along the milk line, from the axilla to the vulva. The accessory tissue usually develops in the axillary region. Around 8 months' gestation, the original epithelial pit should evert and become a nipple. If a nipple fails to elevate above the chest wall, the result is an *inverted nipple* (Figure 5-3).

Breast tissue defects may be unilateral or bilateral and may be caused by drug ingestion, disease, trauma,

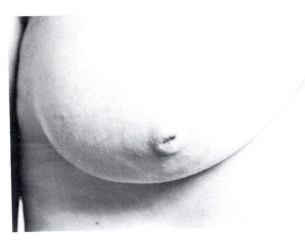

FIGURE 5-3
Nipple inversion. (From Seidel.[96])

or other iatrogenic factors. Bilateral micromastia and macromastia may develop during puberty as a response (or lack of response) to ovarian hormones. The breasts may not develop if estrogen production is inadequate or if the mammary tissue is unable to respond to this hormone. Micromastia may be related to injury of the breast tissue. Children who regularly eat estrogen-infiltrated meat show breast enlargement and formation of ovarian cysts.

It may be difficult to distinguish between *amastia* and *micromastia* (hypoplasia); however, during pregnancy hypoplastic breasts enlarge. Hormonal factors cannot influence absent breast tissue (amastia). Pubertal or *juvenile macromastia* (hyperplasia) is caused by an abundance of glandular growth in young women 14 to 20 years of age. Another form of hyperplasia is *trunk breasts*, a deformity caused by an enlarged areola with herniation of the anterior parenchyma. An increase in fatty tissue, or *adipose hyperplasia*, occurs in women between 35 and 50 years of age.

Premature thelarche refers to breast development that occurs before other signs of sexual maturation as a result of endogenous or exogenous causes. Adolescent,

juvenile, or virginal *hypertrophy* refers to breast tissue that continues to grow after puberty. Male breast development and female drug-induced breast development (gynecomastia) may also occur. Unilateral *micromastia* and *aplasia* occur when only one breast develops normally. The undeveloped breast may be the result of defective muscles and bones in that pectoral area or of a deficiency of regional blood vessels. *Symmastia*, a midline webbing, is an infrequent finding usually associated with symmetrically large breasts.

CLINICAL MANIFESTATIONS

The clinical manifestations of congenital and developmental breast anomalies are numerous and varied. They may include absence of one or both breasts, absence of one or both nipples, presence of more than two breasts or nipples, asymmetric breasts, abnormally small or large breasts, and back discomfort associated with heavy breasts.

COMPLICATIONS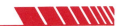

Ineffective breast-feeding (with absence of breast tissue or nipples)
Inflammation
Psychosocial disturbances related to malformation

DIFFERENTIAL DIAGNOSIS

The following conditions may have similar signs and symptoms and should be ruled out:
Muscle or bone deformities
Hormonal imbalances
Tumors or cysts
Hamartomas (resemble neoplasms)
Klinefelter's syndrome
Turner's syndrome
Associated diseases (pulmonary, liver tuberculosis; bronchitis)
Trauma

DIAGNOSTIC STUDIES AND FINDINGS

Diagnostic test	Findings
Measurement of mammotropic hormones, estrogen levels	To identify underlying hormonal imbalances or pathologic abnormalities
Ultrasonography, biopsies	To assess for central nervous system (CNS), adrenal, and ovarian tumors
Drug, chromosome analyses	To determine exogenous (amphetamines, teratogens) and endogenous pathologic conditions

MEDICAL MANAGEMENT

DRUG THERAPY

Hormonal drugs are administered as needed.

SURGERY

Reconstructive surgery may be done to reduce or enlarge breasts. Breasts may be augmented with saline prostheses. Extra nipples may be removed, or a nipple may be reconstructed.

NURSING CARE

See pages 78 to 81.

Fibrocystic Changes

Fibrocystic changes are breast nodules that are related to the menstrual cycle. Other names associated with cystic conditions are *benign mastopathy, chronic cystic mastitis, epithelial* and *fibrocystic mastopathy, fibrocystic disease, fibroadenosis, cystic disease, cystic mammary hyperplasia* or *dysplasia, cystic mastopathy, cyclic nodularity, hyperplastic cystic disease, Schimmelbusch's disease,* and *blue dome cysts.*

Fibrocystic changes make up the most common breast condition of women in their childbearing years (Figure 5-4). Approximately 50% of all women have palpable breast masses, and 90% show irregularities on scanning studies or histologic tests. In general, 70% of breast biopsies are nonproliferative lesions, and 26% are proliferative lesions without atypia (benign growing cells). Biopsies have shown that 50% to 70% of women have fibroadenomas. The cystic condition known as Bloodgood's, Schimmelbusch's, or blue dome disease is characterized by cysts larger than 3 mm in diameter that usually occur in women 45 to 55 years of age. Epithelial duct hyperplasia is more common in women 35 to 45 years old.

PATHOPHYSIOLOGY

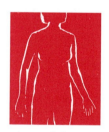

Hyperplastic, fibrotic, and cystic disorders generally have been referred to as fibrocystic conditions. Cyst formation may involve an excess of fibrous stroma (basic breast tissue) or a proliferation of epithelial cells. Different classification systems have been used to describe cyclic nodularities, such as *aberrations* of *normal development* and *involution* (ANDI). These commonly found breast "disorders" can be microscopically identified as *nonproliferative* lesions (limited growth), *proliferative lesions without atypia,* and *atypical hyperplasia.* Nonproliferative lesions include epithelial-related calcifications, papillary apocrine changes, and mild hyperplasia. Proliferative lesions without atypia include florid hyperplasias, intraductal papillomas, and sclerosing adenosis. Sclerosing adenosis usually is a unilateral proliferation of intralobular fibrosis and small acini. Atypical hyperplasia includes ductal and lobular hyperplasias. Epithelial hyperplasia describes ill-defined masses of the ducts. The risk of carcinoma increases with an increase in atypical hyperplasia.

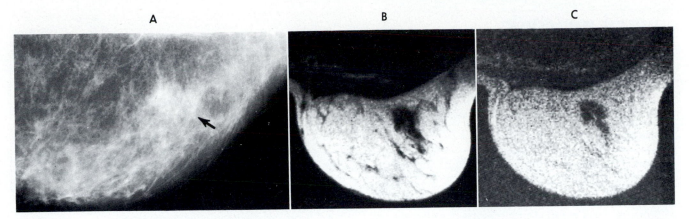

FIGURE 5-4
Typical fibrocystic condition in right breast. (From Stark, Bradley.[100b])

Fibrocystic changes typically are associated with palpable, tender breast lumps that change during the menstrual cycle. Monthly variations in estrogen and progesterone levels may facilitate changes in breast tissue. For example, an excess of estrogen and a reduction in progesterone during the luteal phase of the menstrual cycle may facilitate morphologic changes in breast tissue.

Increased levels of female hormones cause blood vessels to swell. The breast retains water, and milk glands and ducts enlarge. Swollen mammary glands may become painful and lumpy. After menstruation, the breasts decrease in size and are less tender. This monthly swelling and reducing cycle may cause breast tissue to become firm with cysts (sacs or pockets of fluid) in the enlarged or obstructed milk ducts. Fibrocystic characteristics often subside after menopause.

CLINICAL MANIFESTATIONS

Symptoms of fibrocystic changes usually develop about 1 week before menstruation and subside about 1 week after menstruation. Several palpable, regularly shaped nodules (lumpy breast tissue) commonly appear. The nodules normally are round, smooth, bumpy (or form a lump), and mobile without retractions. They may be firm or soft. Occasionally a single, delineated lump appears. The area is tender or painful and sensitive to the touch. The patient may describe sensations such as burning, dull aching, fullness, or heaviness. Several pockets of fluid accumulate. Fibrous rubbery tissue (mammary dysplasia) may develop.

COMPLICATIONS
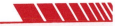

Infection
Pain that interferes with activities of daily living
Development into cancer (from atypical hyperplastic cells, though this rarely occurs)

DIFFERENTIAL DIAGNOSIS

The following conditions may have similar signs and symptoms and should be ruled out:
Carcinoma
Inflammation

NURSING CARE

See pages 78 to 81.

DIAGNOSTIC STUDIES AND FINDINGS

Diagnostic test	Findings
Mammography, ultrasonography	To determine underlying pathologic condition
Biopsy, needle aspiration, and histologic examination	To detect fibrosis, cystic cells, or pathology

MEDICAL MANAGEMENT

GENERAL MANAGEMENT

Local heat applications; support bra (be sure bra is large enough); limiting dietary caffeine (coffee, sodas, tea, chocolate) to decrease cyclic adenosine monophosphate (cAMP).

DRUG THERAPY

Pain medications (such as aspirin and ibuprofen), vitamin E, danazol, tamoxifen.

SURGERY

Subcutaneous mastectomy may be performed to minimize discomfort and the need for biopsies.

Benign Breast Masses

Several types of benign tumors can develop in the breasts, skin, and accessory glands, the most common being *fibroadenomas*. A variety of other tumors may also be found, such as *papillomas* and *leiomyomas*.

Fibroadenomas are common breast tumors in young women (Figure 5-5). These solid masses may occur in women from 15 to 60 years of age, although they most often appear between 21 and 25 years of age. Fibroadenomas are the third most common neoplasm of the breast, after carcinoma and fibrocystic breast changes. As many as 20% of women over 70 years of age may have intraductal papillomas. They are found most often in women 35 to 45 years of age.

PATHOPHYSIOLOGY

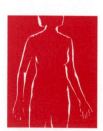

A *fibroadenoma* is a single, solid tumor consisting of glandular and fibrous tissue. It can be moved when palpated. These neoplasms usually are asymptomatic. They do not typically respond to monthly hormonal changes, although some premenstrual tenderness may occur. These tumors grow slowly, and they may stop expanding after reaching 2 to 3 cm in diameter. Either fibroadenomas

COMMON MANIFESTATIONS OF BREAST MASSES

Fibroadenoma

Single, delineated, solid lump
Not usually cyclic
Unilateral, occasionally multiple
Round shape, lobular
Usually firm, may be soft
Mobile, slips without retractions
Not usually tender or symptomatic

Lipomas

Soft
Movable
Well delineated

Fibrous histiocytomas

Firm
Nodular

Intraductal papilloma or florid adenoma

Single or multiple mass
Mass near subareolar ducts
Nipple discharge, serous or bloody

Fat necrosis

Local irritation
Firm, irregular mass
Discoloration often present

Mondor's disease

Thrombophlebitis
Firm, nodular cord under skin

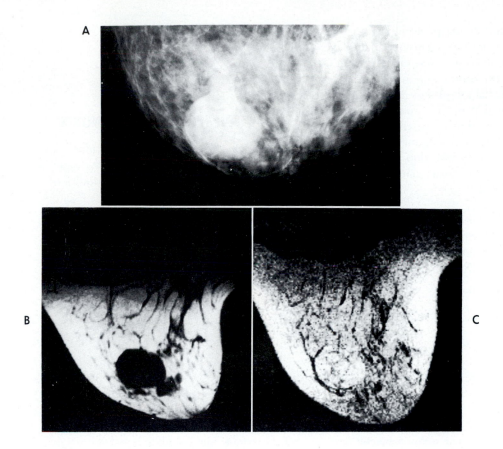

FIGURE 5-5
Fibroadenoma in right breast. (From Stark, Bradley.[100b])

or prominent mammary lobules may develop and then disappear in teenagers, a phenomenon more common in young women taking oral contraceptives.

A tan-yellow, straw-colored, or bloody discharge from the nipple may indicate the presence of an *intraductal papilloma*. Intraductal papillomas are small, nonpalpable tumors usually found in a subareolar collection duct. This neoplasm poses little risk of a cancerous condition if the papilloma is a solitary tumor.

There are a number of tumors described by their diagnostic type that require medical diagnosis. *Multiple florid papillomas (cystadenomas* or *intracystic papillomas)* suggest a 25% chance of malignancy. *Cystosarcoma phyllodes (phyllodes tumor)* is an aggressive tumor that usually is benign. These tumors are large, firm, and nodular. Cystosarcomas may occur during adolescence.

A *florid adenoma of the nipple (subareolar duct papillomatosis)* appears as a well-defined, single lump or nodule, 1 to 2 cm in diameter, in the areola. A serosanguineous nipple discharge or ulceration and crusting may be present. A florid adenoma may resemble Paget's disease. (See Chapter 6, "Breast Malignancies, page 84, for a discussion of Paget's disease.)

Tubular adenomas and *adenomas of the ducts* are rare. *Lactating adenomas* and *lactating fibroadenomas* infrequently occur unaccompanied by pregnancy. *Granular cell tumors* may resemble carcinoma. *Pleomorphic adenomas* are also rare and may be confused with malignant tumors.

There are several types of rare, benign, nonepithelial neoplasms. *Mesenchymoma (hamartoma, angiomyolipoma)* tumors occur in subcutaneous tissue and consist mostly of fat. Mesenchymomas are difficult to distinguish from lipomas, although mesenchymomas are more gray. *Fibrous histiocytomas*, which are firm, nodular neoplasms, develop in the skin and may infiltrate the breast tissue.

Leiomyomas in the breast may develop from the smooth muscles of blood vessels *(vascular leiomyomas)* or from the smooth muscles of skin *(superficial leiomyomas)*. A *lipoma* is a more common solitary lesion that usually develops in older women. Lipomas usually are well delineated, soft, and movable. *Adenolipomas* are lipomas consisting of fat and epithelial lobules.

Granular cell tumors are firm, fixed, well-circumscribed neoplasms that may be confused with early signs of carcinoma. These tumors may attach themselves to the underlying pectoral fascia. *Neurofibromatosis* (small pigmented skin lesions) may develop in the skin and subcutaneous tissue of the breast. It is more often found in the nipple and areola areas.

A few epithelial neoplasms of the skin and accessory glands may develop in the breasts. Squamous cell epitheliomas are rare, but *basal cell epitheliomas* may develop. Pigmented or nonpigmented *moles* may occur, and *melanomas* may develop in the breast region. *Mixed tumors* of the sweat glands may develop in the dermis of the breast.

CLINICAL MANIFESTATIONS

The primary clinical manifestation of benign breast masses is a unilateral, single, firm lump that usually is not painful. Nipple discharge may be present.

NURSING CARE

See pages 78 to 81.

COMPLICATIONS

Carcinoma
Inflammation

DIFFERENTIAL DIAGNOSIS

The following conditions may have similar signs
 and symptoms and should be ruled out:
Pseudoeczematous condition
Malignancy
Structural defect
Fibrocystic changes

DIAGNOSTIC STUDIES AND FINDINGS

Diagnostic test	Findings
Mammography, ultrasonography, magnetic resonance imaging	To determine cause of mass or lesion
Complete blood count (CBC)	To identify inflammation
Cultures	For nipple discharge, if infection is suspected
Histochemistry, flow cytometry, needle aspiration	To detect hormonal and cellular indications of pathologic condition
Biopsy and cytologic tests for histologic examination	To determine underlying pathology

MEDICAL MANAGEMENT

GENERAL MANAGEMENT

Regular observation of benign masses that do not require surgical intervention.

SURGERY

Excisional biopsy or wedge tissue removal of breast mass; surgical removal of epithelial neoplasms.

Inflammation and Trauma of the Breast

Inflammatory conditions of the breast include *mammary duct ectasia* (also called *stale milk mastitis, comedomastitis, plasma cell mastitis, varicocele tumor,* and *mastitis obliterans*) and *abscesses. Tuberculosis, fungal infections,* and *Mondor's disease* (thrombophlebitis of the breast and chest wall) cause inflammatory reactions. **Traumatized breast tissue** may result from mechanical or chemical factors. *Sulfur granules* and *amyloid pseudotumor* can be caused by irritants. *Granulomatous mastitis* and *sarcoidosis* are granulomas that occur without organisms, probably as a result of an immunologic process. *Fat necrosis* usually is caused by trauma and may resemble an abscess.

Breast infections are more common in lactating women. Mammary duct ectasia occurs most often in women past menopause. A nipple discharge and nipple retraction develop in 20% of women who have this disorder. Older women also may have more fat necrosis as a result of falls or breast trauma. Fat necrosis rarely causes tumors.

PATHOPHYSIOLOGY

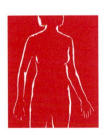

Symptoms of *mammary duct ectasia* appear in the subareolar area in older women. The collecting ducts dilate, causing fibrosis, inflammation, and discharge. Cellular debris and lipidlike material may distend the ducts to 3 to 5 mm and give the ducts a blue color.

Fat necrosis is caused by trauma to the fatty breast tissue. Most patients with fat necrosis have large breasts with ecchymoses or reddened skin areas. The inflammatory lesions are superficial and usually are located in the areolar region.

CLINICAL MANIFESTATIONS

Mammary duct ectasia may cause a serous, blood-tinged, puslike, or thick nipple discharge; in rare cases it may produce a thick, firm, round, fixed tumor. Fat necrosis may resemble an abscess.

COMPLICATIONS
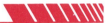

Systemic infection
Vascular disorders (e.g., phlebitis)

DIFFERENTIAL DIAGNOSIS

The following conditions may have similar signs and symptoms and should be ruled out:
Carcinoma
Structural defect
Tissue necrosis

DIAGNOSTIC STUDIES AND FINDINGS

Diagnostic test	Findings
Complete blood count (CBC)	Elevated white blood count may indicate infection
Biopsy	To identify underlying pathologic condition
Culture of tissue or nipple discharge	To determine organism causing the inflammation
Mammography, ultrasonography, magnetic resonance imaging	To detect cysts or tumors

MEDICAL MANAGEMENT

GENERAL MANAGEMENT

Cold application (for fresh, small hematomas); heat treatment (for older bruising); good hygiene, especially around nipples; warm compresses for mastitis due to breast feeding (continue to nurse and massage clogged ducts).

DRUG THERAPY

Antibiotics (as needed).

Supervised anticoagulant therapy (especially if breast necrosis appears secondary to anticoagulant therapy).

Topical antibacterial drugs (with irritated nipple).

SURGERY

Incision and drainage of abscesses; excisional biopsies as indicated.

---

1 ASSESS*

ASSESSMENT	OBSERVATIONS			
	CONGENITAL AND DEVELOPMENTAL ANOMALIES	FIBROCYSTIC CHANGES	BENIGN MASSES	INFLAMMATION AND TRAUMA
History	Endocrine function, precocious or delayed development	Monthly breast changes, child-bearing age, diet, stress, smoking habits	Use of oral contraceptives, age of onset of neoplasms 18 to 35, family incidence of breast masses	Accidents, assault, use of anticoagulants, postmenopause, mastitis
Mammary glands	Development, size, symmetry, duplication, function (lactation if applicable)	Symmetry, multiple masses, usually cysts in upper outer quadrants	Unilateral mass (firm mobile, nodular), inverted nipple, nipple discharge	Abscess, edema, ecchymosis, hematoma, phlebitis, subareolar firm mass, nipple dimpling or retraction
Comfort	Back pain possible with large breasts; underlying herniation	Breasts periodically tender or painful	Breasts nontender	Breasts may be painful or nontender
Psychosocial	Anxiety associated with breast condition and diminished self-esteem			

*Nursing care should be well documented in the patient's permanent health care record.

2 DIAGNOSE

NURSING DIAGNOSIS	SUBJECTIVE FINDINGS	OBJECTIVE FINDINGS
Body image disturbance related to breast condition	Reports shame, altered sense of femininity or sexual attractiveness	Social withdrawal, avoids interaction or intimacy, avoids looking at or touching breasts, hides body part
Pain or discomfort related to breast or nipple disorder	Describes location, sensation, and aggravating and relieving factors	Grimacing, altered muscle tone, diaphoresis, elevated vital signs, dilated pupils
Knowledge deficit related to cause and/or diagnosis of breast condition	Expresses concern about breast symptoms, admits lack of knowledge about condition	May be talkative or withdrawn; requests information about disorder
Fear/anxiety related to treatment and prognosis	Expresses anxiety about long-term consequences of breast deformity, tumor, or ailment	Elevated vital signs, diaphoresis, dilated pupils, increased muscle tone
Decisional conflict related to treatment options	Indecision about treatment options or delayed decision making	Irritable, withdrawn or restless

3 PLAN

Patient goals

1. The patient will have a positive body image.
2. The patient's pain will be relieved.
3. The patient will understand the cause and diagnosis of her breast condition.
4. The patient's fears about the treatment and prognosis will be resolved.
5. The patient will select and undergo the appropriate treatment.

4 IMPLEMENT

NURSING DIAGNOSIS	NURSING INTERVENTIONS	RATIONALE
Body image disturbance related to breast condition	Assess patient's feelings about her body image.	To clarify patient's feelings.
	Respect need for temporary denial or withdrawal.	To facilitate coping mechanisms.
	Encourage problem solving (e.g., cosmetic surgery, clothing choices).	To provide external support.

➜ ❯ ❯

NURSING DIAGNOSIS	NURSING INTERVENTIONS	RATIONALE
Pain or discomfort related to breast or nipple disorder	Evaluate character and severity of pain.	To assess pain patterns.
	Provide information on pain control (e.g., heat, clothing options, analgesics, dietary options).	To enable patient to minimize pain.
	Collaborate with physician and health team to ensure effective pain control.	To enhance pain control through team approach.
Knowledge deficit related to cause and/or diagnosis of breast condition	Encourage patient to ask questions; assess readiness to learn.	To clarify patient's understanding.
	Use a variety of educational methods and materials; use nonjudgmental methods to assess learning.	To promote retention of information.
	Involve family in learning process as appropriate.	To promote support for patient.
Fear/anxiety related to treatment and prognosis	Validate patient's fears; identify and correct misconceptions.	To help patient clarify fears.
	Discuss patient's past coping strategies.	To promote patient's self-confidence.
	Collaborate with health team to present medical and surgical options.	To alleviate patient's fear.
Decisional conflict related to treatment options	Discuss procedures and their advantages, risks, and possible outcomes with patient and family.	To help patient make an informed choice.

5 EVALUATE

PATIENT OUTCOME	DATA INDICATING THAT OUTCOME IS REACHED
Patient has a positive body image.	Patient expresses acceptance of body with or without cosmetic changes. Patient's nonverbal behavior shows increased acceptance of her breasts.
Patient's pain has been relieved.	Patient reports pain is under control and shows no nonverbal evidence of pain.
Patient understands the cause and diagnosis of her breast condition.	Patient can describe the cause of her breast condition.

PATIENT OUTCOME	DATA INDICATING THAT OUTCOME IS REACHED
Patient's fears about treatment and prognosis have resolved.	Patient understands prognosis and treatment options for her disease.
Patient has selected and is undergoing appropriate treatment.	Patient and family have made an informed choice and are pursuing treatment.

PATIENT TEACHING

GENERAL

1. Explain the causes and frequency of breast variations specific to the patient.
2. Explore possible treatment options. Inform the patient (and family when appropriate) that surgical correction of breast variations and medical treatment for endocrine disorders are often successful.
3. Provide information on counseling if needed to help the patient regain a positive body image.

CONGENITAL AND DEVELOPMENTAL ANOMALIES

1. Provide information and support through diagnostic procedures; ask patient and family questions to assess their learning and/or emotional needs.
2. Provide extra learning materials, such as brochures and pictures that the patient/family may keep; genetic information may be particularly difficult to comprehend and accept.
3. Perform preoperative teaching, when corrective surgery is indicated, and/or assist patient with selecting appropriate health care referrals, such as a cosmetic surgeon.
4. Assess patient's self-concept; explain that body image disturbance may persist even after corrective surgery, and refer to counseling as needed.

FIBROCYSTIC CHANGES

1. Explain that limiting coffee, tea, and chocolate (methylxanthines) may help decrease breast size, additional cyst formation, and discomfort. Provide information about cyclic adenosine monophosphate (cAMP) and cyclic guanosine monophosphate (cGMP), if the patient would benefit from learning about how increased levels of these nucleotides cause her symptoms.
2. Discuss the use of oral vitamin E, which may reduce fibrocystic symptoms.
3. Help the patient identify ways to reduce stress and smoking, which may facilitate cystic discomfort.
4. Explain the reasons for using oral contraceptives, danazol, or other drugs to treat the patient's condition.
5. Explain the reasons for excisional biopsies or wedge resections.

BENIGN BREAST MASSES

1. Explain that a biopsy or wedge resection will provide a diagnosis of the mass; surgery can be performed to remove the mass.
2. Refer the patient to support groups and other sources of aid to help her cope with the long-term consequences of her breast disorder.

INFLAMMATION AND TRAUMA

1. Teach the patient the signs and symptoms of infection, i.e., change in skin color or temperature, broken skin, nipple discharge.
2. Help the patient explore ways to prevent infection and trauma.
3. Explain the treatments used for these conditions (e.g., broad-spectrum antibiotics).
4. Explain that good hygiene, treatment, and prevention usually correct nipple drainage, fistulas, hematomas, and abscesses.
5. Refer the patient for counseling in cases involving abuse.

CHAPTER 6

Breast Malignancies

There are several different types of breast cancer. These malignancies have different cellular and structural variations, as well as different rates of metastatic growth. Cancer of the breast can be defined in the strictest sense as an uncontrolled growth of anaplastic cells in the tissue of the breast. It might also be defined as the disease most feared by women because of the accompanying psychologic trauma. Society has a preoccupation with women's breasts as a symbol of femininity and sexuality. Loss or mutilation of a breast as a result of cancer can have far-ranging effects on a woman's self-image and her perceptions of her sexual desirability.

Breast cancer is the most common major cancer among women in the United States, and its incidence is on the rise, particularly among black women. Women over 65 years of age have double the reported number of cases found in the 45 to 64 age-group. Older women are also more likely than younger women to have metastatic disease at the time of initial diagnosis. The American Cancer Society has estimated that 182,000 women will be diagnosed with breast cancer in 1993 and that 46,300 women will die of the disease. The Cancer Society also estimates and that 1 in 9 women will be diagnosed with breast cancer during her lifetime. However, the mortality rate is fairly stable despite the rising incidence, which can be attributed in part to early detection and a wider range of treatment options.

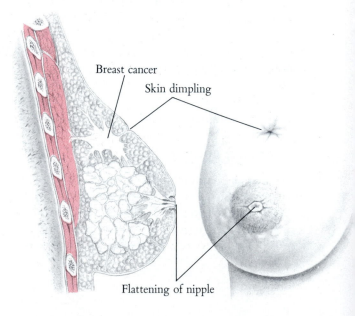

Clinical signs of breast cancer: nipple retraction and dimpling of skin. (From Belcher.[9a])

PATHOPHYSIOLOGY

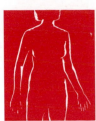

The cause of breast cancer is unknown; however, a number of factors appear to correlate with an increased incidence of the disease. It should be noted that all known factors are associated with only 25% to 30% of diagnosed cases. Approximately 70% of women diagnosed with breast cancer have no evident risk factors.

Cancer occurs when certain cells proliferate without organization and with little or no differentiation. One theory holds that certain stimuli, which have yet to be definitively identified, initiate this proliferation by overpowering the normal mechanisms that control growth. The result is uninhibited growth, uncontrolled function, and rapid motility, which permits the cancer to spread to other parts of the body by invading adjacent tissues or by migrating through the blood or lymph systems. The migration process is called *metastasis*. The primary site of a malignancy (cancer cell growth) is the site of original growth. A secondary site occurs when cells migrate and colonize in an additional body site.

There are three major classifications of breast cancer by histopathologic type: ductal, lobular, and nipple (Paget's disease) (Figure 6–1). Tumors are also com-

POSSIBLE RISK FACTORS FOR BREAST CANCER

Age >40 years
Familial history of breast cancer (risk is increased if affected relative is mother or sister, if disease develops in both breasts and/or develops before menopause)
Early menarche/late menopause
Nulliparity or first child after age 30
Exposure to ionizing radiation (particularly if exposure occurs before age 35)
Personal history of cancer (breast, colon, ovarian, endometrial, thyroid)
Personal history of atypical hyperplasia
Excessive alcohol consumption
High-fat diet and obesity, especially after menopause

monly identified as in situ or invasive. Breast cancers sometimes show histopathologic characteristics of more than one tumor type, and a large percentage of in situ tumors, if left untreated, become invasive.

Ductal carcinoma originates in the lactiferous ducts, which drain the mammary glands. Most breast cancers are classified as invasive ductal tumors. These tumors are also commonly labeled as "not otherwise

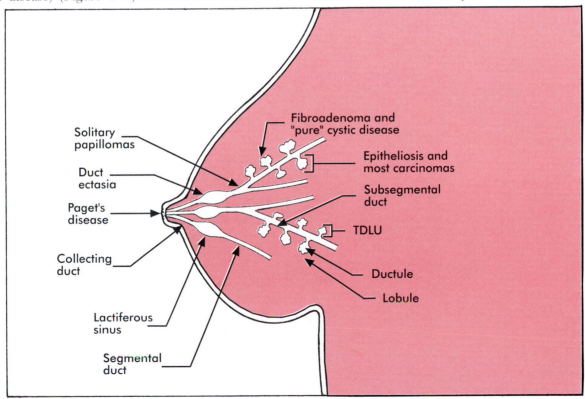

FIGURE 6-1
Correlation between anatomic structures and pathologic processes in the breast. (Redrawn from Isaacs.[63])

specified" breast cancer. This tumor type forms a dense fibrotic core and radiates tentacles that invade and distort surrounding breast structures. The tumor mass generally is painless, nonmobile, solid, irregularly shaped, poorly defined, and unilateral.

A **comedo ductal tumor,** such as the medullary, papillary, and mucinous subtypes, often manifests as a well-defined mass of medium consistency with slight mobility. Inflammatory comedo ductal tumors are associated with skin erythema, edema, and induration.

Lobular carcinoma originates in the lobules of the breast and is unique to women. It is rarely palpable in situ and often is found incidentally through a biopsy for some other benign breast condition. It is bilateral, occurs more frequently in the premenopausal period, and shows a high incidence of hormone receptors in invasive lesions.

Nipple carcinoma, or **Paget's disease,** originates in the nipple complex and often is manifested in conjunction with invasive ductal carcinoma. Crusting, oozing, and bleeding from the nipple are common signs of nipple carcinoma. Nipple erosion is also possible.

CLINICAL MANIFESTATIONS

The most common presenting sign of breast cancer is a lump, mass, or thickening in the breast. About one quarter of all detected masses are diagnosed as cancerous. The cancerous lump most often (50%) is located in

---

HISTOPATHOLOGIC CLASSIFICATIONS OF BREAST CANCER

Ductal

   Ductal carcinoma in situ
   Invasive (predominantly intraductal)
   Invasive

Comedo

   Inflammatory
   Medullary
   Mucinous
   Papillary
   Scirrhous
   Tubular

Lobular

   In situ
   Invasive (predominantly in situ)
   Invasive

Nipple

   Paget's disease
   Paget's disease with intraductal cancer
   Paget's disease with invasive ductal cancer

---

the upper outer quadrant of the breast (Figure 6-2). Nipple discharge may be present, although it usually is associated with benign breast conditions. Unilateral serosanguineous or bloody discharge of recent onset should be viewed suspiciously. Pain and tenderness are rarely present until the disease has reached an advanced stage. Other signs and symptoms of advanced disease may include nipple or skin dimpling and retraction, changes in breast size, shape, and color; fixed nodular lumps in the axilla; and frank skin ulcerations (Figure 6-3).

The complications associated with advanced forms of breast cancer occur primarily as a result of tumor infiltration or metastasis or both. Common infiltration sites are the opposite breast, axilla, and brachial plexus; common metastatic sites are the lungs, liver, and bones.

COMPLICATIONS

Metastatic breast cancer
Ascites
Pathologic fracture
Spinal compression
Pleural effusion
Brachial plexopathy

DIFFERENTIAL DIAGNOSIS

Benign breast masses, such as fibrocystic changes

DIAGNOSTIC STUDIES
Screening

Three major screening methods are used to detect breast cancer: breast self-examination (BSE), clinical physical examination, and various imaging techniques. The American Cancer Society has issued guidelines for use of these screening techniques (see the box on page 85).

Currently about 90% of all palpable breast tumors are detected by the woman or a significant other in her life. This makes BSE a very powerful self-screening tool for women who want to participate actively in their health care. BSE should be performed monthly, immediately after a woman's menstrual period ends. Postmenopausal women should choose a consistent time for examination each month. (See BSE teaching guide, page 85.)

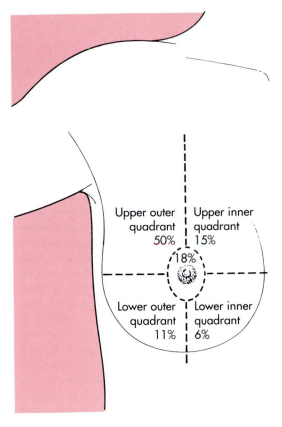

A woman should have a clinical examination by a qualified physician or nurse as recommended by the American Cancer Society's guidelines, as well as any time she detects a change in her breast through self-examination. The clinical examination is also important for detecting the 10% to 15% of tumors that are missed by mammography. Approximately 26% of cancers are found by physical examination.

Imaging techniques are used to detect tumors that as yet are clinically undetectable. A number of techniques have been tried, but the two most successful are mammography and ultrasonography (ultrasound). Mammography, the recommended technique, has been found to have an 85% to 90% success rate. However, ultrasound is helpful in distinguishing between cysts and solid tumors and for women with dense breasts.

FIGURE 6-2
Location of breast cancer. (From Belcher.[9a])

SCREENING GUIDELINES

Breast self-exam:	Monthly—20 years of age and over
Clinical exam:	Every 3 yrs—Age 20 to 40
	Yearly—Over 40 years of age
Mammography:	Screening exam—By age 40
	Every 1 to 2 years—Age 40 to 49
	Yearly—Age 50 and over
MRI:	For questionable mammography findings

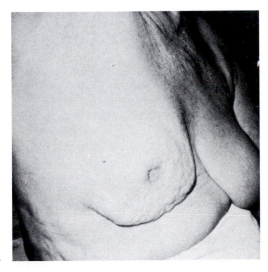
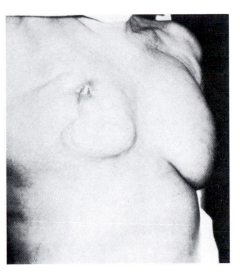

FIGURE 6-3
A, Locally advanced carcinoma. Note nipple retraction, skin edema, and dimpling. **B,** Locally advanced cancer. Note fixation and deformity of contour. (From Gallagher.[36a])

Once screening tests indicate the possibility of breast cancer, a definitive diagnosis is needed through histologic examination of tissue obtained by biopsy. Mammography is also being used to localize lesions more precisely for biopsy and to confirm biopsy success. Other procedures can be used as diagnostic adjuncts.

PROGNOSIS

Staging of breast cancer provides a prognosis, guides treatment, and allows comparison of the effectiveness of various types of treatment. A number of staging methods have been described in the literature, but the TNM system, which describes the primary tumor (T), lymph node involvement (N), and degree of metastasis (M), is universally accepted. The box to the right defines the symbols used in the TNM staging system. The box below describes the various stages of cancerous breast tumors. Figure 6-4 illustrates the stages of breast cancer.

The staging is the most definitive prognostic tool available. The 5-year survival rate of cancer diagnosed and treated at stage 0 (in situ cancer) approaches 100%. Treated stage I disease has a 5-year survival rate of 85% to 95%, depending on the size of the primary tumor.

The prognosis falls progressively with an increasing number of involved lymph nodes (Figure 6-5). Involvement of one to three nodes reduces the 5-year survival rate to about 50%. Women with 10 or more involved nodes have a survival rate equal with that of untreated cancer. With *no* nodal involvement, the chance of remaining disease free is 70% to 75%.

STAGING FOR BREAST CARCINOMA

Stage	T	N	M
Stage 0	T_{is}	N_0	M_0
Stage I	T_1	N_0	M_0
Stage IIA	T_0	N_1	M_0
	T_1	N_1	M_0
	T_2	N_0	M_0
Stage IIB	T_2	N_1	M_0
	T_3	N_0	M_0
Stage IIIA	T_0	N_2	M_0
	T_1	N_2	M_0
	T_2	N_2	M_0
	T_3	N_1	M_0
	T_3	N_2	M_0
Stage IIIB	T_4	Any N	M_0
	Any T	N_3	M_0
Stage IV	Any T	Any N	M_1

STAGING DEFINITIONS FOR BREAST CARCINOMA

Primary tumor (T)

T_X Primary tumor cannot be assessed
T_0 No evidence of primary tumor
T_{is} Carcinoma in situ
T_1 Tumor ≤2 cm in greatest dimension
 T_{1a} ≤0.5 cm
 T_{1b} >0.5 cm and <1 cm
 T_{1c} >1 cm and <2 cm
T_2 Tumor >2 cm and <5 cm
T_3 Tumor >5 cm
T_4 Tumor of any size with direct extension to chest wall or skin
 T_{4a} Extension to chest wall
 T_{4b} Edema (including peau d'orange) or ulceration of skin or satellite skin nodules confined to same breast
 T_{4c} Both T_{4a} and T_{4b}
 T_{4d} Inflammatory carcinoma

Regional lymph nodes (N)

N_X Regional nodes cannot be assessed
N_0 No regional node metastasis
N_1 Metastasis to movable, ipsilateral axillary lymph nodes
 N_{1a} Only micrometastasis (none larger than 0.2 cm)
 N_{1b} Metastasis to nodes larger than 0.2 cm
  N_{1bi} Metastasis in 1 to 3 nodes, >0.2 cm and <2 cm
  N_{1bii} Metastasis to 4 or more nodes, >0.2 cm and <2 cm
  N_{1biii} Extension of tumor beyond the capsule of a lymph node metastasis <2 cm
  N_{1biv} Metastasis to a node ≥2 cm
N_2 Metastasis to ipsilateral axillary lymph nodes that are fixed to one another or to other structures
N_3 Metastasis to ipsilateral internal mammary lymph nodes

Distant metastasis (M)

M_X Presence of distant metastasis cannot be assessed
M_0 No distant metastasis
M_1 Distant metastasis, including metastasis to ipsilateral supraclavicular lymph nodes

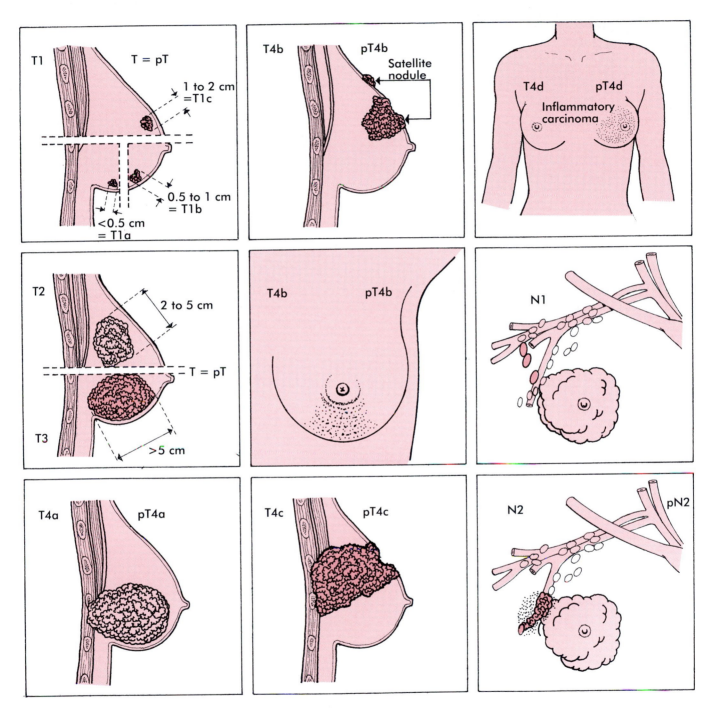

FIGURE 6-4
Staging of breast cancer according to TNM classification. (Redrawn from Spiessl et al.[100a])

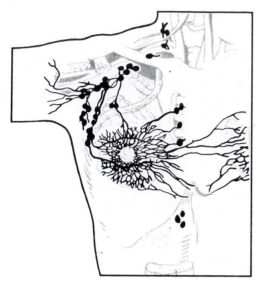

FIGURE 6-5
Lymphatic spread of breast cancer. (From Bobak.[13])

DIAGNOSTIC STUDIES AND FINDINGS

Diagnostic test	Findings
Primary disease	
Biopsy (needle, excision)	
Lesion	Evidence of malignant cells
Axillary nodes	Evidence of malignant cells
Estrogen/progestin receptors	<3 fmol/mcp*—negative; >10 fmol/mcp—positive
Metastasis	
Tumor markers	
Carcinoembryonic antigen	Elevated—liver metastasis
Liver function studies	Evidence of liver metastasis
Bone scan	Evidence of bone metastasis
Chest x-ray	Evidence of lung metastasis
Computed tomography (CT) scan	Evidence of brain metastasis

*Femtomoles per milligram of cytosol protein.

MEDICAL MANAGEMENT

Medical management of diagnosed carcinoma of the breast includes surgery, radiation therapy, and adjuvant therapy such as chemotherapy and hormone treatments. The choice of management techniques is based on the type, size, and extent of the carcinoma and research studies of treatment efficacy. Surgery often is the primary treatment choice for removing the tumor, with radiation therapy, hormone therapy, and/or chemotherapy added after surgery. Radiation therapy is also used to control pain, to prevent pathologic fractures, and to treat cerebral metastases in advanced stages of the disease.

DRUG THERAPY

Chemotherapy: Use of combinations of cytotoxic drugs for cell destruction; usually recommended for premenopausal, node-positive women.

Hormone therapy: Use of hormones such as estrogens, androgens (used infrequently); progestins or hormone antagonists, such as antiestrogens for cell destruction for postmenopausal, node-positive and/or receptor-positive (responsive to hormonal treatment) women; tamoxifen.

Complications: Chemotherapy may lead to hair loss, anemia, and bone marrow depression. Approximately 82% of patients experience radiation fatigue, and 75% have changes in breast sensation.

SURGERY

Lumpectomy: Wide excision and removal with margin of healthy tissue.

Partial mastectomy: Excision of tumor with wider margin of healthy tissue than with lumpectomy.

Quadrantectomy: Removal of one quarter of the breast.

Mastectomy:

Subcutaneous: Removal of as much breast tissue as possible while preserving overlying skin and the nipple-areolar complex.

Total: Complete removal of all breast tissue and the axillary tail of Spence.

Modified radical: Removal of all breast tissue and axillary lymph nodes.

Radical: Removal of breast tissue, axillary lymph nodes, and underlying pectoral muscles.

Superradical: Removal of breast tissue, axillary lymph nodes, pectoral muscles, and internal mammary lymphatic chain.

Breast reconstruction: Replacement of lost breast tissue by expanders, implants, or muscle flaps.

Complications: Surgical complications include infection of the incision line, sloughing of the nipple and areola, lymphedema, seroma (in 15% of patients), nerve injury, impaired range of motion in the shoulder joint, and injury to the brachial plexus. Complications of breast reconstruction include infection of the prosthesis pocket, hematomas under skin flaps, necrosis of the skin, deflation or leakage of implants, fixation of the implant to the chest wall, or migration of silicone (commonly used until recently) from leaking implants, leading to systemic complications.

RADIATION THERAPY

Bradytherapy: Implantation of radioactive sources.

Teletherapy: Use of an external photon/electron beam.

Complications: Radiation may lead to skin ulceration, lymphedema, fibrosis, and pneumonitis. (See the box on page 88 for instructions on skin care.)

1 ASSESS*

ASSESSMENT	OBSERVATIONS
Primary care and prevention	
Medical history	Family history of breast cancer, past cancer, early menarche, late menopause, exposure to ionizing radiation, nulliparous, age over 40
Risk factors	High-fat diet, obesity
Breast	Mass, changes in shape, enlarged axillary nodes, bloody nipple discharge, dimpling, nipple retraction
Self-care practices	History of BSE, record of previous clinical examinations/mammography
Acute care	
Surgical incision	Redness, warmth, tenderness, drainage (serous, serosanguineous), pus
Skin	Edema, flaking, peeling of axilla or arm on affected side, erythema, ulceration, discoloration of radiation site
Extremities	Loss of sensation and impaired function of arm on affected side
Pain	Report of pain in incision, heaviness or pain in axilla or arm of affected side
Vital signs	Increased heart rate, elevated blood pressure, altered respiratory rate
Psychosocial	Fear, anxiety, denial, altered sleep patterns, inability to comprehend, difficulty in decision making
Long-term care	
Respiratory	Chronic cough, hoarseness, sputum, chest pain, frequent upper respiratory infections (URI)
Extremities	Bone/joint pain, fracture
Neurologic	Headache, dizziness, abrupt mood change
Abdomen	Edema, ascites, prominent veins on abdominal wall, tenderness in right upper quadrant, palpation of liver ridge
Nutritional status	Loss of appetite, nausea and vomiting, weight loss
Skin	Jaundice, bruising, petechiae
Breast (remaining)	Mass, change in shape, enlarged axillary nodes, bloody discharge, dimpling, nipple retraction
Psychosocial	Withdrawal from significant others, anger, avoids intimacy, avoids discussing experience

*Nursing care should be well documented in the patient's permanent health care record.

2 DIAGNOSE

NURSING DIAGNOSIS	SUBJECTIVE FINDINGS	OBJECTIVE FINDINGS
Primary care and prevention		
Knowledge deficit of breast screening measures related to lack of information, lack of custom or habit, decreased sense of susceptibility or seriousness	Reports misconceptions	No regular BSE, clinical examination, or mammography schedule; unable to demonstrate BSE
Acute care		
Decisional conflict related to number of and controversy about treatment options	Reports uncertainty, vacillation, delay of decisions; appears self-absorbed	Physical signs of stress and tension, irritability, restlessness
Fear related to diagnosis of cancer, loss of breast	Reports apprehension, panic, "fight or flight" reaction	Diaphoresis, dilated pupils, increased pulse and respirations
Impaired skin integrity related to surgery and/or radiation	Complains of itching, heaviness of arm, tenderness, pain	Redness, swelling, warmth, and drainage at incision; elevated temperature; lymphedema; discoloration and flaking at radiation site
Pain related to surgery, advanced stage of disease	Reports pain and factors that aggravate or relieve it	Guarding, grimacing, increased pulse and respirations
Anticipatory grieving related to diagnosis, loss of breast	Expresses denial, disbelief, shock; anger; bargaining; self-absorption; empty feeling	Tears, flushing, shortness of breath, sighing, hostile actions, distancing from others
High risk for infection related to cancer process and/or surgical treatment	Complains of signs and symptoms of infection	Broken skin; change in body fluids, nutrition, and immunity
Body image disturbance related to altered/lost breast	Reports feeling hopeless and depersonalized, unfeminine and sexually undesirable; preoccupied with loss	Avoids intimacy and intercourse; refuses to view breast; takes no interest or excessive interest in appearance
Ineffective family coping related to diagnosis/prognosis	Woman and family describe inability to share; feeling overwhelmed; unable to discuss or deal with cancer-related issues	Arguing, conflict; abuse or neglect of woman; rejection or abandonment by loved one

NURSING DIAGNOSIS	SUBJECTIVE FINDINGS	OBJECTIVE FINDINGS
Fear related to diagnosis, treatment, and prognosis	Expresses desire to detect metastases early; expresses desire for more information about cancer and resources	Keeps follow-up appointments; performs monthly BSE; has mammogram
High risk for sexual dysfunction related to disease process and treatment	Expresses concern about dyspareunia	Dry vaginal mucosa

3 PLAN

Patient goals

Primary care and prevention

1. The patient will understand the recommendations for breast cancer screening and follow those recommendations, including BSE.
2. The patient will recognize her personal risk factors.
3. The patient will adopt a diet low in fat and high in fiber.

Acute care

1. The patient will make informed treatment decisions in an appropriate time frame and will accept the decisions made.
2. The patient's fear will be reduced or eliminated.
3. The patient's skin will be intact and free of infection, and circulation will be maintained.
4. The patient will have no pain.
5. The patient will express feelings of loss appropriately and will use sources of help and support.
6. The patient will be free of infection.

Long-term care

1. The patient will accept the change in her body and will incorporate it into her self-concept.
2. The patient and family will demonstrate effective coping patterns and healthy interpersonal interactions.
3. The patient will demonstrate improved health behaviors.

4 IMPLEMENT

NURSING DIAGNOSIS	NURSING INTERVENTIONS	RATIONALE
Primary care and prevention		
Knowledge deficit of breast screening measures related to lack of information, lack of custom or habit, decreased sense of susceptibility or seriousness	Develop teaching plan for screening procedures, BSE demonstration, available resources, diet, and activities.	To improve health behaviors, increase likelihood of early detection, and increase knowledge and decision-making ability.

NURSING DIAGNOSIS	NURSING INTERVENTIONS	RATIONALE
Acute care		
Decisional conflict related to number of and controversy about treatment options	Provide accurate, readily understood options; check what patient is hearing; serve as advocate with physician and other health care providers; encourage use of support systems; allow time for decision making.	To enable patient to make a decision, to verify patient's understanding, and to provide support.
Fear related to diagnosis of cancer, loss of breast	Encourage patient to express her feelings, and validate those feelings; facilitate use of coping strategies; include patient as active participant in her own care; keep her informed of progress.	To dispel or reduce patient's fear and encourage self-care.
Impaired skin integrity related to surgery and/or radiation	Keep skin clean and dry; monitor dressings and skin integrity; elevate arm.	To prevent infection, impaired circulation, and tissue sloughing.
Pain related to surgery, advanced stage of disease	Monitor type of pain; use pain-relief measures as appropriate; encourage diversional activities.	To decrease or eliminate pain.
Anticipatory grieving related to diagnosis, loss of breast	Encourage patient to express her feelings, and validate those feelings; facilitate use of coping strategies.	To facilitate grieving process and allow patient to confront diagnosis and loss.
High risk for infection related to cancer process and/or surgical treatment	Monitor patient's temperature, skin condition; use sterile technique for incision care following surgery.	To detect and treat early signs of infection, especially following surgery.
Long-term care		
Body image disturbance related to altered/lost breast	Encourage patient to express her feelings and validate those feelings; encourage patient to look at and touch altered body part; encourage her to take an interest in her appearance; encourage spousal interactions; refer for couples, counseling and to support groups.	To facilitate incorporation of body change into self-concept.
Ineffective family coping related to diagnosis/prognosis	Encourage expression and sharing of feelings; encourage family counseling.	To help family members resume normal roles and functions.
Fear related to diagnosis, treatment, and prognosis	Provide adequate information about diagnosis, treatment, and prognosis, and review their benefits; encourage questions.	To promote knowledge about health and to relieve fear about breast cancer, treatment, and prognosis.

NURSING DIAGNOSIS	NURSING INTERVENTIONS	RATIONALE
High risk for sexual dysfunction related to disease process and treatment	Help patient and couple explore feelings; refer to counseling as needed.	To provide support if changes in sexuality occur.

5 EVALUATE

PATIENT OUTCOME	DATA INDICATING THAT OUTCOME IS REACHED
Patient understands recommendations for breast cancer screening and follows those recommendations.	Patient gives correct feedback as to time schedule for BSE, clinical physical examination, and mammography; patient follows age-appropriate screening guidelines.
Patient recognizes her personal risk factors.	Risk profile is correct.
Patient can describe prevention techniques.	Patient verbalizes understanding of risk reduction; e.g., adoption of low dietary fat and high fiber intake.
Patient makes informed treatment decisions in an appropriate time frame and accepts decisions made.	Decisions reached are timely and appropriate for this patient and her value system; patient states acceptance of decision and consequences.
Patient's fear has been reduced or eliminated.	Patient has no diaphoresis; pupils are not dilated; vital signs are normal; patient feels no apprehension.
Patient's skin is intact and free of infection; circulation is maintained.	Skin is clean, dry, warm, and of normal color and turgor; dressing is dry, and temperature is normal.
Patient has no pain.	Vital signs are within normal limits; patient shows no grimacing or guarding and states she feels no pain.

PATIENT OUTCOME	DATA INDICATING THAT OUTCOME IS REACHED
Patient expresses feelings of loss appropriately and uses sources of help and support.	Patient accepts her loss, and uses support systems.
Patient is free of infection.	Patient shows no signs of inflammation; WBC is within normal range; vital signs are within normal range.

Long-term care

Patient has accepted body change and has incorporated change into her self-concept.	Patient expresses acceptance of her body and herself; she has resumed her usual sexual activity and takes an interest in her appearance.
Patient and family demonstrate effective coping patterns and healthy interpersonal interactions.	Family displays ability to communicate; usual roles and functions have been resumed.
Patient demonstrates improved health behaviors.	Patient keeps appointments, performs BSE, has mammograms, and knows early signs of metastasis.

PATIENT TEACHING

1. Emphasize the importance of continuing participation in screening procedures (i.e., clinical breast examination, mammography, and breast self-examination).
2. Teach the patient how to perform breast self-examination, and evaluate her performance.
3. Clarify and reinforce the physician's explanation of the diagnosis, prognosis, and treatment options.
4. Explain the rationales for treatment plans; discuss specific treatment procedures and their effects.
5. Teach the patient hand and arm care for the affected side.
6. Provide information about available community resources (e.g., Reach for Recovery, the American Cancer Society, and other support groups, home health care, and hospice care).
7. If the patient has had a mastectomy, teach her how to perform self-examination of the incision site and assessment of the lymph nodes, and evaluate her ability to do so.
8. Teach the patient self-care at all levels of the care continuum, from primary care and screening to acute and long-term follow-through after diagnosis and medical treatment for breast cancer.

CHAPTER 7

Gynecologic Conditions and Benign Variations

A variety of nonmalignant conditions affect women's reproductive organs. *Congenital anomalies* and *acquired structural conditions* may have anatomic and physiologic consequences. *Reproductive tissue growth*, apart from pregnancy, includes the proliferation of endometrial cells, the formation of benign cysts, and the growth of neoplasms. Trauma may cause *injury and inflammation* of the external and internal reproductive organs.

Congenital and Acquired Structural Disorders

Defects of the reproductive tract cover a wide spectrum of minor to severe malformations. Reproductive defects may result from teratogenic or unknown causes. Malformations may be **congenital** (e.g., ambiguous genitalia) or **acquired** (prolapsed uterus, vaginal fistula).

Müllerian fusion defects are the most common congenital uterine anomaly, occurring in about 0.1% to 0.4% of women (Figure 7-1). Longitudinal vaginal septum is the most common congenital vaginal defect. Congenital malformations of the uterine tubes and ovaries are uncommon. Bladder exstrophy occurs in about 1 in 40,000 births. Pelvic floor weakness is associated with birth interventions and other pathologic conditions.

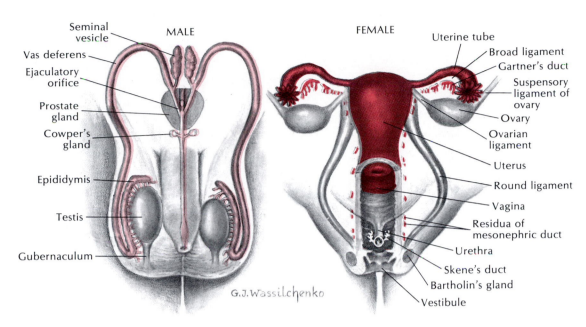

FIGURE 7-1
Homologues of internal genitals. Müllerian duct defects may result in congenital malformations of the female reproductive organs. (From Bobak.[13])

PATHOPHYSIOLOGY

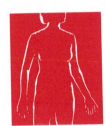

Chromosomal abnormalities may result in gonadal deformities. There are a variety of uterine, vaginal, and bladder deformities that are a result of müllerian tract defects. Uterine malformations include *rudimentary uterus, uterus didelphys, bicornis bicollis (bicornuate uterus)*, and *unicolis (unicornuate uterus)* (Figure 7-2). A missing uterus is rare, except when the vagina is also missing. In these conditions the vaginal septum may be incomplete or complete and either a single or a double cervix may be present.

Longitudinal septum malformation results from incomplete müllerian duct division and vaginal formation in the fetus. *Transverse septum* and *imperforate hymen* may also arise from the failure of early vaginal mem-

brane resorption of the fetus. *Vaginal atresia* (membrane above the hymen) may result from faulty congenital development of the paramesonephric duct or müllerian caudal portions. A *septate vagina* is caused by incomplete müllerian duct fusion, resulting in complete or partial vaginal duplication.

Congenital remnants from the mesonephric and paramesonephric duct may cause cystic pelvic masses. Remnants of Gartner's duct may lead to cyst formation in lateral vaginal walls, or it may result in a connection between the vagina and ureter.

Exstrophy occurs when the midline fails to fuse in the fetus. Associated disorders such as an imperforate anus or duplicate ureters may also be present. Ambiguous genitalia is a chromosomal disorder arising from endogenous or exogenous causes. Diethylstilbestrol (DES) exposure

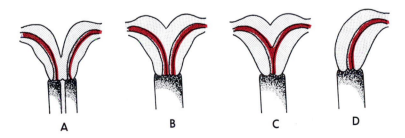

FIGURE 7-2
Abnormal uteri. **A,** Uterus didelphys bicollis (separate vagina). **B,** Uterus bicornis bicollis (vagina simplex.) **C,** Uterus bicornis unicollis (vagina simplex). **D,** Uterus unicornis. (Modified from Wilson, Carrington.[107a])

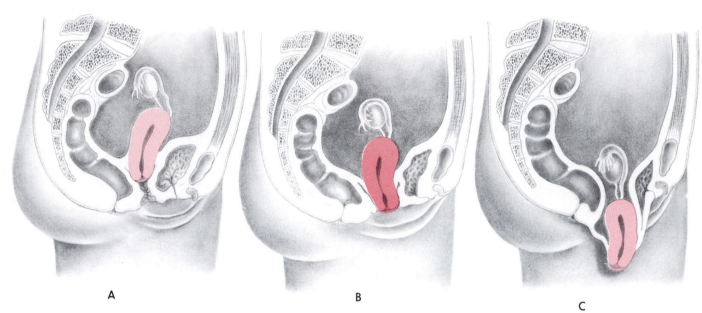

FIGURE 7-3
Uterine prolapse. **A,** First degree. **B,** Second degree. **C,** Complete prolapse. (From Seidel.[96])

while in utero has also produced a variety of defects including cervical and uterine structural abnormalities.

Acquired structural problems of the internal and external genitalia may be caused by trauma, laceration, infection, tumors, atrophy (from genetic factors or decreased estrogen), and vascular disorders. *Pelvic relaxation* may involve the pelvic diaphragm (levator ani and coccygeus muscles) or ligaments (cardinal and uterosacral), or the endopelvic fascia. Injury during childbirth may result in fistulas and trauma to adjacent organs such as the rectal, bladder, and urethral areas. *Uterine displacement* (wandering womb) may occur.

Urethroceles result when the paravaginal fascia, the fascial layer between the vagina and urethra, is weakened. The urethra bulges, or herniates, into the vagina, which may result in pressure sensations. Urethroceles may be confused with urethral diverticula. *Cystoceles* result when the paravaginal and pubocervical fasciae lose their integrity, and sometimes when the levator ani muscle gives insufficient support. As a result, the bladder bulges into the vagina. *Rectoceles* may develop from loss of tone in either or both the paravaginal and pararectal fasciae within the rectovaginal septum. The posterior rectal wall bulges into the vagina, causing pressure sensations and difficulty with evacuating the bowel. *Enterocele* is the bulging of the peritoneal sac into the rectovaginal septum as a result of pelvic relaxation.

Uterine prolapse is the result of diminished tone of the supporting structures of the uterus, which causes displacement of the uterus and vaginal pressure (Figure 7-3). Uterine prolapse frequently is associated with a cystocele and rectocele. The prolapse may be charac-

terized as first degree (mild), second degree (marked), or third degree (complete). *Vaginal vault prolapse* may occur secondary to a hysterectomy or may be associated with uterine prolapse. *Genital fistulas* involve urinary and enterovaginal tears or separations. These fistulas may be located in the urethrovaginal, vesicovaginal, or ureterovaginal areas (Figure 7-4). Enterovaginal fistulas are found most often in the large bowel and occasionally in the small bowel. They often are associated with fourth-degree obstetric lacerations.

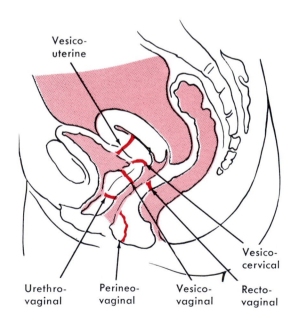

FIGURE 7-4
Types of fistulas that may develop in vagina, uterus, and rectum. (From Phipps.[88])

CLINICAL MANIFESTATIONS

The clinical manifestations of congenital structural defects may include the following:

Longitudinal septum—dyspareunia with coitus
Transverse septum—adolescent cyclic lower abdominal pain; blood distending upper vagina because of no opening for discharge of menses
Adenosis (with or without DES exposure)—increased mucus
Vaginal discharge; beefy red upper vagina

The clinical manifestations of acquired structural defects may include bulging of the organ into the vagina, rectum, or urethral areas, especially during straining. Uterine displacement is also possible. Incontinence, urinary frequency, or dysuria may occur with frequent bladder infections. Constipation or the need for manual pressure with a finger in the vagina may occur with rectocele.

COMPLICATIONS

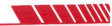

Cysts, fistulas, infection
Bladder and bowel dysfunction
Organ malformation
Infertility resulting from malformation

DIFFERENTIAL DIAGNOSIS

The following conditions may have similar signs and symptoms and should be ruled out:
Neoplasms
Chromosomal disorders
Pathologic conditions of the musculoskeletal system

NURSING CARE

See pages 108 to 111.

MEDICAL MANAGEMENT

GENERAL MANAGEMENT

Perineal exercises such as Kegel exercises and bowel training are used to decrease straining (for pelvic relaxation disorders).

Pessary therapy (supporting rings, bulbs, and devices worn in vagina) is used if surgery is not an option.

DRUG THERAPY

Hormones: Topical estrogen (for relaxation due to low estrogen level).

Antibiotics: For bladder infection.

Stool softeners

SURGERY

Reconstruction for appearance and for decreasing urinary tract infections (bladder exstrophy).

Surgical correction of ambiguous genitalia to male or female, as determined by chromosome testing.

Surgical creation of vagina (for atresia).

Surgical division of uterine septum (most frequently required procedure); cesarean section may be required following repair and pregnancy (for müllerian fusion defects).

Surgical repair of prolapsed uterus, cystocele, rectocele, or enterocele; hysterectomy.

DIAGNOSTIC STUDIES AND FINDINGS

Diagnostic test	Findings
Pelvic examination	To assess observable and palpable structures
Biochemical tests	Urinary steroid excretion may signify adrenal cortical syndromes
Hysteroscopy, laparoscopy	To determine existence of müllerian fusion defects
Hysterosalpingography	
Intravenous pyelogram (IVP), X-rays, ultrasonography	To identify genitourinary or gastrointestinal condition

Endometriosis

Endometriosis is the development of stroma (connective tissue) and endometrial glands (identical to uterine tissue) *outside* the uterus. This ectopic endometrial tissue may form cysts that contain altered blood.

Approximately 20% to 25% of women may have endometriosis sometime during their lives. Endometriosis may affect 1% to 3% of women of childbearing age, and the incidence of the disorder among premenopausal women has been reported as 7% to 10%. Although teenagers and postmenopausal women may have endometriosis, it is most common during the reproductive years and rare in women over 50 years of age. Endometriosis is diagnosed in 30% to 60% of infertile women. The known incidence of the disorder has increased since endoscopic procedures came into use. Endometriosis is found in 8% to 30% of pelvic laparotomies and in 20% of gynecologic surgeries. In 10% of the cases there is cervical, vaginal, and bowel involvement; ovarian involvement occurs in 65% of the cases.

PATHOPHYSIOLOGY

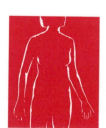

The cause of endometriosis is not clearly understood, but the disorder may be related to retrograde or regurgitated menstruation (*transportation* theory), dissemination via vascular or lymphatic routes, *metaplasia* (tissue transformation), or a combination of transportation and metaplasia (*induction*). Fragments of endometrial mucosa from the oviduct or uterus may travel into the peritoneal cavity with menstrual flow. Lymphatic or vascular metastasis may occur, since endometriosis may involve any mucosal surface, including the nasal mucosa, lungs, pleura, bowel, bladder, kidneys, umbilicus, episiotomy scars, arms, thighs, legs, and vertebral space.

The most common sites of ectopic endometrium are the uterosacral ligaments, sigmoid colon, rectovaginal septum, round ligaments, pelvic peritoneum, ovaries, cul-de-sac, and urinary bladder (Figure 7-5). Pelvic pain may be caused by edema, blood pooling, and migration of menstrual debris into tissues outside the uterus. Because ectopic endometrial tissue responds to the hormonal fluctuations of the menstrual cycle, it may proliferate and bleed throughout the menstrual cycle. *Chocolate cysts*, a common characteristic of endometriosis, result from encapsulated old blood from ovarian endometriosis. Cystic spaces may enlarge to 8 to 10 cm. Endometriosis has been classified as mild (implants *not* associated with scarring or retraction), moderate (usually involving ovaries with scarring and retraction), and severe (involving adhesions, ligaments, and organs of elimination).

Although endometriosis is a progressive, chronic disease, it may never become symptomatic, and it may disappear after menopause. Women with endometriosis may have polyclonal V cell activation, which is associated with autoimmune disease.

CLINICAL MANIFESTATIONS

The major symptom of endometriosis is secondary dysmenorrhea, although the patient may be asymptomatic.

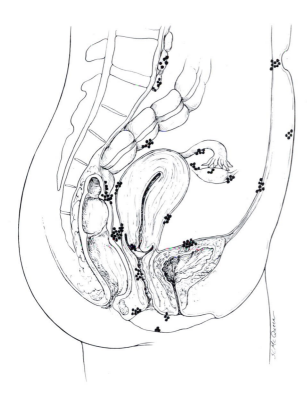

FIGURE 7-5
Common sites of endometriosis. (From Droegemueller.[31])

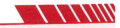

COMPLICATIONS

Infertility
Spontaneous abortions
Adhesions that distort the pelvic structure

DIFFERENTIAL DIAGNOSIS

The following conditions may have similar signs
and symptoms and should be ruled out:
Anovulatory bleeding
Ectopic pregnancy
Miscarriage
Appendicitis
Cysts
Pelvic inflammatory disease (PID)
Urinary tract infection (UTI)

NURSING CARE

See pages 108 to 111.

Abnormal uterine bleeding and dyspareunia (pain during sexual intercourse) may also be present. The physical examination may reveal a tender, fixed, retroverted uterus with a nodular posterior cul-de-sac; nodular thickening and tenderness of uterosacral ligaments and the uterine surface; narrowing and scarring of the posterior vaginal fornix; and adnexal tenderness, enlargement, or mass. Endometriosis may cause more intense menstrual cramps or lower abdominal pain associated with elimination. A full bladder, constipation, or a full colon may cause discomfort until urination or a bowel movement is achieved. Cramps may last for a short period of time, or they may continue or recur. Intestinal discomfort, nausea, and vomiting may also relate to endometriosis.

DIAGNOSTIC STUDIES AND FINDINGS

Diagnostic test	Findings
Pelvic examination, Pap smear, pregnancy tests, complete blood count, urinalysis	To identify any underlying disorder or pathologic condition
Laparoscopy and biopsy	To confirm presence of endometrial tissue outside the endometrium

MEDICAL MANAGEMENT

DRUG THERAPY

Oral contraceptives composed of estrogen and progestin: To cause pseudopregnancy and decidual necrosis and absorption.

Progestins: To produce endometrial atrophy.

Gonadotropin-releasing hormone (GnRH) agonists: To cause estrogen to decrease to levels similar to those of women who have had the ovaries removed.

Danazol or testosterone: To suppress ovarian function, which causes pseudomenopause and discourages endometrial growth.

SURGERY

Laparoscopy to visualize and remove implants.

Electrocauterization or laser ablation to remove endometriotic tissue implants and capsules and to lyse adnexal lesions.

Cautery or resection of endometrial lesions.

Surgery for acute rupture and compromised urinary or bowel function.

Total abdominal hysterectomy and bilateral salpingo-oophorectomy.

Presacral neurectomy, excision of uterosacral ligaments, and anterior uterine suspension to decrease pain.

Benign Masses

Benign gynecologic masses may appear as neoplasms (new growths), cysts (sacs with fluid or semisolid material), leiomyomas (nonencapsulated tumors), or polyps (bulging growths). Cysts may develop in the vulva, vagina, or ovaries. Leiomyomas usually appear in the vulva or uterus. Polyps are more commonly found on the cervix and in the endometrium.

Leiomyomas are the most common pelvic neoplasm. They occur in about 20% to 25% of women over age 35. Leiomyomas are more common in black women than in white women in the United States. Pelvic masses are most often found in the ovaries. Polyps are the most common lesions of the cervix and usually occur during the reproductive years. Endometrial polyps usually appear around menopause. Ovarian cysts usually develop between puberty and menopause. Bartholin's gland cysts are associated with gonorrhea in 10% to 50% of the cases.

PATHOPHYSIOLOGY

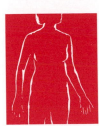

Leiomyomas are also called *myomas* (muscular tissue), *fibromyomas* (fibrous tissue), *fibromas* (connective tissue), or *fibroids* (an older term referring to fibrous tissue) (Figure 7-6). Leiomyomas of the uterus (connective tissue and smooth muscle) may be *intramural* (in the uterine wall), *subserosal* (beneath the perineal membrane), or *submucous* (below the endometrium).

A *parasitic leiomyoma* refers to the attachment of a tumor to the omentum or viscera with a secondary blood supply. *Cervical leiomyomas* and *intraligamentous leiomyomas* may also develop. Leiomyomas grow in response to increased estrogen levels associated with birth control pills and pregnancy, and they regress after menopause. Leiomyomas may degenerate into hyaline, cystic, or calcified tissue. Hemorrhage into a tumor may result in aseptic necrosis and red-colored degeneration.

Benign growths of the vulva include *sebaceous cysts* (usually between the labia majora and minora), *pigmented nevi, glomus tumors* (dermis), *leiomyomas* (smooth muscle), *fibromas* (mesodermal), and *lipomas* (adipose). *Bartholin's cysts* are caused by obstruction of Bartholin's duct, edema, and the accumulation of mucus. Bartholin's cysts usually are unilateral and may be associated with infection such as gonorrhea. Vaginal cystic lesions include Gartner's duct cysts, adenosis (nodular), and endometriosis.

Strictly speaking, several ovarian cysts are not considered neoplastic, since they grow from existing rather than new tissue (Figure 7-7). *Functional ovarian cysts* include *corpus luteum cysts, follicle cysts,* and *theca lutein cysts.* Functional cysts are associated with ovulation. A follicular cyst usually is asymptomatic and transient. However, follicular cysts may be associated with

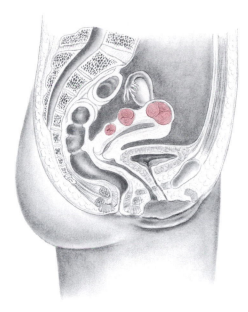

FIGURE 7-6
Myomas of the uterus (fibroids). (From Seidel.[96])

polycystic ovary (PCO) syndrome, resulting in ovarian enlargement from hyperplasia. Leaking or ruptured corpus luteum cysts cause symptoms resembling those of appendicitis, such as pain, leukocytosis, and low-grade fever.

Theca lutein cysts are associated with conditions such as hydatidiform mole and gonadotropin therapy. Lutein cysts may be associated with amenorrhea or delayed menses. They may rupture and require surgery.

Inflammatory cysts develop in the ovaries and uterine tubes after an infection. *Endometrial cysts* are associated with endometriosis, and they usually are filled with old blood *(chocolate cysts)*. *Inclusion cysts* usually are asymptomatic cysts that develop after an infection or menopause. *Parovarian cysts* develop between the

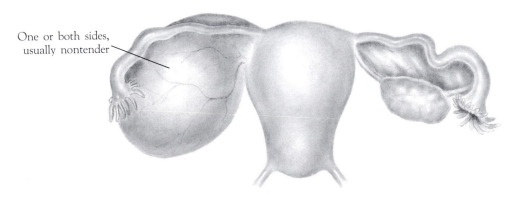

One or both sides, usually nontender

FIGURE 7-7
Ovarian cyst. (From Seidel.[96])

ovary and fallopian tube in postpubertal girls and in women.

Neoplastic polyps may protrude into the cervix or endometrium. *Cervical polyps* usually are soft and red and located near the cervical os. They often are associated with inflammation and vascular congestion. *Endometrial polyps* are often associated with endometrial hyperplasia and leiomyomas. Polyps frequently regress if oral contraceptives were used and are then discontinued.

CLINICAL MANIFESTATIONS

Leiomyomas may cause pressure, pain, and excessive or prolonged menses. They may also cause constipation or urinary frequency. Large leiomyomas may cause hypertension and polycythemia. Lutein ovarian cysts may cause pain, tenderness, amenorrhea, or delayed menses. A degenerating tumor may result in an elevated temperature. Corpus luteum cysts may cause mild leukocytosis and a low-grade fever.

Irregular, firm palpable nodules in lower abdomen or an irregular abdominal contour may be felt.

Bleeding of polyps may occur after douching or coitus.

COMPLICATIONS

Infection
Tumor hemorrhage
Ruptured cyst
Torsion (twisted adnexa)
Infarcted tissue
Adhesions
Infertility

DIFFERENTIAL DIAGNOSIS

The following conditions may have similar signs and symptoms and should be ruled out:
Malignancy
Pregnancy, hydatidiform mole
Colonic disease, diverticulitis
Renal stone, urinary tract infection (UTI)
Endometriosis
Pelvic infection
Appendicitis

Figure 7-8 illustrates one method of evaluating a pelvic mass.

NURSING CARE

See pages 108 to 111.

DIAGNOSTIC STUDIES AND FINDINGS

Diagnostic test	Findings
Pregnancy test	Usually negative; positive with hydatidiform mole
Laparoscopy	Polycystic ovaries
Ultrasonography	Visualization of functional versus neoplastic cysts; adnexal masses
Abdominal x-rays	Visualization of functional versus neoplastic cysts
Laboratory studies	Leukocytosis with generating tumor
Urine analysis (UA), urine culture,	Infection; elevated with STDs, inflammatory cyst, or PID
Complete blood count (CBC)	
Culdocentesis	Increased with theca lutein cysts
Human chorionic gonadotropin (HCG) hormone	Old blood from cyst may be present in the culture fluid.
Pelvic and rectal examinations	Palpation of cyst
Dilation and curettage	Submucosal leiomyomas, endometrial polyps

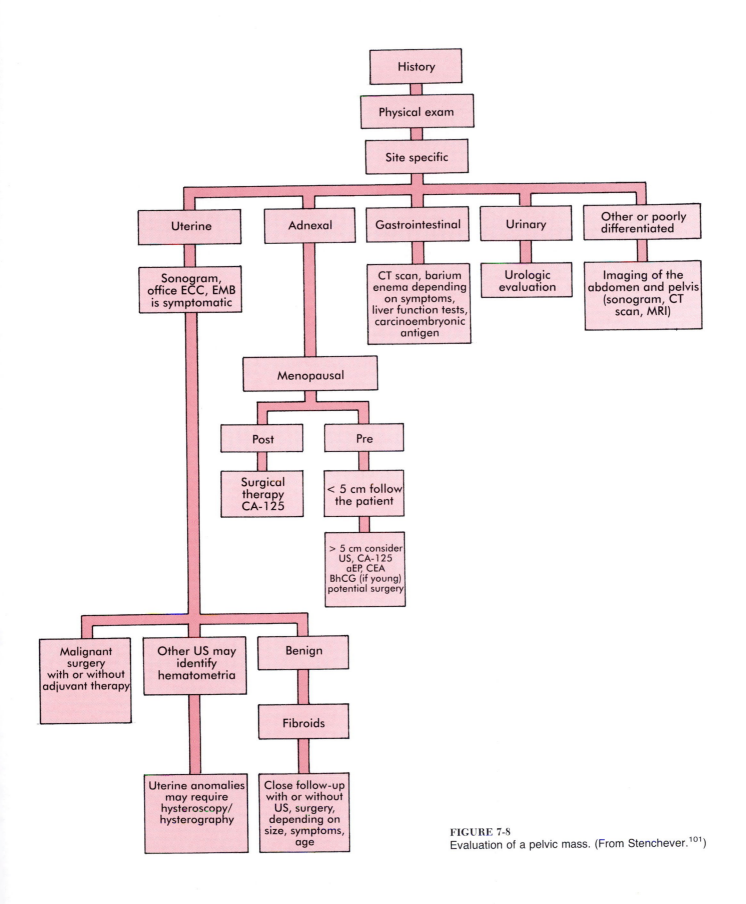

FIGURE 7-8
Evaluation of a pelvic mass. (From Stenchever.[101])

MEDICAL MANAGEMENT

GENERAL MANAGEMENT

Regular gynecologic examinations to monitor leiomyomas.

DRUG THERAPY

Analgesics; oral contraceptives.

SURGERY

Cryosurgery for cervical polyps; cystectomy; myomectomy; total hysterectomy.

Inflammation and Trauma

Injury and inflammation (secondary to trauma or irritants) may result in gynecologic disorders of the perineum and pelvic organs.

Perineal injuries resulting from bicycle accidents are more common in children. The incidence of pelvic trauma from automobile accidents is unknown. Trauma from insertion of a foreign body is rare, apart from tampon-related injuries.

PATHOPHYSIOLOGY

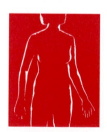

Trauma and inflammation other than from sexually transmitted diseases and assault may result from a number of different situations such as accidents, exercise-related mishaps, or chemical irritants from hygiene products. Different irritants may cause burning, pain, itching, or blistering.

CLINICAL MANIFESTATIONS

The clinical manifestations of inflammation and trauma may include perineal lacerations, edema, abscesses, or ulcers; bleeding, ecchymosis, or hematomas; lichenifi-

cation (leathery skin from chronic inflammation or scratching); and red or white patches. The physical examination may reveal urethral trauma and bowel or pelvic girdle defects.

COMPLICATIONS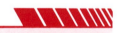

Infection
Acquired structural defects
Hemorrhage

DIFFERENTIAL DIAGNOSIS

The following conditions may have similar signs and symptoms and should be ruled out:
Sexual assault
Foreign body in vagina or rectum
Sexually transmitted diseases
Contact dermatitis
Vigorous sexual intercourse
Spermicidal products
Condoms
Douches or deodorant sprays

KEGEL EXERCISES

Perineal exercises help strengthen the pubococcygeus
muscle, which rims the vagina.

During urination, tighten muscles and stop the flow
in midstream. There will be a sensation of pulling
upward into the vagina, and the buttocks will be
squeezed together.

Repeat this stopping and starting of the urinary flow.
Stop urination for 3 to 5 seconds, then relax and start
the flow again. Repeat this sequence 12 to 24 times
or more during urination.

To be effective, Kegel exercises should be performed
at least four times a day.

DIAGNOSTIC STUDIES AND FINDINGS

Diagnostic test	Findings
Cultures; Potassium hydroxide (**KOH**) scrapings of vulvar skin	Underlying pathologic condition, such as sexually transmitted disease, versus structural defect.
Darkfield preparations	

MEDICAL MANAGEMENT

GENERAL MANAGEMENT

Ice for recent minor injuries; heat for older ecchymotic areas.

Education regarding contact with chemicals.

Determine etiologic agent.

DRUG THERAPY

Antibiotics; analgesics; tetanus booster (for trauma, if patient has not been immunized within 7 years).

SURGERY

Suturing of lacerations; incision and drainage; correction of structural damage.

1 ASSESS*

OBSERVATIONS

ASSESSMENT	STRUCTURAL DEFECTS	ENDOMETRIOSIS	BENIGN MASSES	INFLAMMATION AND TRAUMA
History	Childbearing complications, pelvic trauma, previous laboratory studies (chromosomal, endocrine), previous tumors, drug exposure, elimination problems	Dysmenorrhea, chronic pelvic or lower back pain or pressure (less pain after menses), dyspareunia, infertility, spontaneous abortions	Race, infertility or pregnancy, excessive or long menses, noncyclic bleeding, elimination problems, pain, fever, change in size or shape of uterus	Accidents, assault, use of anticoagulants, use of hygiene products, factors that aggravate or relieve pain, bleeding, edema, itching
Reproductive organs	Development, size, symmetry, duplication, position, function; uterine displacement or prolapse, urethrocele, cystocele, rectocele, enterocele, vaginal vault prolapse	Symmetry, multiple masses; cysts usually in upper outer quadrants; nodular thickening along uterosacral ligaments; structural induration and fixation; scarring or narrowing of posterior vaginal fornix	Irregular, firm, lower abdominal nodules; irregular abdominal shape; signs of other system involvement (CNS, GI, GU)	Vulvar lesions, redness, fistulas, foreign body, ecchymosis, hematomas, lacerations
Pain/discomfort	Pelvic pressure, elimination disfunction, dyspareunia and altered sexual function	Worsening dysmenorrhea, dyspareunia, tiredness or weakness	Pain in vulva, abdomen, or ovarian region	Irritation, tenderness, urticaria, dyspareunia
Psychosocial	Anxiety associated with gynecologic condition, knowledge deficit, and/or self-concept disturbance			

*Nursing care should be well documented in the patient's permanent health care record.

2 DIAGNOSE

NURSING DIAGNOSIS	SUBJECTIVE FINDINGS	OBJECTIVE FINDINGS
Self-esteem disturbance related to gynecologic condition	Reports feeling less sexually attractive; expresses low self-esteem due to abuse, infertility, or discomfort	Social withdrawal, avoidance of intimacy, lack of eye contact, excessive passivity, work history problems

NURSING DIAGNOSIS	SUBJECTIVE FINDINGS	OBJECTIVE FINDINGS
Pain (or discomfort) related to gynecologic disorder	Describes location, sensation, and aggravating and relieving factors	Facial expressions of pain or discomfort, altered muscle tone, diaphoresis, elevated vital signs, dilated pupils
Knowledge deficit related to cause and/or diagnosis of gynecologic condition	Expresses concern about gynecologic symptoms; requests information about condition	May be talkative or withdrawn; shows interest through active facial expressions and gestures
Anxiety related to treatment and prognosis	Expresses anxiety about long-term consequences of gynecologic tumor, deformity, or ailment	Elevated vital signs, diaphoresis, dilated pupils
Decisional conflict related to treatment options	Shows indecision about treatment options or delays decision making	Irritable, withdrawn or restless, tense

3   PLAN

Patient goals

1. The patient will regain her self-esteem.
2. The patient's pain will be relieved.
3. The patient will understand the diagnosis.
4. The patient's anxiety about the treatment and prognosis will be resolved.
5. The patient will select and implement the appropriate treatment.

4   IMPLEMENT

NURSING DIAGNOSIS	NURSING INTERVENTIONS	RATIONALE
Self-esteem disturbance related to gynecologic condition	Assess patient's feelings about her self-image; respect her need for temporary denial or withdrawal.	To clarify patient's feelings and facilitate coping mechanisms.
	Encourage problem solving such as surgery, abuse counseling, or other treatment as needed.	To provide support.
Pain (or discomfort) related to gynecologic disorder	Evaluate character and severity of pain.	To assess pain patterns.
	Provide information about pain control measures, such as analgesics.	To enable patient to minimize pain.
	Document and collaborate with physician and health team to ensure effective pain control.	To enhance pain control with team approach.

→ > >

NURSING DIAGNOSIS	NURSING INTERVENTIONS	RATIONALE
Knowledge deficit related to cause and/or diagnosis of gynecologic condition	Encourage patient to ask questions.	To clarify patient's understanding.
	Assess patient's readiness for learning; use a variety of educational methods and materials; use nonjudgmental methods to assess learning.	To facilitate learning.
	Involve family in learning process as appropriate.	To promote support for patient.
Anxiety related to treatment and prognosis	Validate patient's anxiety; identify and correct misconceptions.	To help patient clarify fears.
	Discuss patient's past coping strategies.	To promote patient's self-confidence.
	Collaborate with health team to present medical and surgical options.	To help reduce patient's anxiety.
Decisional conflict related to treatment options	Discuss procedures, advantages, risks, and possible outcomes; help patient and family with choices.	To enable patient to make an informed choice.

5 EVALUATE

PATIENT OUTCOME	DATA INDICATING THAT OUTCOME IS REACHED
Patient has regained her self-esteem.	Patient acknowledges self-confidence, and her nonverbal behavior shows acceptance of her gynecologic condition.
Patient's pain has been relieved.	Patient states that pain has been relieved and shows no nonverbal evidence of pain.
Patient understands the cause and diagnosis of her gynecologic condition.	Patient can describe the cause of her gynecologic condition.
Patient's anxiety has resolved.	Patient states that her anxiety has abated.
Patient has selected and implements appropriate treatment.	Informed choice about treatment has been made by the patient and her family, as appropriate.

PATIENT TEACHING

GENERAL

1. Explain the pathophysiology and frequency of gynecologic variations specific to the patient.
2. Explore possible treatment options. Inform the patient (and family when appropriate) that surgical correction of gynecologic variations and medical treatment of endocrine disorders often are successful.
3. Provide information on counseling if needed for resolution of low self-esteem.
4. Discuss sexual dysfunction, if appropriate. Explain corrective procedures for gynecologic conditions, such as prolapse, that may interfere with intercourse.

CONGENITAL AND STRUCTURAL DEFECTS

1. Reassure the patient that many congenital and acquired defects may be surgically corrected.
2. Describe nonsurgical treatment options as appropriate, such as Kegel exercises to increase muscle tone.

ENDOMETRIOSIS

1. If pregnancy is desired, discuss the possible recession of endometriosis after pregnancy.
2. Help the patient identify pain-relieving measures for dysmenorrhea and dyspareunia; explain that dysmenorrhea secondary to endometriosis usually worsens.
3. Help the patient identify any tiredness or weakness that may be secondary to anemia; explain the need for dietary and vitamin supplements.

4. Discuss pharmacotherapy options, such as danazol and progestin-estrogen therapy; explain that these medications relieve symptoms but do not cure the condition, and side effects are severe.
5. Discuss the use of laparoscopy for removing endometriomal capsules and endometriotic implants and for lysis of lesions of the ovaries and fallopian and uterine tubes; answer questions about resection or cautery for visible lesions.
6. Give preoperative instructions as needed for total abdominal hysterectomy and bilateral salpingo-oophorectomy

BENIGN MASSES

1. Discuss the importance of regular examinations if observation, rather than treatment, of a mass is indicated.
2. As appropriate, describe myomectomy for removing leiomyomas and preserving the uterus for pregnancy.
3. Explain the use of laparotomy for removing cysts and for controlling bleeding from ruptured cysts.

INFLAMMATION AND TRAUMA

1. Explore ways to prevent inflammation and/or trauma.
2. Teach the patient the signs and symptoms of infection.
3. Refer the patient to counseling as needed.

CHAPTER 8

Gynecologic Malignancies

A gynecologic cancer is an uncontrolled growth of anaplastic cells in the tissues of the female genital organs, which are the uterus, fallopian tubes, ovaries, vagina, and vulva. Cancer of the genital organs is second only to breast cancer as a cause of morbidity and mortality in women. A woman's perception of her sexuality and female self-identity often is profoundly affected by the diagnosis and treatment of gynecologic cancers. The incidence of these cancers is increasing; they account for approximately 15% of all cancer in women. The American Cancer Society has estimated that more than 71,500 women will be diagnosed with genital cancer in 1993 and that approximately 24,400 women will die of the disease. These figures do not include the 45,000 cases of carcinoma in situ of the cervix expected to be diagnosed.

Cervical Cancer

Cancer of the cervix begins as a neoplastic change in the junction between the exocervix (the outer surface of the cervix), which is covered with squamous epithelium, and the endocervix (the inside of the cervical canal), which is covered with columnar epithelium. Cervical intraepithelial neoplasm is the precursor of cervical cancer.

More than two thirds of cervical cancers are now diagnosed in the preinvasive stage, and mortality rates have dropped sharply, largely because of widespread and effective screening techniques. Cervical cancer is more common among women of lower economic status, and the age of the woman at diagnosis is decreasing. Deaths among women in underdeveloped countries remain high.

PATHOPHYSIOLOGY

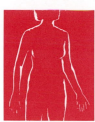

Cervical cancer now is generally considered a sexually transmitted disease (STD). Probable agents are human papillomaviruses, with the herpes simplex virus as a possible cofactor. There are many different strains of genital warts, or condylomata, but strains 16 and 18 seem to be associated with the development of cervical cancer.

Research suggests a possible dietary link, with deficiencies in vitamin A and C and folic acid contributing to cancer of the cervix. There is no evidence of any link to endocrine dysfunction or hormone imbalance. Family history and menstrual history also show no correlation to prevalence of cervical cancer.

Cervical cancers are predominantly squamous cell carcinomas (90%). A few cases of adenocarcinoma are thought to be related to in utero exposure to diethylstilbestrol (DES). Cervical cancer begins as a neoplastic change in the cervical epithelium and eventually involves the full thickness of the epithelium (Figure 8-1). An invasive tumor forms in a cauliflower shape or as an exophytic, endophytic, or ulcerative lesion with a friable texture and a hard, nodular edge.

CLINICAL MANIFESTATIONS

Cervical cancer usually has no characteristic or typical sign or symptom. Bleeding develops with blood-tinged discharge that may progress to spotting and frank bleeding. The bleeding is caused by ulceration of the epithelial surface; however, some tumors spread without ulceration and thus with no bleeding. Other possible indicators are prolonged menstrual periods or an increase in number of periods, and bleeding immediately after intercourse.

COMPLICATIONS

Anemia (from chronic bleeding in advanced disease)

Persistent backache or leg pain (from invasion of the pelvic side wall)

Hematuria, urgency, and voiding difficulties (from invasion of the bladder)

Rectal bleeding and tenesmus (from invasion of the rectal wall)

DIAGNOSTIC STUDIES

Screening

The Papanicolaou (Pap) smear is a highly effective screening device when performed correctly in conjunction with a thorough physical and bimanual pelvic examination. How often a woman should have a Pap

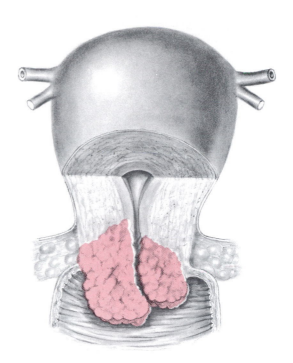

FIGURE 8-1
Advanced cervical cancer. (From Belcher.[13])

RISK FACTORS FOR CERVICAL CANCER

Onset of intercourse before age 20
Multiple sex partners
Infections with human papillomavirus (HPV)
Cigarette smoking
Low socioeconomic status

---

smear is a matter of debate. Current guidelines recommend that a woman start having Pap smears at age 18 or at the onset of sexual activity, whichever occurs first. Women with a high-risk profile should have an annual Pap smear, whereas others may be screened less frequently after three or more examinations with negative results.

When a Pap smear reveals atypical cells, a definitive diagnosis is made through histologic examination of tissue obtained by colposcopy and biopsy. Other procedures, such as cervicography, may be used as diagnostic adjuncts or to determine whether the tumor has spread.

PROGNOSIS

Staging of the cancer provides a prognosis, guides treatment, and allows comparison of the effectiveness of various types of treatment. The two most commonly ac-

FIGURE 8-2
Examples of staging definitions for cervical cancer. **A,** *TNM T2b/FIGO IIB* staging of tumor with parametrial invasion. **B,** *TNM T3b/FIGO IIIB* staging of tumor that extends to pelvic wall and/or causes hydronephrosis or nonfunctioning kidney. **C,** *TNM T4/FIGO IVA* staging of tumor that invades the bladder mucosa or rectum and/or extends beyond the true pelvis.

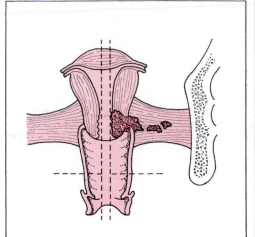

A

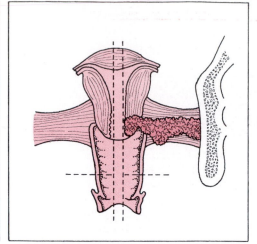

B

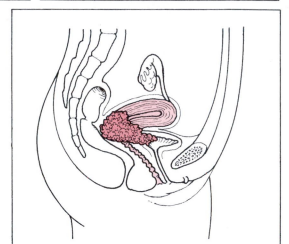

C

cepted staging systems are the TNM system (*t*umor size, axillary lymph *n*ode involvement, and absence or presence of *m*etastases) and the FIGO (Federation International of Gynecology and Obstetrics) system. The boxes below and at right incorporate both systems, define the symbols, and illustrate the various stages for cervical cancer (Figure 8-2).

For years staging of cervical cancer was based on the clinical examination alone. However, in the 1970s interest emerged in surgical staging, which has been shown to be more accurate than clinical staging in about 40% of cases. Treated Stage 0 and Stage Ia squamous cell disease has a survival rate after 5 years approaching 100%. Treated Stage IB disease has a 5-year survival rate of 90%. The prognosis falls steadily as the stage goes higher; stage IV disease has a mortality rate of 95%. Adenocarcinoma has a poorer prognosis at any stage.

NURSING CARE
See pages 128 to 133.

STAGING FOR CERVICAL CARCINOMA

TNM				FIGO
Stage 0	T_{is}	N_0	M_0	
Stage I	T_1	N_0	M_0	Stage I
Stage IA	T_{1a}	N_0	M_0	Stage IA
Stage IA$_1$	T_{1a_1}	N_0	M_0	Stage IA1
Stage IA$_2$	T_{1a_2}	N_0	M_0	Stage IA2
Stage IB	T_{1b}	N_0	M_0	Stage IB
Stage II	T_2	N_0	M_0	Stage II
Stage IIA	T_{2a}	N_0	M_0	Stage IIA
Stage IIB	T_{2b}	N_0	M_0	Stage IIB
Stage IIIA	T_{3a}	N_0	M_0	Stage IIIA
Stage IIIB	T_1	N_1	M_0	Stage IIIB
	T_2	N_1	M_0	
	T_{3a}	N_1	M_0	
	T_{3b}	Any N	M_0	
Stage IVA	T_4	Any N	M_0	Stage IVA
Stage IVB	Any T	Any N	M_1	Stage IVB

STAGING DEFINITIONS FOR CERVICAL CARCINOMA

Primary tumor (T)

TNM	FIGO	
T_X		Primary tumor cannot be assessed
T_0		No evidence of primary tumor
T_{is}		Carcinoma in situ
T_1	I	Cervical carcinoma confined to uterus
$T1_a$	IA	Preclinical invasive carcinoma, diagnosed by microscopy only
T_{1a_1}	IA1	Minimal microscopic stromal invasion
T_{1a_2}	IA2	Tumor with invasive component 5 mm or less in depth taken from base of epithelium, and 7 mm or less in horizontal spread
T_{1b}	IB	Tumor larger than T_{1a_2}
T_2	II	Cervical carcinoma invades beyond uterus but not to pelvic wall or lower end of vagina
T_{2a}	IIA	Tumor without parametrial invasion
T_{2b}	IIB	Tumor with parametrial invasion
T_3	III	Cervical carcinoma extends to pelvic wall and/or lower third of vagina and/or causes hydronephrosis or nonfunctioning kidney
T_{3a}	IIIA	Tumor involves lower third of vagina, no extension to pelvic wall
T_{3b}	IIIB	Tumor extends to pelvic wall and/or causes hydronephrosis or nonfunctioning kidney
T_4	IVA	Tumor invades mucosa of bladder or rectum and/or extends beyond the true pelvis
M_1	IVB	Distant metastasis

Regional lymph nodes (N)

N_X	Regional nodes cannot be assessed
N_0	No regional lymph node metastasis
N_1	Regional lymph node metastasis

Distant metastasis (M)

M_X	Presence of distant metastasis cannot be assessed
M_0	No distant metastasis
M_1	Distant metastasis

DIAGNOSTIC STUDIES AND FINDINGS

Diagnostic test	Findings
Primary disease	
Colposcopy with endocervical curettage	Evidence of malignant cells
Magnetic resonance imaging (MRI)	Estimated tumor volume
Metastasis/spread	
Lymphangiography/needle aspiration	Involvement of lymph channels
Computed tomography (CT) scan of abdomen	Involvement of retroperitoneal lymph nodes
Supraclavicular node biopsy	Involvement of supraclavicular nodes
Excretory urography, cystoscopy, intravenous pyelogram (IVP)	Evidence of spread to bladder
Chest x-ray	Evidence of spread to lung
Proctosigmoidoscopy, barium enema	Evidence of spread to rectum

MEDICAL MANAGEMENT

Medical management of diagnosed carcinoma of the cervix includes surgery, radiation, and adjuvant chemotherapy. Treatment is determined primarily by the stage. Women with stage 0 through stage IIA disease usually are treated surgically, whereas women with stage IIB through stage IIIB disease are treated with radiation therapy. Radiation also is commonly used to treat recurrences and as a palliative measure. Chemotherapy currently is prescribed on an experimental basis in late-stage disease.

SURGERY

Conization: Excision of the mucous membrane of the cervix, maintaining the integrity of the cervical os.

Cryotherapy: Freezing of the cervical lesion with a cautery.

Electrocautery: Burning of the lesion with an electric cautery.

Laser ablation: Vaporization of the lesion with a laser beam.

(*Note:* All of above are used to treat in situ disease in women of childbearing age.)

Hysterectomy: Abdominal or vaginal removal of the uterus and cervix, usually leaving the ovaries intact.

Pelvic exenteration: Nodal dissection and removal of the bladder, urethra, uterus, cervix, vagina, rectum, and all lateral supporting tissues; performed for advanced disease.

Complications: Immediate complications of conization, ablation, and cautery include hemorrhage and uterine perforation. Delayed complications include cervical stenosis or incompetence, infertility, and increased incidence of low-birth-weight babies. Complications of hysterectomy include hemorrhage, pelvic infection, ureteral or rectovaginal fistulas, and bowel obstruction. Possible complications include exenteration, hemorrhage, sepsis, bowel obstruction, pulmonary embolus or edema, cerebrovascular accident, and myocardial infarction.

RADIATION THERAPY

Internal radiation therapy (brachytherapy): Directed at primary tumor site.

Intracavity: A radium applicator is fitted with colpostats and placed in the uterus through the vagina.

Interstitial: Radium implants are inserted into 18-gauge, hollow needles and placed in the parametrium; technique is used when the vaginal anatomy is distorted and intracavity treatment is precluded.

External beam therapy: An external radiation beam is aimed to reach the upper end of the fifth lumbar vertebra; this technique is used to treat extension of the tumor into the extrauterine pelvic soft tissue.

Complications: Radiation may lead to skin ulceration, cystitis, and enteritis, as well as delayed complications such as fistulas, ulcers, and strictures of the bladder or rectum.

DRUG THERAPY

Adjuvant chemotherapy: Use of cytotoxic drugs for cell destruction; experimental treatment for stage III and stage IV disease.

Complications: Chemotherapy may lead to hair loss, anemia, and bone marrow depression.

Endometrial Cancer

Endometrial hyperplasia is associated with the development of endometrial cancer. Malignant cell types include adenocarcinoma, adenoacanthoma, clear cell carcinoma, and squamous cell carcinoma. Endometrial cancer is more likely to metastasize than cervical cancer.

Endometrial cancer is the most common gynecologic malignancy and is one of the six leading causes of death attributed to cancer (Figure 8-3). Fortunately, the cure rate is about 87% because the tumors tend to be localized and well differentiated. This cancer is found primarily in perimenopausal and postmenopausal women between 55 and 60 years of age. These women tend to be of higher socioeconomic status and from industrialized countries. The prevalence of endometrial cancer has increased sharply in recent years. Adenomatous hyperplasia is a precursor to endometrial cancer and when left untreated progresses to invasive cancer about 25% of the time.

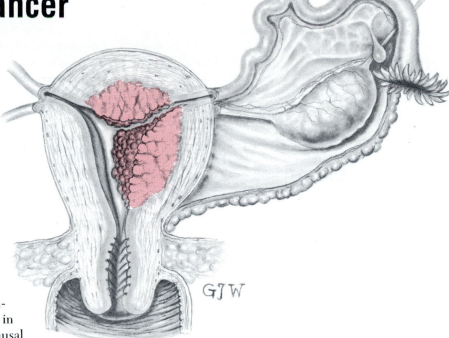

FIGURE 8-3
Endometrial cancer. (From Belcher.[13])

PATHOPHYSIOLOGY

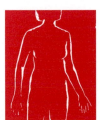

The cause of endometrial cancer has not been firmly delineated, although a link to hormone-related disorders has long been established. However, approximately 40% of endometrial tumors appear to have no known etiology.

Endometrial hyperplasia may be the first sign of developing carcinoma. Hyperplasia may progress to adenocarcinoma, which usually is diagnosed in women age 50 or older. Most endometrial cancers are adenocarcinomas, which begin in the fundus of the uterus and spread to the entire endometrium. The tumor may extend down the endocervical canal and involve the cervix. Other tumor types include adenoacanthoma and clear cell and squamous cell tumors. Squamous cell carcinomas grow rapidly and tend to affect women in their forties or early fifties.

Lower levels of estrogen in postmenopausal women may cause an increase in androstenedione. Obesity and hepatic disease are also associated with higher androstenedione levels. Androstenedione is converted into

---

RISK FACTORS FOR ENDOMETRIAL CANCER

Large body frame and obesity
High-fat diet
Nulliparity
Infertility
Menstrual irregularities (anovulation)
Late menopause
Dysfunctional bleeding during menopause
Prolonged therapy with unopposed exogenous estrogen (estrogen given without concurrent progestins)
Adenomatous hyperplasia of the endometrium
History of breast, colon, or ovarian cancer
History of diabetes and/or hypertension
Family history of endocrine cancers

---

estrone, a postmenopausal estrogen and potential carcinogen. Hyperestrogenism results from the stimulation of the unopposed estrogen, causing endometrial hyperplasia and subsequent endometrial cancer.

CLINICAL MANIFESTATIONS

The most significant clinical sign of endometrial cancer is bleeding. Approximately one third of postmenopausal women who experience such bleeding have endometrial cancer. Bleeding in women who menstruate is unlikely to be a symptom of an endometrial tumor. Later-stage disease that extends beyond the uterus to the parametrium and fallopian tubes and ovaries, and then progresses to the pelvic wall, pelvic and paraaortic lymph nodes, and bladder and bowel, gives rise to corresponding signs and symptoms.

DIFFERENTIAL DIAGNOSIS

Nonmalignant conditions, such as endometriosis, trauma, or benign tumors.

DIAGNOSTIC STUDIES

Screening

Screening for endometrial cancer seems worthwhile because of the clearly defined risk factors. Screening through clinical examination should be directed toward detection and treatment of precursor lesions and well-differentiated, noninvasive tumors. Preventive measures should include restricting prolonged use of unopposed exogenous estrogen (estrogen given without concurrent progestins).

PROGNOSIS

Screening methods for endometrial cancer detection are usually not as successful as those used to detect cervical cancer. Treatment and prognosis depend on the extent of the disease (Figure 8-4).

NURSING CARE

See pages 128 to 133.

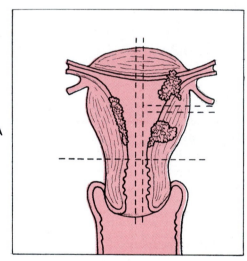

A

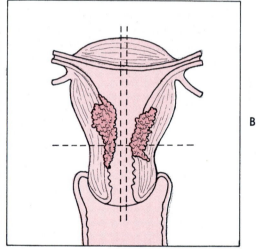

B

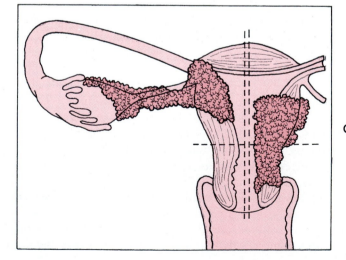

C

FIGURE 8-4
Examples of staging definitions for endometrial (uterine) cancer. **A,** *TNM T_{1a}/FIGO IA* staging of tumor limited to the endometrium; *TNM T_{1b}/FIGO IB* staging of tumor that invades approximately one-half of the myometrium; *TNM T_{1c}/FIGO IC* staging of tumor that invades more than half of myometrium; **B,** *TNM T_{2a}/FIGO IIA* staging of invasion limited to endocervical glandular involvement; *TNM T_{2b}/FIGO IIB* staging of invasion of the cervical stroma; **C,** *TNM T_{3a}/FIGO IIIA* staging of tumor that involves serosa and/or adnexa; *TNM T_{3b}/FIGO IIIB* staging of vaginal involvement.

STAGING FOR ENDOMETRIAL CANCER

TNM				FIGO
Stage 0	T_{is}	N_0	M_0	
Stage I	T_1	N_0	M_0	Stage I
Stage IA	T_{1a}	N_0	M_0	Stage IA
Stage IB	T_{1b}	N_0	M_0	Stage IB
Stage IC	T_{1c}	N_0	M_0	Stage IC
Stage II	T_2	N_0	M_0	Stage II
Stage IIA	T_{2a}	N_0	M_0	Stage IIA
Stage IIB	T_{2b}	N_0	M_0	Stage IIB
Stage III	T_3	N_0	M_0	Stage III
Stage IIIA	T_{3a}	N_0	M_0	Stage IIIA
Stage IIIB	T_{3b}	N_0	M_0	Stage IIIB
Stage IIIC	T_1	N_1	M_0	Stage IIIC
	T_2	N_1	M_0	
	T_{3a}	N_1	M_0	
	T_{3b}	N_1	M_0	
Stage IVA	T_4	Any N	M_0	Stage IVA
Stage IVB	Any T	Any N	M_1	Stage IVB

Stage 0 carcinoma has a 5-year survival rate approaching 100%, and stage I disease has a 5-year survival rate of 77%. The survival rate of late stages decreases as the stage increases. Most endometrial cancer is slow growing with a long and well-defined noninvasive stage.

STAGING DEFINITIONS FOR UTERINE (ADVANCED ENDOMETRIAL) CANCER

Primary tumor (T)

TNM	FIGO	
T_X		Primary tumor cannot be assessed
T_0		No evidence of primary tumor
T_{is}		Carcinoma in situ
T_1	I	Tumor confined to corpus uteri
T_{1a}	IA	Tumor limited to endometrium
T_{1b}	IB	Tumor invades up to or less than one half of myometrium
T_{1c}	IC	Tumor invades more than one half of myometrium
T_2	II	Tumor invades cervix but does not extend beyond uterus
T_{2a}	IIA	Endocervical glandular involvement only
T_{2b}	IIB	Cervical stromal invasion
T_3	III	Local and/or regional spread
T_{3a}	IIIA	Tumor involves serosa and/or adnexa (direct extension or metastasis) and/or cancer cells present in ascites or peritoneal washings
T_{3b}	IIIB	Vaginal involvement (direct extension or metastasis)
N_1	IIIC	Metastasis to pelvic and/or paraaortic lymph nodes
T_4	IVA	Tumor invades bladder mucosa and/or bowel mucosa
M_1	IVB	Distant metastasis

Regional lymph nodes (N)

N_X	Regional nodes cannot be assessed
N_0	No regional lymph node metastasis
N_1	Regional lymph node metastasis

Distant metastasis (M)

M_X	Presence of distant metastasis cannot be assessed
M_0	No distant metastasis
M_1	Distant metastasis

DIAGNOSTIC STUDIES AND FINDINGS

Diagnostic test	Findings
Menstrual history	Irregularities in cycle
Papanicolaou (Pap) smear (detects endometrial cancer in about 50% of cases)	
Pelvic examination	Masses and irregularities
Endocervical aspiration and curettage	Premalignant or malignant cells
Fractional dilation and curettage	Premalignant or malignant calls
Laparotomy with sample of peritoneal fluid or scraping of histologic fragments	Malignant cells
Endometrial biopsy (if risk factors are present)	Premalignant or malignant tissue

MEDICAL MANAGEMENT

Management focuses on identifying and treating hyperplasia by correcting hormonal imbalances. Surgery is a last resort for these lesions.

DRUG THERAPY

Hormone therapy and chemotherapy are used to treat recurrent lesions and to reduce metastases. Chemotherapy seems most effective in poorly differentiated tumors that are not hormone dependent.

Chemotherapy: Use of cytotoxic drugs for cell destruction.

Hormone therapy: Use of hormones such as progestin to induce regression of metastases.

Complications: Chemotherapy may lead to hair loss, anemia, and bone marrow depression.

SURGERY

Once cancer has been diagnosed, surgery is the treatment of choice; it often is used in combination with radiation therapy given either before or after surgery.

Hysterectomy: Abdominal removal of the uterus and cervix with bilateral salpingo-oophorectomy with pelvic and paraaortic lymph node biopsies.

Complications: Hysterectomy complications include hemorrhage, pelvic infection, ureteral/rectovaginal fistulas, and bowel obstruction.

RADIATION THERAPY

Intracavity therapy: Tubes of radium are placed in the endometrial cavity to achieve irradiation of the vaginal vault.

External beam therapy: External radiation beam is aimed at the entire pelvic area.

Complications: Radiation may lead to skin ulceration, cystitis, and enteritis, as well as delayed complications such as fistulas, ulcers, and strictures of the bladder or rectum.

Ovarian Cancer

Malignant ovarian tumors develop from cells present during embryonic ovarian development. The ovaries are also susceptible to metastases.

Ovarian cancer is the sixth most common form of cancer in women and the fourth leading cause of death from cancer (Figure 8-5). The incidence of ovarian cancer, which is rising, is highest in Western industrialized nations, especially among Caucasian women of Northern European descent who are 50 years of age or older.

PATHOPHYSIOLOGY

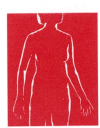

The cause of ovarian cancer has not been established, but the common occurrence of ovarian tumors in the same time frame as breast, colon, and/or endometrial cancer suggests a common etiology. Ovarian cancer is the most difficult gynecologic tumor to cure, because it is seldom detected before the tumor reaches Stage III (see pages 122 to 123 for staging systems).

Most ovarian carcinomas (75%) are epithelial in origin; these tumors include serous cystadenocarcinoma and mucinous, endometroid, and clear cell tumors. Germ cell tumors account for fewer than 5% of all can-

---

RISK FACTORS FOR OVARIAN CANCER
Age (≥ 50 years)
Family history of ovarian cancer (risk increases twentyfold if mother or a sister has had the disease)
More than 40 years of active ovulation
Nulliparity or first pregnancy after age 30
High-fat, low-fiber, vitamin A–deficient diet
Prolonged exposure to asbestos and talc

cerous ovarian tumors, but in women under 20 years of age, they represent 65% of diagnosed ovarian cancers. Germ cell tumors grow rapidly and frequently produce tumor markers.

CLINICAL MANIFESTATIONS

Early ovarian cancer often has no symptoms or only mild ones associated with other common problems, such as vague abdominal discomfort, dyspepsia, bloating, flatulence, and digestive disturbances. Later-stage signs and symptoms include an enlarged abdomen with ascites, abdominal and/or pelvic pain, abdominal and/or pelvic masses, persistent gastrointestinal symptoms, urinary complaints, and menstrual irregularities. Hem

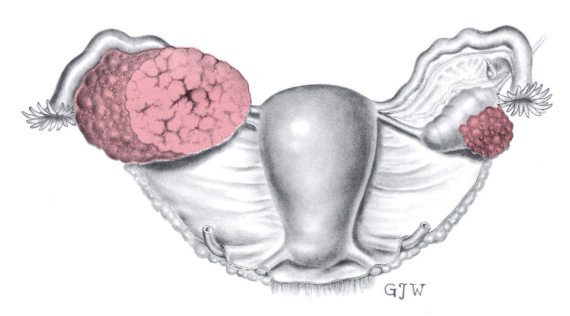

FIGURE 8-5
Cancer of the ovaries. (From Belcher.[13])

orrhage, sepsis, nausea, vomiting, and cachexia may also occur.

DIFFERENTIAL DIAGNOSIS

Nonmalignant conditions, such as benign ovarian cysts.

DIAGNOSTIC STUDIES

Screening

Screening should include regular and thorough abdominal and pelvic examinations, particularly among women who are high risk (see box on page 121). Pelvic ultrasonography with vaginal probe is a useful screening technique.

The 5-year survival rate for ovarian cancer is not promising. Stage I disease has only a 70% survival rate, and the rate for stage II drops below 40%. Since most tumors are not detected until stage III, the prognosis is grim.

PROGNOSIS

The boxes below and at right illustrate how staging of ovarian cancer provides a prognosis, guides treatment, and facilitates comparison of the effectiveness of various treatments.

NURSING CARE

See pages 128 to 133.

STAGING DEFINITIONS FOR OVARIAN CANCER

Primary tumor (T)

TNM	FIGO	
T_X		Primary tumor cannot be assessed
T_0		No evidence of primary tumor
T_1	I	Tumor limited to ovaries
T_{1a}	IA	Tumor limited to one ovary; capsule intact, no tumor on ovarian surface, no ascites
T_{1b}	IB	Tumor limited to both ovaries; capsule intact, no tumor on ovarian surface, no ascites
T_{1c}	IC	Tumor extends to one or both ovaries with any of the following: capsule ruptured, tumor on ovarian surface, ascites, or peritoneal wash with malignant cells
T_2	II	Tumor involves one or both ovaries with pelvic extension
T_{2a}	IIA	Extension or implants on uterus or tubes
T_{2b}	IIB	Extension to other pelvic tissues
T_{2c}	IIC	Extension with malignant cells in ascites or peritoneal wash
T_3	III	Involvement of one or both ovaries with peritoneal metastasis outside pelvis and/or regional lymph node metastasis
T_{3a}	IIIA	Microscopic peritoneal metastasis beyond pelvis
T_{3b}	IIIB	Macroscopic peritoneal metastasis beyond pelvis 2 cm or less in greatest dimension
N_1	IIIC	Peritoneal metastasis beyond pelvis larger than 2 cm in dimension and/or regional lymph node metastasis
M_1	IV	Distant metastasis

Regional lymph nodes (N)

N_X	Regional nodes cannot be assessed
N_0	No regional lymph node metastasis
N_1	Regional lymph node metastasis

Distant metastasis (M)

M_X	Presence of distant metastasis cannot be assessed
M_0	No distant metastasis
M_1	Distant metastasis

STAGING FOR OVARIAN CARCINOMA

TNM				FIGO
Stage 0	T_{is}	N_0	M_0	
Stage I	T_1	N_0	M_0	Stage I
Stage IA	T_{1a}	N_0	M_0	Stage IA
Stage IB	T_{1b}	N_0	M_0	Stage IB
Stage IC	T_{1c}	N_0	M_0	Stage IC
Stage II	T_2	N_0	M_0	Stage II
Stage IIA	T_{2a}	N_0	M_0	Stage IIA
Stage IIB	T_{2b}	N_0	M_0	Stage IIB
Stage IIC	T_{2c}	N_0	M_0	Stage IIC
Stage III	T_3	N_0	M_0	Stage III
Stage IIIA	T_{3a}	N_0	M_0	Stage IIIA
Stage IIIB	T_{3b}	N_0	M_0	Stage IIIB
Stage IIIC	T_{3c}	N_0	M_0	Stage IIIC
	Any T	N_1	M_0	
Stage IV	Any T	Any N	M_1	Stage IV

DIAGNOSTIC STUDIES AND FINDINGS

Diagnostic test	Findings
Laparoscopy with biopsy	To detect malignant cells
Lymphangiography	To detect malignant cells in retroperitoneal nodes
Cancer antigen 125	To detect elevation
Alpha-fetoprotein/human gonadotropin	Elevated in germ-chorionic cell tumors
Paracentesis	To detect malignant cells in fluid

MEDICAL MANAGEMENT

The treatment of choice is surgery with postoperative radiation therapy or chemotherapy. Relapse is common in these patients, particularly if the tumor is poorly differentiated or large or if the tumor is stage II or higher.

DRUG THERAPY

Chemotherapy: Use of single or combination cytotoxic drugs for cell destruction.

SURGERY

Bilateral salpingo-oophorectomy: Removal of ovaries and fallopian tubes.

Hysterectomy: Abdominal removal of the uterus and cervix with bilateral salpingo-oophorectomy and omentectomy.

RADIATION THERAPY

Intracavity therapy: Chromic phosphate injected intraabdominally via peritoneal catheter.

External beam therapy: External radiation beam aimed at the entire abdominal area or at abdominal segments in a strip technique.

Vaginal Cancer

Squamous cell carcinoma and clear cell adenocarcinoma may be found in the vaginal area. Primary tumors of the vagina are rare, since most vaginal tumors spread from the cervix or endometrium.

Vaginal cancer accounts for approximately 1% of all genital cancers. Women over 50 years of age are most frequently affected, particularly when the tumor is a squamous cell carcinoma. A small but significant number of women in their late teens and early twenties have been diagnosed with a clear cell adenocarcinoma of the vagina. However, they generally had mothers who took diethylstilbestrol (DES) during pregnancy.

PATHOPHYSIOLOGY

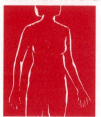

The cause of primary vaginal tumors is unknown, but they are thought to be triggered by genital viruses or chronic irritation. Other risk factors include hysterectomy and previous radiation therapy for cancer of the cervix or rectum.

The 5-year survival rate for carcinoma in situ, which is confined to the intraepithelium, approaches 100%. The rate for stage I tumors, which are limited to the vaginal wall, ranges from 65% to 90%. The rate drops precipitously as the stage rises.

CLINICAL MANIFESTATIONS

Vaginal bleeding usually is the presenting sign; it may be accompanied by vaginal discharge and pelvic discomfort. Some women have no signs or symptoms. The most common tumor site is the upper third of the vaginal posterior wall.

NURSING CARE

See pages 128 to 133.

DIAGNOSTIC STUDIES AND FINDINGS

Diagnostic test	Findings
Vaginal Pap smear; clinical pelvic examination; colposcopy with biopsy	To detect premalignant or malignant cells

MEDICAL MANAGEMENT

DRUG THERAPY

None; chemotherapy currently is ineffective in treating most vaginal lesions.

SURGERY

Carbon dioxide laser therapy: Often used to treat in situ tumors.

Vaginectomy: Sometimes used to treat stage I disease.

Radical hysterectomy with lymphadenectomy or pelvic exenteration: May be used to treat extensive or recurrent disease.

RADIATION THERAPY

The major treatment modality is internal or external radiation therapy.

Vulvar Cancer

Vulvar intraepithelial neoplasms may develop into cancerous conditions over time. Premalignant cells are similar to premalignant vaginal and cervical cells.

Three to five percent of all gynecologic cancers involve the vulva (Figure 8-6). Although a variety of growths and tumors can appear on the vulva, few are cancerous. However, the incidence of vulvar intraepithelial neoplasia, a preinvasive disease, is increasing, particularly in women between 20 and 40 years of age. However, older women, particularly those age 65 or older, are at greatest risk for cancer of the vulva. Invasive vulvar tumors develop on the labia in 70% of cases and on the clitoris in 13%. Other locations include the vaginal and urethral openings or perineal areas.

PATHOPHYSIOLOGY

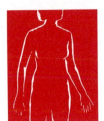

The cause of vulvar cancer is unknown, although long-term pruritus is a significant risk factor, and the human papillomavirus may play a causal role. Most vulvar cancers are squamous cell carcinomas. Older women in low socioeconomic groups seem more at risk, suggesting that age and hygiene may be associated with vulvar cancer. The 5-year survival rate for women with no lymph node involvement is about 85%. As the disease progresses to the nodes and beyond, the survival rate drops dramatically.

CLINICAL MANIFESTATIONS

The presenting signs and symptoms include pruritus, pain, and a vulvar lump or mass. Vulvar carcinoma may result in a lymph node spread pattern.

DIFFERENTIAL DIAGNOSIS

Benign tumors, cysts or lesions; sores associated with sexually transmitted diseases.

NURSING CARE

See pages 128 to 133.

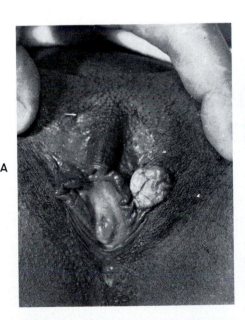
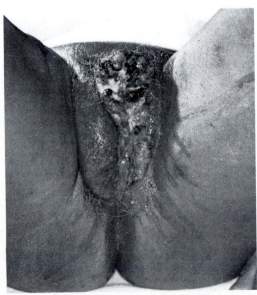

FIGURE 8-6
A, Well-differentiated carcinoma of the vulva. **B,** Advanced carcinoma of the vulva, involving the entire vagina, urethra, and rectum. (From Seidel.[96])

DIAGNOSTIC STUDIES AND FINDINGS

Diagnostic test	Findings
Vaginal Papanicolaou (Pap) smear Clinical pelvic examination Vulvar biopsy with a Keyes dermatologic punch	To detect pathologic conditions.

MEDICAL MANAGEMENT

DRUG THERAPY

Chemotherapy: Used as palliative therapy in advanced disease.

SURGERY

Cautery, laser, cryosurgery: For premalignant vulvar lesions.

Surgery: The major mode of treatment; usually is confined to wide local incision for carcinoma in situ.

Vulvectomy: Used for invasive disease with inguinal lymphadenectomy when there is node involvement.

RADIATION THERAPY

Radiation therapy has been used as palliative therapy in advanced disease.

Uterine Tube Cancer and Gestational Trophoblastic Neoplasms

Cancer of the uterine (fallopian) tubes is the rarest of all gynecologic cancers. Gestational trophoblastic neoplasms (GTNs) are all neoplastic disorders that arise from the placenta, such as hydatidiform mole, invasive mole, placental site tumor, and gestational choriocarcinoma.

The incidence of uterine tube cancer peaks in women in their fifties, although it has been found in women of all ages. The 5-year survival rate has been reported as high as 90% in early disease, but the disease usually is not detected in an early stage, and the overall survival rate is about 40%. Data are insufficient to establish a predictable pattern of recurrence.

Hydatidiform mole, a benign form of gestational choriocarcinoma, is the most common of these tumors, occurring in approximately 1 in 1,500 live births in the United States. Women over 40 years of age have a higher incidence of the disorder. Between 15% and

30% of molar pregnancies lead to choriocarcinoma. The 5-year survival rate for nonmetastatic disease and metastatic disease to sites other than the liver or brain nears 100%. The prognosis is extremely poor if the disease metastasizes to the liver and brain.

PATHOPHYSIOLOGY

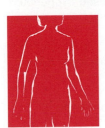

The risk factors and cause of uterine tube cancer and gestational trophoblastic neoplasms are unknown. Most uterine tube neoplasms are papillary adenocarcinomas.

Gestational trophoblastic neoplasms have a unique feature in that they contain paternal chromosomal markers. This malignant tumor of the trophoblast tends to grow rapidly and metastasize widely to the vagina, oral cavity, lungs, brain, or liver.

CLINICAL MANIFESTATIONS

The clinical signs and symptoms of uterine tube cancer are pelvic or colicky pain and vaginal discharge or bleeding.

DIFFERENTIAL DIAGNOSIS

Normal pregnancy and psychogenic symptoms may need to be ruled out.

DIAGNOSTIC STUDIES AND FINDINGS

Diagnostic test	Findings
Uterine tube carcinoma is difficult to diagnose; the disorder frequently is confused with ovarian or uterine cancer.	
Surgery, ultrasonography, suction curettage	Adnexal mass or evidence of choriocarcinoma cells
Beta subunit chorionic gonadotropin levels, serum human chorionic gonadotropin	Elevated (secreted by trophoblastic tumors)

MEDICAL MANAGEMENT

SURGERY

Radical hysterectomy with bilateral salpingo-oophorectomy: Treatment of choice for uterine tube carcinoma.

Simple hysterectomy: Recommended following GTN.

DRUG THERAPY

Chemotherapy: Has been used after surgery, but evaluation of success is uncertain because of the small number of cases of uterine tube cancer. Chemotherapeutic treatment is used for GTN, and maintenance chemotherapy often is used to try to prevent recurrence of GTN.

RADIATION THERAPY

Radiation has been used after surgery, but evaluation of success is uncertain because of the small number of cases of uterine tube cancer.

1   ASSESS*

ASSESSMENT	OBSERVATIONS
Primary care	
Medical history	Family history of cancer; report of endometrial hyperplasia, past cancer, infertility, menstrual irregularities, early menarche, late menopause; exposure to unopposed exogenous estrogen therapy, ionizing radiation, asbestos, or talc; nulliparity, pregnancy before age 20 or after age 40
Risk factors	High-fat, low-fiber diet, vitamin A deficiency, heavy alcohol consumption, smoking, early intercourse, multiple sex partners, obesity
Vulva/vagina	Mass, growth, mole; malodorous watery or bloody discharge; pruritus; pain, aching
Self-care practices	History of vulvar self-examination, record of previous clinical examinations and Pap smears
Acute care	
Surgical incision	Redness, warmth, tenderness, drainage, pus
Skin	Edema, flaking, peeling of axilla or arm on affected side, erythema, ulceration, discoloration of radiation site
Vulva/vagina	Pruritus, discharge, swelling, redness, bleeding, odor
Renal	Urgency, hematuria, difficulty voiding
Abdomen	Distension, edema
Gastrointestinal	Rectal tenesmus, bleeding
Pain	Pain in incision, groin, lower back, abdomen
Vital signs	Increased heart rate, elevated blood pressure, altered respiratory rate
Psychosocial	Fear, anxiety, denial, altered sleep patterns, inability to comprehend, difficulty making decisions
Long-term care	
Respiratory	Chronic cough, hoarseness, sputum, chest pain, frequent upper respiratory infection (URI)
Extremities	Bone or joint pain, fracture
Neurologic	Headache, dizziness, abrupt mood change
Abdomen	Edema, ascites, prominent veins on abdominal wall, tenderness in right upper quadrant, palpation of liver ridge
Nutritional status	Loss of appetite, nausea and vomiting, weight loss
Skin	Jaundice, bruising, petechiae
Psychosocial	Withdrawal from significant others, anger, avoids intimacy, refuses to discuss experience

*Nursing care should be well documented in the patient's permanent health care record.

2 DIAGNOSE

NURSING DIAGNOSIS	SUBJECTIVE FINDINGS	OBJECTIVE FINDINGS
Primary care		
Knowledge deficit of cancer screening measures related to lack of information; lack of custom or habit; decreased sense of susceptibility or seriousness	Has misconceptions about health behaviors	No regular vulvar self-examination, Pap smear, or clinical bimanual examination
Acute care		
Decisional conflict related to treatment options	Expresses uncertainty; vacillates; delays making decisions; is self-absorbed	Physical signs of stress and tension, irritability, restlessness
Fear related to diagnosis of cancer, loss of uterus, loss of childbearing capacity	Reports apprehension, panic, "fight or flight" reaction	Diaphoresis, dilated pupils, increased pulse and respirations
Impaired skin integrity related to surgery and/or radiation	Reports itching, tenderness, discomfort, pain	Redness, swelling, warmth, drainage in incision; elevated temperature; discoloration, flaking of radiation site
Impaired skin integrity related to vaginal discharge	Reports pruritus	Bleeding or discharge, redness, swelling, odor
Pain related to surgery, advanced stage of disease	Reports pain and factors that aggravate and relieve it	Guarding, grimacing, increased pulse and respirations
Anticipatory grieving related to diagnosis, loss of uterus/ovaries	Denial, disbelief, shock; anger; bargaining; self-absorption; empty feeling	Tears, flushing, shortness of breath, sighing, hostile actions, distances herself from others
Long-term care		
Body image disturbance related to lost uterus/ovaries	Reports feeling helpless, hopeless, depersonalized, unfeminine, and sexually undesirable; preoccupied with loss	Avoids intimacy or intercourse; shows withdrawal, isolation behavior; takes no interest or excessive interest in appearance
Altered sexuality patterns related to anatomic and functional changes caused by disease/treatment	Reports rejection or avoidance by either partner; diminished sensation, pain, lack of orgasm	Vaginal dryness, itching or bleeding with coitus

ASSESSMENT	OBSERVATIONS	
Ineffective family coping related to diagnosis/prognosis	Woman and family report inability to share, feeling overwhelmed, are unable to discuss or deal with cancer-related issues	Arguing, conflict; abuse or neglect of woman; rejection or abandonment
Knowledge deficit related to treatment and prevention of malignancy	Expresses desire to detect metastases early; expresses desire for more information about cancer and sources of support	Keeps follow-up appointments; performs monthly vulvar self-examination

3 PLAN

Patient goals

Primary care

1. The patient will understand the recommendations for gynecologic cancer screening and will follow those recommendations.
2. The patient will recognize her personal risk factors.

Acute care

1. The patient will make informed treatment decisions in an appropriate time frame and will accept the decisions made.
2. The patient's fear will be reduced or eliminated.
3. The patient's skin will be intact and free of infection.
4. The patient's perineal area will be clean and odor free.
5. The patient will have no pain.
6. The patient will express feelings of loss appropriately and will use sources of help and support.

Long-term care

1. The patient will accept the change in her body and will incorporate the change into her self-concept.
2. The patient will resume a mutually satisfying pattern of sexual relations with partner.
3. The patient and family will demonstrate effective coping patterns and healthy interpersonal interactions.
4. The patient will demonstrate improved health behaviors.

4 IMPLEMENT

NURSING DIAGNOSIS	NURSING INTERVENTIONS	RATIONALE
Primary care		
Knowledge deficit of cancer screening measures related to lack of information; lack of custom or habit; decreased sense of susceptibility or seriousness	Develop teaching plan for screening procedures, vulvar self-examination, and available resources.	To improve health behaviors, increase likelihood of early detection, and increase knowledge and decision-making ability.
Acute care		
Decisional conflict related to treatment options	Provide accurate, readily understood options; check what patient is hearing; serve as advocate with physician; encourage use of support systems; allow time for decision making.	To enable patient to make an informed decision.

NURSING DIAGNOSIS	NURSING INTERVENTIONS	RATIONALE
Fear related to diagnosis of cancer, loss of uterus, loss of childbearing capacity	Encourage patient to express her feelings, and validate those feelings; facilitate use of coping strategies; include patient as active participant in her own care; keep her informed of progress.	To dispel or reduce patient's fear and encourage self-care.
Impaired skin integrity related to surgery and/or radiation	Keep skin clean and dry; monitor dressings and skin for tissue sloughing.	To prevent infection and breakdown.
Impaired skin integrity related to vaginal discharge	Administer perineal care, and monitor drainage.	To promote patient's comfort and protect skin, and to track status of skin integrity.
Pain related to surgery, advanced stage of disease	Monitor type of pain; use pain-relief measures as appropriate; encourage diversional activities.	To decrease or eliminate pain.
Anticipatory grieving related to diagnosis, loss of uterus/ovaries	Encourage patient to express her feelings, and validate those feelings; facilitate use of coping strategies.	To facilitate grieving process and allow patient to confront diagnosis and loss.
Body image disturbance related to lost uterus/ovaries	Encourage patient to express her feelings, and validate those feelings; encourage patient to socialize and to return to her daily routine; encourage her to take an interest in her appearance; encourage spousal interactions; and refer patient to support groups.	To facilitate incorporation of body change into self-concept.
Altered sexuality patterns related to anatomic and functional changes caused by disease/treatment	Encourage patient to express her feelings about loss of uterus; educate her about anatomic changes; refer for sexual counseling.	To enable patient to resume satisfying sexual relations.
Ineffective family coping related to diagnosis/prognosis	Encourage expression and sharing of feelings; encourage family counseling.	To enable family members to resume normal roles and functions.
Knowledge deficit related to treatment and prevention of malignancy	Help structure health behaviors in manageable fashion; provide adequate information about needed behaviors, and review their benefits.	To promote health and prevent complications of gynecologic cancer.

EVALUATE

PATIENT OUTCOME	DATA INDICATING THAT OUTCOME IS REACHED
Primary care	
Patient understands recommendations for cancer screening and follows those recommendations.	Patient gives correct feedback as to time schedule for vulvar self-examination, Pap smear, and clinical physical bimanual examination; patient follows screening guidelines.
Patient recognizes her personal risk factors.	Risk profile is correct.
Acute care	
Patient makes informed treatment decisions in an appropriate time frame and accepts decisions made.	Decisions reached are timely and appropriate for this patient and her value system; patient states acceptance of decision and consequences.
Patient's fear has been reduced or eliminated.	Patient has no diaphoresis or dilated pupils; vital signs are within normal limits; patient feels no apprehension.
Patient's skin is intact and free of infection.	Skin is clean, dry, and warm and of normal color and turgor; dressing is dry, and temperature is normal.
Patient's perineal area is clean and odor free.	Patient has no drainage, bleeding, or odor; patient reports feeling clean and comfortable.
Patient has no pain.	Vital signs are within normal limits; patient shows no grimacing or guarding and states she feels no pain.
Patient expresses feelings of loss appropriately and uses sources of help and support.	Patient accepts her loss and uses support systems.
Long-term care	
Patient has accepted body change and has incorporated change into her self-concept.	Patient expresses acceptance of her body and herself; she has resumed usual daily activities and takes an interest in her appearance.
Patient resumes a mutually satisfying pattern of sexual relations with partner.	Patient has resumed sexual functioning; both partners express satisfaction.

PATIENT OUTCME	DATA INDICATING THAT OUTCOME IS REACHED
Patient and family demonstrate effective coping patterns and healthy interpersonal interactions.	Family displays ability to communicate; usual roles and functions have been resumed.
Patient demonstrates improved health behaviors.	Patient keeps appointments, performs vulvar self-examination, has regular Pap smears and clinical examinations, and knows early signs and symptoms of metastasis.

PATIENT TEACHING

1. Emphasize the importance of continuing participation in screening procedures.
2. Teach the patient how to perform vulvar self-examination, and evaluate her performance.
3. Clarify and reinforce the physician's explanation of the diagnosis, prognosis, and treatment options.
4. Explain the rationales for the treatment plans; discuss specific treatment procedures and their effects.
5. Provide information about available community resources (e.g., the American Cancer Society, home health care, and hospice care).

Sexually Transmitted Diseases and Gynecologic Infections

Because the presence of one sexually transmitted disease predisposes a woman to other organisms, a comprehensive screening regimen should be carried out to detect any additional causative agents.

The sexually transmitted diseases (STDs) encompass several different infections and diseases that are transmitted through sexual contact. Traditionally the term "venereal disease" has referred to gonorrhea, syphilis, and other common infections such as genital warts or herpes. However, the number of venereal diseases classified has grown from five to more than 50. Currently STDs represent a wide range of disorders, from relatively minor inflammatory conditions to eventually lethal diseases. Infections may be local or systemic, and they may be caused by a number of different pathogens such as *viruses*, *bacteria*, *fungi/yeasts*, *protozoa*, and *ectoparasites* (Table 9-1). STDs are spread through vaginal intercourse, oral sex, and anal intercourse. Inflammation may arise from factors other than sexual transmission. For example, pelvic inflammatory disease (PID) may be associated with an intrauterine device (IUD), and urinary tract infections (UTIs) and toxic shock syndrome (TSS) may develop as a result of conditions unrelated to sexual activity. Opportunistic infections occur in people with immunologic disorders.

Acquired Immune Deficiency Syndrome (AIDS)

Acquired immune deficiency syndrome (AIDS) is caused by the *human immunodeficiency virus (HIV)*. AIDS is a cell-mediated immunity defect that causes immunodeficiency. This viral disease may have originated in African green monkeys and probably then spread to human beings from monkey blood that was used during fertility rituals. Human immunodeficiency virus spread from Africa to Haiti and then to the United States.

AIDS, the late manifestation of HIV infection, may develop within a few months to 10 years after infection. The first case of AIDS was reported in 1981; by 1991 more than 200,000 cases had been documented. Over 50% of women with AIDS probably contracted the disease from IV drug use and contaminated needles. The etiology is unknown in about 20% of women with AIDS. Sexual spread of AIDS to women is the third

Table 9-1

CAUSES OF COMMON SEXUALLY TRANSMITTED DISEASES

Classification/disease	Causative agent
Viral	
Acquired immune deficiency syndrome (AIDS)	Human immunodeficiency virus (HIV)
Hepatitis	Types A through E; usually hepatitis B virus (HBV)
Genital herpes	Herpes simplex virus (HSV), types 1 and 2
Genital warts/condylomas (also called condylomata acuminata)	Human papilloma virus (HPV)
Genital papules	Molluscum contagiosum virus (MCV)
Bacterial	
Gonorrhea	*Neisseria gonorrhoeae*
Syphilis	*Treponema pallidum*
Chlamydia	*Chlamydia trachomatis*
Lymphogranuloma venereum (LGV)	
Mucopurulent cervicitis (MPC)	
Bacterial vaginosis	Several causative agents may be seen in combination:
Nonspecific vaginitis	*Gardnerella (Haemophilus) vaginalis*
Gardnerella infection	*Corynebacterium vaginale*
	Mycoplasma hominis
	(Unusual organisms, e.g., *Mobiluncus, Escherichia coli, Streptococcus* species)
Chancroid ulcers	*Haemophilus ducreyi*
Fungal/yeast	
Monilial vaginitis (candidiasis)	*Candida albicans*
Protozoan	
Trichomonas (trichomoniasis)	*Trichomonas vaginalis*
Parasitic	
Pubic lice or crabs	*Pediculus pubis (Pthirus pubis)*
Scabies (mites or itch)	*Sarcoptes scabiei*

most likely route of transmission. The spread of AIDS seems to occur more frequently from males to females than vice versa. About 10% of HIV infections in women have resulted from blood products given during surgery, during childbirth, or for the control of bleeding disorders. An infant born to a woman with HIV has an estimated 30% to 40% chance of having acquired the virus from the mother.

PATHOPHYSIOLOGY

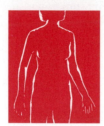

The human immunodeficiency virus is one of the retroviruses, which change their ribonucleic acid (RNA) to deoxyribonucleic acid (DNA) once they invade the body cell, causing a number of cellular changes. HIV invades macrophages and monocytes, which probably allows the virus to be transported throughout the body. The pathophysiologic result is complex. The incubation period varies from 3 to 6 months, although symptoms may be so mild as to be missed. It may be months or years before symptoms appear or HIV infection converts to AIDS. Transmission of the AIDS virus may occur when bodily secretions from an infected person enter another person's body. Semen, blood, feces, vaginal secretions, saliva, and breast milk may serve as media of transmission. Semen is a *known* source of transportation, although other fluids may also transmit HIV, especially if they contain blood. Items such as sex toys (dildo or vibrator) may also become contaminated.

CLINICAL MANIFESTATIONS

The symptoms of HIV infection vary, and some individuals remain asymptomatic for years. Early symptoms often include flulike manifestations: sore throat, rhinitis, and rash. Later symptoms include leukopenia (low WBC count) and idiopathic thrombocytopenia (low platelet count and clotting factors). Other signs may include dermatitis, fever, night sweats, diarrhea, yellowing of the toenails, weight loss, lymphadenopathy, oral hairy leukoplakia (furry white patches in the mouth), and enlarged tonsils. Infections may develop, such as herpes, shingles, molluscum contagiosum, encephalitis, meningitis, enterocolitis, and vaginal candidiasis.

A person with HIV is susceptible to invading organisms that may affect all body systems. More than half of those infected with HIV develop neurologic disorders, including AIDS dementia complex (ADC). Opportunistic infections may involve cerebral and meningeal areas, damaging the central nervous system. Gastrointestinal disorders may occur, and more than 20 infectious organisms may cause diarrhea. Impaired liver function may result in susceptibility to hepatitis viruses. Approximately 60% of people with HIV develop *Pneumocystis carinii* pneumonia (PCP), which leads to the diagnosis of AIDS. Systemic infections and dermatologic disorders commonly develop, caused by such organisms as the herpes virus and staphylococci. Kaposi's sarcoma (KS) develops more in men than in women with AIDS.

NURSING CARE

See pages 155 to 157.

DIAGNOSTIC STUDIES AND FINDINGS

VIRUSES

A virus is a noncellular, submicroscopic, disease-causing agent that usually consists of one type of nucleic acid enclosed by a protein covering. Currently few treatments are available, and the prognosis for viral infections is discouraging. The *human immunodeficiency virus (HIV)* causes *acquired immune deficiency syndrome (AIDS)*. *Hepatitis*, also a virus, often is associated with HIV. Other irritating but usually less serious viral disorders are *herpes virus* infections; *condylomata acuminata*, which are anogenital warts or pointed wartlike growths caused by the *human papilloma virus (HPV)*; and *molluscum contagiosum*, a skin disease characterized by soft tumors or growths with stems, caused by a *poxvirus*. Even the common cold is caused by a virus.

Diagnostic test	Findings
HIV tests	
Enzyme-linked immunosorbent assay (ELISA)	Antibodies to HIV (positive test); run twice to rule out false-positive results
HIV antibody test (traditional AIDS test)	Presence of antibodies means that the body may be trying to fight HIV infection; additional testing required
Western blot test	Used to confirm ELISA or HIV antibody test; negative result means no antibodies are present
P24 antigen test	Circulating HIV antigen yields positive result
Signs of impaired immune system	
Hematocrit (Hct)	Decreased
Erythrocyte sedimentation rate (ESR)	Elevated
CD4 lymphocytes	Decreased
CD4/CD8 lymphocyte ratio	Lowered or reversed ratio (normal, 2:1)
Serum β2 microglobulin	Elevated
Serum neopterin	Elevated
Hemoglobin (Hgb)	Decreased

MEDICAL MANAGEMENT

GENERAL MANAGEMENT

Promote general health and prevent, control, and treat opportunistic infections; restore and maintain equilibrium.

DRUG THERAPY

Antiinfective therapy; prophylaxis of PCP and other infections.

Zidovudine (AZT, Retrovir), analogs to inhibit HIV replication and attachment to CD4 receptors.

Recombinant human erythropoietin (r-HuEPO) to stimulate RBC production.

Hepatitis

There are five types of viral hepatitis. Sexual transmission of hepatitis usually is associated with types B and D.

A woman usually contracts hepatitis B or hepatitis D through parenteral drug use or sex with a bisexual partner. About 90% of cases of hepatitis C are caused by posttransfusion infection.

PATHOPHYSIOLOGY

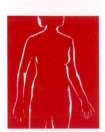

The hepatitis B virus (HBV) is a DNA virus belonging to the hepadnavirus group or family. The presence of an "e antigen" (HB_eAg positive) may increase susceptibility to HBV infection. Active HBV predisposes individuals to delta hepatitis. Sexual transmission of hepatitis A or hepatitis C (non-A, non-B) can occur, although hepatitis A usually is transmitted through fecal-oral contamination, and hepatitis C usually is a bloodborne infection. (Hepatitis E usually is not an STD.) The incubation period for HBV is 45 to 60 days.

Hepatitis infections may cause nausea, vomiting, anorexia, malaise, jaundice, dark urine, and abdominal pain. Arthritis, skin rashes, and arthralgia (joint inflammation) may occur. Acute infections may result in permanent immunity. Approximately 33% to 50% of individuals with acute infections are symptomatic, and 5% to 10% become asymptomatic carriers.

Hepatitis may result in chronic hepatitis (persistent, active), cirrhosis, hepatocellular (liver cell) carcinoma, hepatic failure, and death. Infants born to mothers with hepatitis may develop chronic hepatitis B.

DIAGNOSTIC STUDIES AND FINDINGS

Hepatitis can be diagnosed only with HBV serologic tests.

Diagnostic test	Findings
Hbe antigen (HB_eAg)	Positive result with infection
Antibody to HB surface (or core) antigen (anti-HBc)	Positive result usually relates to previous infection and current immunity
Liver function tests	Usually elevated in all hepatitis infections

NURSING CARE

See pages 155 to 157.

MEDICAL MANAGEMENT

GENERAL MANAGEMENT

Promote general health and prevent, control, and treat opportunistic infections; restore and maintain equilibrium.

DRUG THERAPY

Hepatitis B immune globulin (HBIG) and hepatitis B vaccine may help reduce risk of infection.

Herpes

For pictures of herpes lesions, see Color Plates 5, 6, and 7, page xi.

Herpes labialis (herpes of the lips, mouth, and face) was recognized by the Emperor Tiberius when he placed a ban on public kissing in Rome. There are five major types of herpes simplex virus (HSV). Type 1 **(HSV-1)** usually is found above the waist, and type 2 **(HSV-2)** usually is found below the waist, although orogenital sex may result in cross-contamination of these locations. **Types 3, 4, and 5** generally are not associated with sexual contact.

Eighty percent of HSV-2 is found in the genital region. Approximately 300,000 to 500,000 new cases of genital herpes occur in the United States each year, along with the millions of individuals who have recurring herpes progenitalis symptoms. Although other herpes viruses may not be directly associated with sexual contact, kissing, previous HSV infections, or an impaired immune system may predispose a woman to these infections.

PATHOPHYSIOLOGY

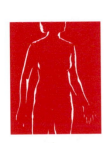

Herpes simplex virus type 1 and type 2 (genital herpes) are large deoxyribonucleic acid (DNA) viruses that require immunotyping for diagnosis. Herpes readily infects the mucosal or surface linings of the mouth and vagina. The incubation period is 3 to 7 days for HSV-1 and 3 to 5 days for HSV-2.

HSV infection may manifest as single or multiple vesicles that rupture and form small, painful ulcers that heal without scarring. The initial infection lasts 14 to 21 days and may involve fever and flulike symptoms. Subsequent infections are less severe and last approximately 8 to 12 days. Viral shedding may occur during the latency period.

The primary symptom of herpes infection is the appearance of single or multiple painful ulcers or blisters in the genital or mouth area. Occasionally herpes sores are found in other body areas. Urination may be painful if the lesions are near the urinary tract. Fever and body aches may occur with the first episode.

Aseptic meningitis is associated with the first outbreak of genital herpes. Neonatal herpes, contracted from the mother, may result in local, systemic, and/or permanent disorders.

NURSING CARE

See pages 155 to 157.

DIAGNOSTIC STUDIES AND FINDINGS

Diagnostic test	Findings
Herpes simplex virus (HSV) cultures	Positive result with presence of multi-nucleated giant cells
Tissue culture from base of lesion using neutralizing solution for fluorescent antibody tests	To differentiate type 1 and type 2 viruses in 24 to 48 hours
HSV serologies	To differentiate HSV from syphilis, chancroid, trauma, or other pathologic condition
Pap smear	

MEDICAL MANAGEMENT

GENERAL MANAGEMENT

Genital herpes: Measures to promote health, e.g., exercise, good nutrition, and stress reduction seem to decrease number of outbreaks.

DRUG THERAPY

Genital herpes: Systemic acyclovir (Zovirax) may decrease symptoms and recurrence. The Centers for Disease Control (CDC) suggests the following regimens:

First episode of genital herpes: Acyclovir, 200 mg PO 5 times a day for 7-10 days or until clinical resolution occurs.

Recurrent episodes: Acyclovir, 200 mg PO 5 times a day for 5 days; *or* acyclovir, 800 mg PO 2 times a day for 5 days.

Genital Warts (Condylomas)

Historically, **condylomas** were called "figs." These wartlike or figlike growths are referred to as condylomata acuminata, or by their causative agent, human papilloma virus (HPV).

In the mid-1970s, HPV was associated with cervical cancer and precancerous conditions. HPV types 16 and 18 are often found among cervical cancer cells and cancers of the vulva and vagina. Of the more than 20 types of HPV, only types 16 and 18 are associated with cancer.

PATHOPHYSIOLOGY

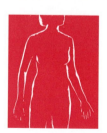

Condyloma acuminatum is the most common type of four virus-producing warts. These warts are pink to brown, elongated lesions that cluster and resemble cauliflower. The incubation period for HPV is 1 to 6 months. The seed or wart growth is facilitated by warm, moist conditions. HPV may infect the oral, cervical, anal, or vaginal mucosa.

NURSING CARE

See pages 155 to 157.

DIAGNOSTIC STUDIES AND FINDINGS

Diagnostic test	Findings
Pap smear, biopsy	To diagnose cervical involvement and rule out malignancy
Gonococcal and chlamydial cultures	To differentiate warts from other pathologic conditions
Rapid plasma reagin (RPR)	To rule out syphilis

MEDICAL MANAGEMENT

GENERAL MANAGEMENT

The goal is to prevent the warts from spreading.

SURGERY

Cautery, laser excision, or cryotherapy (treatment with liquid nitrogen) may be required. The Centers for Disease Control (CDC) suggests the following regimens:

External genital or perianal warts

Recommended: Cryotherapy with liquid nitrogen or cryoprobe.

Alternative: Podophyllin, 10% to 25% in tincture of benzoin. Apply less than 0.5 ml per treatment to an area 10 cm². Wash off in 1-4 hours. Repeat weekly. (Not used during pregnancy.)

Vaginal warts

Recommended: Cryotherapy with liquid nitrogen. Use of cryoprobe in vagina is not recommended because of the risk of perforation and fistula complications.

Alternatives: Trichloroacetic acid (80% to 90%), applied only to warts, then powder talc or sodium bicarbonate (baking soda) to remove acid. Repeat weekly. *Or* podophyllin, 10% to 25% in tincture of benzoin. Skin must be dry, and treatment area must be no larger than 2 cm². Repeat weekly. (Not used during pregnancy.)

Anal warts

Recommended: Cryotherapy with liquid nitrogen.

Alternative: Trichloroacetic acid (80% to 90%) regimen *or* surgical removal.

Oral warts

Recommended: Cryotherapy with liquid nitrogen; *or* electrodesiccation/electrocautery; *or* surgical removal.

Molluscum Contagiosum

Molluscum contagiosum is a benign condition that affects the mucous membranes and skin, producing genital lesions or papules. It is caused by the *molluscum contagiosum virus (MCV)*.

Molluscum contagiosum is more commonly seen as a sexually transmitted disease in girls and young women 10 to 16 years of age, although young children may develop symptoms without sexual transmission.

For a picture of a papule caused by molluscum contagiosum, see Color Plate

PATHOPHYSIOLOGY

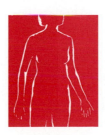

The molluscum contagiosum virus is a poxvirus with an incubation period of 2 to 7 weeks. The lesions cause hyperplastic epidermis and cyst-shaped lobules to form. They vary in color but usually are whitish-pink or tan and dome shaped. Their surfaces form a thick, creamy, umbilicated (indented) appearance.

The lesions are 1 to 5 mm in size. They are shiny and firm and usually appear pearly white. The lesions are most often seen on the trunk and in the anogenital region. Multiple genital lesions appear and then spontaneously clear in 6 to 9 months. Complications may include secondary infection or bleeding of lesions and warts.

NURSING CARE

See pages 155 to 157.

DIAGNOSTIC STUDIES AND FINDINGS

Diagnostic test	Findings
Stain, microscopic examination of cells	Molluscum bodies in epithelial cells

---

MEDICAL MANAGEMENT

GENERAL MANAGEMENT

May require no treatment, or treatment with podophyllin, trichloroacetic acid, or silver nitrate.

SURGERY

Cryotherapy (treatment with liquid nitrogen) may be required.

Gonorrhea

The term *gonorrhea* was coined by the Roman physician Galen. Gonorrheal discharge was believed to contain semen (gonos). It has also been called "clap," which is derived from the word "clappoir," a Parisian house of prostitution during the Middle Ages.

Gonorrhea currently is the most frequently documented STD in the United States, with an annual incidence of 1 million cases. An estimated 1 million to 2 million additional cases are not reported. Pelvic inflammatory disease (PID) occurs in about 20% of women with untreated gonorrhea.

PATHOPHYSIOLOGY

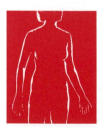

Gonorrhea is caused by the bacterium *Neisseria gonorrhoeae*, a gram-negative diplococcus (Figure 9-1). The organism is oxidase positive and located within polymorphonuclear (PMN) leukocytes. The incubation period is 2 to 10 days, although it can extend to 30 days. Gonorrhea may cause vaginal discharge, dysuria, pelvic or abdominal pain, or abnormal menses. Vaginal burning and itching may be severe. However, many women are asymptomatic.

If left untreated, gonorrhea may result in pelvic inflammatory disease (PID) and disseminated gonococcal infection, including arthritis, septicemia, and dermatitis. *Ophthalmia neonatorum* may occur in newborns if prophylactic treatment is not given. Other infections, such as inflammation of Bartholin's glands, may develop.

NURSING CARE

See pages 155 to 157.

DIAGNOSTIC STUDIES AND FINDINGS

Diagnostic test	Findings
Gonococcal (GC) cultures from vagina, cervix, urethra, anus, uterine tubes, pharynx, or blood	Positive oxidase reaction, Gram's stain morphology, and confirmed sugar fermentation, fluorescent antibody, or coagglutination for GC
Enzyme-linked immunosorbent assay (ELISA)	Positive for GC

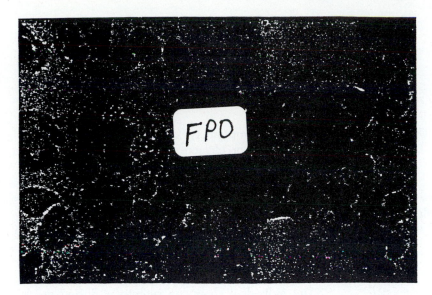

For a picture of a Gram's stain showing cervical gonorrhea, see Color Plate 14, page xiii.

FIGURE 9-1
Neisseria gonorrhoeae: gram-negative intracellular diplococci.
(From Baron and Finegold.[8a])

MEDICAL MANAGEMENT

GENERAL MANAGEMENT

Treatment of bacterial STDs includes tracing and contacting sex partners so that they may be treated also. Barrier devices may help prevent and control the spread of bacterial STDs.

DRUG THERAPY

Gonorrhea: Antibiotics such as cefoxitin, doxycycline, and tetracycline. Cultures should be repeated in 1 week to evaluate results, since some strains are resistant. The Centers for Disease Control (CDC) suggests the following regimens:

Genital gonococcal infection: Ceftriaxone, 250 mg IM once, plus doxycycline, 100 mg PO 2 times a day for 7 days.

Pharyngeal gonococcal infection: Ceftriaxone, 250 mg IM once, plus erythromycin base, 500 mg PO 4 times a day for 7 days.

BACTERIA

Bacteria are minute, unicellular structures with spherical, rod-shaped, or spiral formations. Sexually transmitted bacterial infections include *gonorrhea, chlamydia and lymphogranuloma venereum (LGV), nongonococcal pelvic inflammatory disease, syphilis, chancroid, granuloma inguinale,* and *Gardnerella vaginalis* infection. Some terms indicate the site of infection, such as *pelvic inflammatory disease (PID), salpingitis, vaginitis,* and *urethritis.* PID typically is associated with gonorrhea or chlamydia, or both. Vaginitis may be caused by trichomoniasis, candidiasis, or an allergic reaction.

Syphilis

Syphilis is a chronic systemic disease characterized by a primary lesion. It is both an ulcerative and a systemic condition. The Book of Job in the Bible describes syphilitic-type symptoms, and Christopher Columbus may have encountered syphilis in the West Indies.

Between 1985 and 1990 syphilis increased approximately 75%. The incidence in the United States, which varies from state to state, is about 2 to 7 cases per 100,000 people.

PATHOPHYSIOLOGY

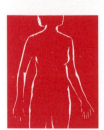 Syphilis is caused by *Treponema pallidum*, a spirochete consisting of six to 14 tight, mobile spirals that give the organism the appearance of a corkscrew (Figure 9-2). *T. pallidum* invades the mucous membranes and migrates to regional lymph nodes and systemic organs. During the incubation period, blood is infectious with *T. pallidum*.

DIAGNOSTIC STUDIES AND FINDINGS

Diagnostic test	Findings
Cultures and serologic tests: rapid plasma reagin (RPR, previously called VDRL) and other treponemal and nontreponemal tests	To detect *T. pallidum*

For pictures of primary and secondary syphilitic lesions, see Color Plates 8, 9, and 10, page xii.

The first symptom typically is a single, firm, painless open sore or chancre at the site of entry on the genitals or mouth. The incubation period lasts anywhere from 10 to 90 days but averages about 3 weeks.

Syphilis progresses through four stages. The primary stage is characterized by painless chancres, or ulcers. The secondary stage involves several symptoms such as skin rash, condylomata and lymphadenopathy. The round, flat, or oval grayish papules of secondary syphilis develop 6 to 12 weeks after the initial infection.

The individual shows no symptoms during the latent stage. During the tertiary, or neurosyphilis, stage, a person may be asymptomatic or may show neurologic symptoms such as ataxia and confusion.

Untreated syphilis progresses to the tertiary stage, resulting in neurologic disorders such as paralysis and insanity. Cardiovascular syphilis may cause destruction of the heart and blood vessels.

NURSING CARE

See pages 155 to 157.

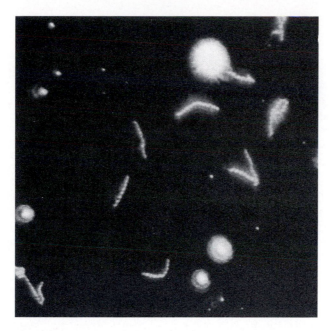

FIGURE 9-2
Treponema pallidum: appearance in a darkfield preparation.
(From Baron and Finegold.[8a])

MEDICAL MANAGEMENT

GENERAL MANAGEMENT

Treatment of bacterial STDs includes tracing and contacting sex partners so that they may also be treated.

DRUG THERAPY

Syphilis usually is treated with penicillin G, benzathine, or probenecid. The Centers for Disease Control (CDC) suggests the following regimens:

Syphilis (primary and secondary and early latent stage of less than 1 year's duration)

Recommended: Penicillin G, 2.4 million U IM in one dose.

Alternatives: Doxycycline, 100 mg PO 2 times a day for 2 weeks; *or* tetracycline, 500 mg PO 4 times a day for 2 weeks.

Late latent syphilis of more than 1 year's duration, gummas, and cardiovascular syphilis

Recommended: Penicillin G, 7.2 million U total, administered as 3 doses of 2.4 million U IM, given 1 week apart for 3 consecutive weeks.

Alternatives: Doxycycline, 100 mg PO 2 times a day for 4 weeks; *or* tetracycline, 500 mg PO 4 times a day for 4 weeks.

Neurosyphilis (at any stage)

Recommended: Aqueous crystalline penicillin G, 12 million to 24 million U, administered 2 million to 4 million U IV q 4 h for 10-14 days.

Alternatives: Procaine penicillin, 2.4 million U IM daily for 10-14 days; *or* probenecid, 500 mg PO 4 times a day for 10-14 days.

Chlamydia

Chlamydia is an intracellular pathogen that is the leading cause of blindness worldwide when the eyes are infected at birth or through poor hygiene. Chlamydial infections include *chlamydial cervicitis, mucopurulent cervicitis (MPC),* and *lymphogranuloma venereum (LGV).*

For a picture of genital elephantiasis caused by chronic lymphogranuloma venereum, see Color Plate 12, page xii.

Lymphogranuloma venereum (LGV) is more common in tropical regions. Approximately 250 new cases are reported each year. Chlamydial infections are associated with gonorrhea in 45% of individuals seeking treatment. An estimated 10% to 20% of sexually active teenage girls have chlamydial infections, and about 1 in 10 to 20 pregnant women is diagnosed with chlamydial endocervical infection. Of the 1 million women with pelvic inflammatory disease (PID), 20% to 40% have PID caused by *Chlamydia trachomatis.* Mucopurulent cervicitis (MPC) may occur, which is the female version of nongonococcal urethritis (NGU) or of the nonspecific urethritis that occurs in men. *C. trachomatis* is the causative agent in 30% to 50% of all cases of cervicitis or NGU.

PATHOPHYSIOLOGY

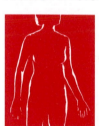

Lymphogranuloma venereum is caused by different strains of *C. trachomatis* and is spread by sexual contact, almost without exception. The incubation period for chlamydial cervicitis is 7 to 21 days. Mucopurulent cervicitis (MPC) is a clinical diagnosis that refers to the presence of yellow mucopurulent endocervical exudate (mucopus). The principal cause of MPC infections is *C. trachomatis,* although they may also be caused by *Neisseria gonorrhoeae, Trichomonas vaginalis,* or the herpes virus.

Chlamydial cervicitis may be asymptomatic. When present, symptoms include a mucopurulent vaginal discharge (mucopus); pelvic, lower back, and abdominal pain; and urethritis, resulting in urinary burning and frequency. The most common sign of LGV is buboes (swollen lymph nodes), which occur more frequently in men.

Chlamydial cervicitis may result in infertility from salpingitis (inflamed uterine tubes). Uterine bleeding, endometritis, urethritis, liver inflammation, and pregnancy and newborn complications may occur. PID may also develop. LGV may cause genital elephantiasis, rectal strictures, abscesses, and fistulas.

NURSING CARE

See pages 155 to 157.

DIAGNOSTIC STUDIES AND FINDINGS

Diagnostic test	Findings
Tissue cultures	Microscopic staining shows presence of elementary bodies
Blood tests	Positive for antibodies against *C. trachomatis*
Monoclonal antibody detection	Positive culture for antibodies
PID (if suspected)	
White blood cell count (WBC)	Elevated
Erythrocyte sedimentation rate (ESR)	Elevated
Laparoscopy, culture	Tubal exudate establishes PID

MEDICAL MANAGEMENT

GENERAL MANAGEMENT

Treatment of bacterial STDs includes tracing and contacting sex partners so that they may also be treated.

DRUG THERAPY

The Centers for Disease Control (CDC) suggests the following regimens:

Chlamydial infections

Recommended: Doxycycline, 100 mg PO 2 times a day for 7 days; *or* tetracycline, 500 mg PO 4 times a day for 7 days.

Alternatives: Erythromycin base, 500 mg PO 4 times a day or equivalent salt for 7 days; *or* erythromycin ethylsuccinate, 800 mg PO 4 times a day for 7 days.

Lymphogranuloma venereum (LGV)

Recommended: Doxycycline, 100 mg PO 2 times a day for 21 days.

Alternatives: Tetracycline, 500 mg PO 4 times a day for 21 days; *or* erythromycin, 500 mg PO 4 times a day for 21 days; *or* sulfisoxazole, 500 mg PO 4 times a day for 21 days (or equivalent sulfonamide course).

Bacterial Vaginosis and Gardnerella Vaginalis

Bacterial vaginosis (BV) has several names and may be caused by different bacteria or a combination of bacteria. The term *nonspecific vaginitis* may be used when the exact causative agent is unclear. Many terms have been used previously to describe vaginitis symptoms, such as **Gardnerella vaginalis,** *Haemophilus vaginalis* vaginitis, Corynebacterium vaginitis, *Mycoplasma hominis,* and *Mobiluncus.* Gardnerella vaginalis is more commonly diagnosed and referred to in health care literature today.

Bacterial vaginosis is the most common cause of vaginal symptoms such as discharge and itching in women of childbearing age. Nonspecific vaginitis frequently occurs in sexually active women. Women with previous infections and those whose sex partners have not been treated are likely to have recurrent vaginitis. The incidence of *Gardnerella vaginalis* is higher in women who use hormonal contraceptives. However, increased incidence is not associated with the hormonal shifts related to the menstrual cycle.

PATHOPHYSIOLOGY

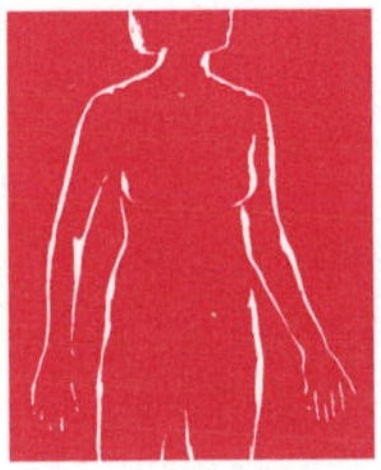

Bacterial vaginosis results in a change or replacement of the lactobacilli of the vagina. These normal vaginal flora often become mixed with *Gardnerella* organisms, anaerobes, or *M. hominis.* Nonspecific vaginitis and *Gardnerella vaginalis* occur with an altered or more alkaline vaginal pH. The organism *Gardnerella vaginalis* will not usually grow in the normal acidic environment of the vagina. The use of hormonal contraceptives may cause an acid and sugar level change in the vagina and predispose the woman to multiple infections. The incubation period for bacterial vaginosis is unknown, since it is often related to an overgrowth of normal vaginal organisms.

Gardnerella vaginalis produces a vaginal discharge resembling flour paste that may be thin and gray and have a fishy odor, without inflammation. Vaginal symptoms may vary. Bacterial vaginosis often is associated with a malodorous vaginal discharge. Leukorrhea (a white discharge) or a thick, grayish yellow discharge may be present. Vaginal irritation and itching are common.

Few complications are associated with *Gardnerella vaginalis*, apart from congenital anomalies from maternal exposure. Postcoital bleeding may occur.

NURSING CARE

See pages 155 to 157.

DIAGNOSTIC STUDIES AND FINDINGS

Diagnostic test	Findings
Vaginal pH	pH >4.5
Culture of vaginal secretions	Microscopic evidence of "clue cells" (epithelial cells coated with bacteria) from vaginal secretions placed in normal saline; presence of *G. vaginalis* organisms
Potassium hydroxide (KOH); whiff test	Positive: fishy odor
Rapid plasma reagin (RPR) and gonococcal culture (GC)	Few lactobacilli or leukocytes found

MEDICAL MANAGEMENT

GENERAL MANAGEMENT

Treatment of bacterial STDs includes tracing and contacting sex partners so that they may be treated also.

DRUG THERAPY

Gardnerella vaginalis usually is treated with metronidazole (Flagyl), although a variety of medications, such as clindamycin and ampicillin, eliminate harmful bacteria. Both (or all) partners should be treated. The Centers for Disease Control (CDC) suggests the following regimens:

Recommended: Metronidazole, 500 mg PO 2 times a day for 7 days.

Alternative: Clindamycin, 300 mg PO 2 times a day for 7 days.

Chancroid

Chancroid is an ulcerative condition that usually occurs in the genital area. It was differentiated from syphilis around 1838.

The incidence of chancroid is increasing. In the early 1980s only 800 cases were reported each year; in 1987 more than 6,000 cases were reported. As with other viral infections, individuals with the human immunodeficiency virus (HIV) are also susceptible to bacterial infections such as tuberculosis.

PATHOPHYSIOLOGY

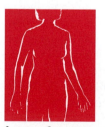

Chancroid is caused by *Haemophilus ducreyi*, a gram-negative, pleomorphic bacillus found in strands of mucus. Since chancres look similar, a painful chancroid may be confused with a painless syphilitic chancre. The incubation period for men is about 1 to 14 days; it is a little longer for women.

For a picture of Gram's stain showing *Haemophilus ducreyi*, see Color Plate 13, page xiii.

Chancroid symptoms include reddish groin areas; one or more irregularly shaped, painful genital ulcers; foul odor with puslike discharge from the ulcers; and edema near the sores. Chancroids typically have erosive, ragged, serpiginous (wavy) borders.

Chancroid complications include relapse, systemic spread, necrotic tissue, and fistulas. Secondary infections result.

NURSING CARE

See pages 155 to 157.

DIAGNOSTIC STUDIES AND FINDINGS

Diagnostic test	Findings
Culture or microscopic examination of exudate from bubo or lesions; tests to rule out other causes of ulcers, particularly syphilis and herpes	Isolation of *H. ducreyi* bacilli (may be difficult to differentiate from other organisms)
Enzyme-linked immunosorbent assay (ELISA)	Positive for *H. ducreyi* bacilli

---

MEDICAL MANAGEMENT

GENERAL MANAGEMENT

Treatment of bacterial STDs includes tracing and contacting sex partners so that they may be treated also.

DRUG THERAPY

Chancroid usually is treated with erythromycin or ceftriaxone. The Centers for Disease Control (CDC) suggests the following regimens:

Recommended: Erythromycin base, 500 mg PO 4 times a day for 7 days; *or* ceftriaxone, 250 mg IM in a single dose.

Alternatives: Trimethoprim/sulfamethoxazole, 160/800 mg (one double-strength tablet) PO 2 times a day for 7 days; *or* amoxicillin (500 mg) plus clavulanic acid (125 mg) PO 3 times a day for 7 days; *or* ciprofloxacin, 500 mg PO 2 times a day for 3 days.

Monilial Vaginitis

Monilial vaginitis (candidiasis) is referred to as a fungal, yeast, or candidal infection. It is caused by *Candida albicans*.

Candidiasis is more common with cancer, obesity, diabetes, immunologic disorders, pregnancy, and the use of hormonal contraceptives. However, approximately 75% of all women have a yeast infection sometime in their lives. Yeast infections are more common in tropical climates. Approximately 30% of women are asymptomatic.

DIAGNOSTIC STUDIES AND FINDINGS

Diagnostic test	Findings
Cultures	Presence of *Candida albicans*
Pap and gonococcal smear	To differentiate other pathology
Urinalysis	To rule out glycosuria and increased bacteria
Potassium hydroxide (KOH) prep	To detect hyphae and *C. albicans* spores and yeast branches and buds
Saline wet mount	To rule out trichomoniasis

PATHOPHYSIOLOGY

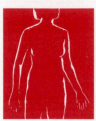

Vulvovaginal candidiasis is caused by *Candida albicans*, an organism that is part of the normal vaginal flora. These organisms prefer warm, moist environments, and overgrowth may occur in a variety of situations, such as with stress or systemic disease. Yeast infections are greatly exacerbated before menstruation and during pregnancy. The incubation period varies from 3 to 28 days.

Candidiasis produces a thick, cheesy discharge. Vaginal or genital burning and itching may be severe, and inflammation and scratch marks may be visible. However, women frequently are asymptomatic.

For a picture of Gram's stain showing vaginal candidiasis, see Color Plate 13, page xiii.

Candidiasis may cause secondary infections in internal or external genitalia through bacterial contamination. Thrush or oral infection may occur from oral-genital sex or neonatal exposure during birth. Immunocompromised individuals are at risk for monilial infections and the spread of candidal infection to the central nervous system, lungs, heart, joints, and other body areas.

NURSING CARE

See pages 155 and 157.

MEDICAL MANAGEMENT

DRUG THERAPY

Antifungal products (e.g., miconazole, nystatin) are used. The Centers for Disease Control (CDC) suggests the following regimens:

Recommended: Miconazole nitrate vaginal suppository, 200 mg at bedtime for 3 days; *or* clotrimazole vaginal tablets, 200 mg at bedtime for 3 days; *or* butoconazole 2% cream, 5 g intravaginally at bedtime for 3 days; *or* terconazole, 80 mg suppository or 0.4% cream intravaginally at bedtime for 3 days.

Alternatives: Miconazole nitrate vaginal suppository, 100 mg, or 2% cream, 5 g at bedtime for 7 days; *or* clotrimazole vaginal tablets (100 mg) *or* clotrimazole 1% cream, 5 g at bedtime for 7 days.

Trichomoniasis

Trichomoniasis is a vaginal inflammation that may involve the labia and vulva. It is caused by *Trichomonas* organisms, which are one-celled, flagellated protozoa.

Trichomoniasis is most common in women 16 to 35 years of age, with a higher incidence in pregnant women. Other less common protozoal infections also may result from sexual contact. For example, the protozoal diseases amebic dysentery and giardiasis are more common in individuals who practice anal sex.

PATHOPHYSIOLOGY

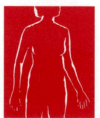

Trichomoniasis usually is caused by sexual activity (Figure 9-3). It may also be contracted by swimming in contaminated water, sitting in hot tubs, or using contaminated towels, and the infection may extend to the urogenital region. The incubation period varies from 3 to 28 days. Trichomoniasis is exacerbated during and after menstruation.

Trichomoniasis produces a frothy or bubbly, heavy, greenish-gray discharge. The genitalia may be red with scratch marks and/or edema, and vaginal bleeding may be present. Itching and burning are intense, but 25% of women may be asymptomatic.

Trichomoniasis may predispose women to other infections, and neonates may acquire trichomoniasis from maternal exposure.

NURSING CARE

See pages 155 to 157.

For a picture of a wet mount showing vaginal trichomoniasis, see Color Plate 15, page xiii.

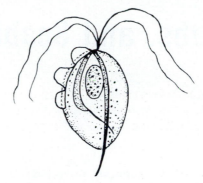

FIGURE 9-3
Trichomonas vaginalis: note the characteristic flagella and the undulating membrane. (From Baron and Finegold.[8a])

VULVOVAGINITIS

Vulvovaginitis is an inflammation of the mucous membranes of the vagina and vulva. Superficial tissue is irritated, and a purulent exudate usually is present. Vulvovaginitis is similar to bacterial vaginosis or nonspecific vaginitis; these are all terms describing an inflammatory process. Various combinations of organisms may cause these symptoms. The agents most responsible for vulvovaginitis are *Trichomonas vaginalis* (protozoan), *Candida albicans* (yeast or fungus), and *Gardnerella* (bacteria). Ectoparasites (pinworms and lice) and allergies may also cause vulvovaginitis. As with pelvic inflammatory disease (PID), vulvovaginitis may or may not be caused by a sexually transmitted organism.

DIAGNOSTIC STUDIES AND FINDINGS

Diagnostic test	Findings
Pap smear; urine, discharge specimens	Staining; microscopic examination to detect *Trichomonas* organisms
Wet smear with normal saline	Presence of mobile trichomonads or moving protozoa
Potassium hydroxide (KOH) smear	To rule out *Candida* organisms
Urinalysis	To rule out bacteria

MEDICAL MANAGEMENT

DRUG THERAPY

Trichomoniasis usually is treated with metronidazole. The Centers for Disease Control (CDC) suggest the following regimens:

Recommended: Metronidazole, 2 g PO in a single dose.

Alternative: Metronidazole, 500 mg 2 times a day for 7 days.

Lice, Crabs, and Scabies

Parasitic infections usually involve louse or nit (louse egg) infestations of pubic areas. Common parasitic infections are caused by *Pediculus pubis (Pthirus pubis)* and *Sarcoptes scabiei.*

The itch mite (scabies) first appears in records in 1687, which may be the first example of the discovery of a known cause for human disease. Scabies and pthiriasis outbreaks occur in crowded or poor hygienic living conditions, as well as through sexual contact. Crab lice appear most often in the 15 to 19 age group, and more often in women than men.

PATHOPHYSIOLOGY

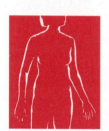 An *ectoparasitic infection* is caused by mites that burrow into the skin. Scabies is caused by a number of *hominis* parasites. The incubation period for scabies is 4 to 6 weeks (Figure 9-4). *Pthiriasis (Pthirus pubis* or crab louse) are lice parasites that infest the eyes, genitals, and armpits. The incubation period for crabs is 4 to 5 weeks.

Scabies produces irregular skin marks and burrows, usually on the breasts or abdomen or in the genital area. Intense itching that worsens at night is typical. Blisters near the end of burrows may be visible. Crabs

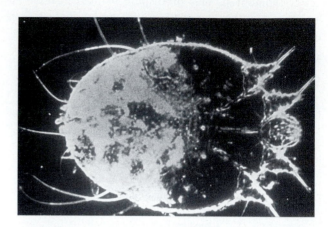

FIGURE 9-4
Photomicrograph of scabies mite. (Courtesy of the Centers for Disease Control.[21])

manifest as sky-blue marks on the genitals, thighs, and/or torso. Scratch marks may appear over infested areas.

Ectoparasitic infections may facilitate other bacterial infections as a result of scratching and general skin breakdown.

NURSING CARE

See pages 155 to 157.

MEDICAL MANAGEMENT

GENERAL MANAGEMENT

All clothing, bedding, and towels used during the infestation period must be laundered or dry cleaned.

DRUG THERAPY

Miticides or scabicides (e.g., Nix, Rid, Kwell) are used to treat infestations. The Centers for Disease Control (CDC) suggests the following regimens:

Ectoparasitic pediculosis pubis

Permethrin 1% creme rinse, applied to affected area and washed off after 10 minutes; *or* pyrethrins and piperonyl butoxide, applied to the affected area and washed off after 10 minutes; *or* lindane 1% shampoo, applied for 4 minutes and then thoroughly washed off (not to be used for pregnant or lactating women).

Scabies

Recommended: Lindane 1%, 1 ounce of lotion or 30 g of cream applied thinly to all areas of the body from neck down and washed off thoroughly after 8 hours (not to be used for pregnant or lactating women).

Alternative: Crotamiton 10%, applied to entire body from neck down for 2 nights and washed off thoroughly 24 hours after the second application.

Inflammation Unrelated to STDs

Toxic shock syndrome (TSS) usually is caused by *Staphylococcus aureus* and results in an acute bacterial infection. The use of tampons is associated with this syndrome. **Urinary tract infections (UTIs)** and **pelvic inflammatory disease (PID)** may or may not be related to sexual activity.

Toxic shock syndrome develops in 1 of every 20,000 women who menstruate, although this rate may be falling since the removal of some tampons from the market. TSS also has occurred in some individuals after surgery. Pelvic inflammatory disease and urinary tract infection often are associated with factors other than sexual activity, such as underlying immunologic or kidney problems or structural disorders (prolapse).

PATHOPHYSIOLOGY

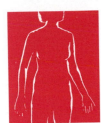

Staphylococcus aureus may grow more rapidly in the body when blood-soaked material is present, such as tampons, nasal packing, or surgical dressings. TSS seems to occur with breakdown of the skin and/or mucous membrane. The incubation period for TSS varies, but it usually develops within 7 days and usually during menses. Urinary tract infections (UTIs) may be caused by a number of pathogens such as *Escherichia coli*, *Staphylococcus saprophyticus*, group B streptococci, and *Klebsiella* organisms.

Symptoms of TSS include sudden high fever, vomiting, diarrhea, head and throat pain, dizziness, malaise, edema in the extremities, muscle cramps, and skin rash with desquamation (peeling). Nonpurulent inflammation of the conjunctivae and hyperemia of the oropharynx and/or vagina may occur.

Symptoms of UTI include dysuria, urgency, frequency, and suprapubic pain. Fever, chills, nausea, vomiting, and genital discharge may also develop.

OTHER SEXUALLY TRANSMITTED INFECTIONS

The number of infections transmitted by sexual contact exceeds the list of "common" STDs. For example, the mononucleosis and Epstein-Barr viruses may be spread by kissing. Cytomegalovirus (CMV) may be contracted by sexual activity. *CMV* may cause jaundice, swollen lymph nodes, fever, headaches, malaise, and muscle pain. Like most sexually transmitted diseases, CMV is particularly dangerous if spread from a woman to her newborn baby. *Retroviruses* cause several kinds of cancers and are also associated with the human immunodeficiency virus (HIV) and human T-cell lymphotropic virus (HTLV-II). As with most viral infections, there is virtually no treatment, or treatment focuses on relieving symptoms.

Less common bacterial infections can also arise. *Granuloma inguinale*, for example, is more common outside the United States. The symptoms are single or multiple painless, beefy, red, coarse sores that have a strong, sour odor. Granuloma inguinale may cause narrowing, scarring, and swelling of the vagina, and the sores may spread to other areas such as the throat, face, and chest. Granuloma inguinale is treated with antibiotics.

The symptoms of TSS may progress to life-threatening disorders. The woman may experience loss of consciousness, disorientation, hypotension, and impaired renal function. UTI left untreated may result in renal disorders such as pyelonephritis.

DIAGNOSTIC STUDIES AND FINDINGS

Diagnostic test	Findings
Physical examination	Physical examination findings of fever, genital discharge, and possible shock.
Toxic shock syndrome	
White blood cell count (WBC)	Increased
Blood urea nitrogen (BUN), creatinine, bilirubin	Increased
Enzyme studies: serum glutamic oxaloacetic transaminase (SGOT) and serum pyruvic transaminase (SGPT), creatinine phosphokinase (CPK)	Increased
Platelets	Decreased
Urinary tract infection	
Complete blood count (CBC) with differential	Elevated WBC; left shift of polys to bands
Urine analysis (UA) with Gram's stain	Pathogen group identified greater than or equal to 1 to 2 bacteria per unspun specimen

MEDICAL MANAGEMENT

DRUG THERAPY

TSS

Medical management of TSS includes antiinfective agents such as cefoxitin, cefazolin, penicillin-resistant agents, antistaphylococcal agents, and corticosteroids.

UTI

Treatment for UTI may be aimed at correcting cystitis or the source of infection. Prophylaxis against recurrent UTI may be needed with medications such as Septra or Macrodantin.

PID

Treatment for PID may differ, according to the causative organism. The Centers for Disease Control (CDC) suggests the following regimens:

Cefoxitin, 2 g IM plus probenecid, 1 g PO concurrently; *or* ceftriaxone, 250 mg IM, or equivalent cephalosporin; *or* erythromycin, 500 mg PO 4 times a day for 10-14 days (to substitute for doxycycline/tetracycline) **plus** Doxycycline, 100 mg PO 2 times a day for 10-14 days; *or* tetracycline, 500 mg PO 4 times a day for 10-14 days.

1 ASSESS*

	OBSERVATIONS			
ASSESSMENT	VIRUSES (AIDS, HEPATITIS, HERPES, MCV)	BACTERIA (GONORRHEA, CHLAMYDIA, SYPHILIS, CHANCROID)	FUNGI/YEASTS, PROTOZOA, ECTOPARASITES	INFLAMMATION UNRELATED TO STD
History	Sexual activity without protection (oral, rectal, genital); multiple partners or known viral transmission; previous STD	Sexual activity without protection (oral, rectal, genital); multiple partners or known bacterial transmission; previous STD	Sexual activity without protection (oral, rectal, genital); multiple partners or known transmission of infection; previous STD	Use of IUD or tampons; pregnancy and childbearing data; predisposition to UTI
Typical symptoms	Lesions or crusts; *MCV:* cyst-shaped papules, complains of burning, pruritus; fever, chills, headaches, malaise, joint pain, urinary tract or abdominal discomfort	*GC:* urinary tract or rectal discomfort (women may be asymptomatic with GC and chlamydial infections); *syphilis:* single, painless papule with enlarged inguinal lymph nodes; *chancroid:* painful lesion; elongated lesions with warts; *trichomoniasis:* odor, frothy yellow-green vaginal discharge	*Candidiasis:* vaginal and labial irritation, severe itching; *protozoa and ectoparasites:* rashlike skin irritation and pruritus; *mites:* possible red blister–type reaction	*Staphylococcal infections and TTS:* fever, rash, genital edema, inflamed vagina; *UTI:* dysuria, urgency, frequency, back pain, fever symptoms; *PID:* elevated WBC and ESR, pelvic or back pain
Psychosocial	Anxiety associated with STD or gynecologic infection, knowledge deficit, and/or self-concept disturbance.			

*Nursing care should be well documented in the patient's permanent health care record.

2 DIAGNOSE

NURSING DIAGNOSIS	SUBJECTIVE FINDINGS	OBJECTIVE FINDINGS
Knowledge deficit related to cause, treatment, and prevention of STDs and non-STD infections	Reports previous infection; lacks correct information about condition	Diagnosis of STD or non-STD infection; history of STD
High risk for infection related to inflammatory processes such as impaired skin and organ integrity	Reports persistent or worsening symptoms such as fever and severe back or pelvic pain	Fever, signs of advanced infection (e.g., large area of mite or wart infestation), skin breakdown; signs of systemic complication (e.g., elevated WBC and vital signs, nonclotting blood); abscesses or purulent exudate
Pain (discomfort) related to infection	Describes symptoms of burning, itching, pain, or interruption of daily activities	Inflamed areas, edema, discharge, lesions
High risk for sexual dysfunction related to fear of infection	Reports sexual difficulties, changes in activities, or inability to achieve a satisfactory relationship	Withdrawn; little or no eye contact; physical signs of infection that may alter body image

› › ›

3 PLAN

Patient goals

1. The patient will understand the cause of her condition and how to prevent further infection; the patient and her partner or partners will be free of infection.
2. The patient's infection will resolve or be brought under control without complications.
3. The patient will have no pain or discomfort.
4. The patient will have a healthy sexual relationship, and patients with viral infections (e.g., herpes, AIDS) will understand the potential for transmitting the disease.

4 IMPLEMENT

NURSING DIAGNOSIS	NURSING INTERVENTIONS	RATIONALE
Knowledge deficit related to cause, treatment, and prevention of STDs and non-STD infections	Discuss transmission, treatment, and prevention of infection; provide teaching materials concerning treatment and ways to minimize risks (e.g., contraceptive barriers, preventing renal infections).	To provide information that will help patient and partner to prevent infections and/or practice safe sex.
	Refer to health care specialists as needed for treatment of viral symptoms.	To provide support for individuals with viral infections that cannot be eliminated.
High risk for infection related to inflammatory processes such as impaired skin and organ integrity	Discuss importance of treatment regimen and follow-up care; monitor vital signs, laboratory test results; assist patient in observing for signs of worsening condition or systemic complication.	To promote healing and prevent infection.
Pain (discomfort) related to infection	Help patient minimize discomfort with prescribed treatment; reassure patient that most symptoms will subside.	To promote comfort.
High risk for sexual dysfunction related to fear of infection	Encourage patient and partner to express their feelings.	To promote problem solving and recognition of risk factors for infection.

5 EVALUATE

PATIENT OUTCOME	DATA INDICATING THAT OUTCOME IS REACHED
Patient and partner understand the cause, treatment, and prevention of infection.	Patient and partner can describe how infection occurred, treatment options, and methods for minimizing future infection.
Infection has resolved or been brought under control, and inflammatory and immunologic risks have been minimized.	Cultures are negative; there are no physical signs of inflammation such as edema, redness, or discharge; laboratory results are within normal range.

PATIENT OUTCOME	DATA INDICATING THAT OUTCOME IS REACHED
Patient has no pain or discomfort.	Patient shows no signs of irritation and reports she is free of pain.
Patient and partner experience sexual satisfaction, and/or patient accepts need for safe sex or abstinence to reduce risk of transmitting the disease.	Patient reports resolution of feelings of sexual dysfunction.

PATIENT TEACHING

General guidelines

1. Review the patient's health and sexual history to identify treatment needs and the risk of reinfection.
2. Discuss the reasons for completing all treatment protocols.
3. Encourage the patient to ask questions about sexual health, and provide information about sexually transmitted diseases and ways of practicing safe sex, such as abstinence or using condoms.

Viruses

1. Assess the impact of the viral infection on the patient and family; discuss the patient's life-style and risk behaviors, and refer for counseling as needed.
2. If the patient has herpes or HIV, provide information about the risks and management of pregnancy with these infections.
3. Explain the need for sex partners to be tested and treated.
4. Describe the treatment plans and the need for follow-up with molluscum and condyloma infections; discuss the importance of a Pap smear for all women with anogenital warts.

Bacteria

1. Describe the use of antibacterial agents to treat infection.
2. Explain the importance of full treatment and why complications occur from untreated bacterial infections such as gonorrhea and syphilis; assist with appropriate prenatal screening as indicated.
3. Discuss why sexual activity should be limited until the treatment regimen has been completed.

4. Describe why good hygiene practices are important, especially keeping genital secretions away from the face and eyes.

Fungi, yeast, protozoa, ectoparasites

1. Teach the patient good hygiene practices, such as wiping from front (mons) to back after urinating or defecating.
2. Discuss ways to decrease moisture or irritation in the genital area, such as wearing cotton underwear and avoiding the use of sprays, deodorants, or other chemicals in that area.
3. Help the patient and family devise ways to minimize chances of recontamination.

Infections unrelated to STDs

1. Describe methods for reducing the risk of infection, such as using tampons properly, or using sanitary pads instead; if recommended, avoiding douching or baths (if showers are recommended), or using an alternative means of contraception (if IUD is removed).
2. Explain the drug regimen for the patient's condition, especially the need to take all prescribed medications regularly.
3. Discuss ways to prevent infection; for example, preventive measures for urinary tract infections include adequate fluids, proper emptying of the bladder, appropriate diet, exercise, and rest.
4. Help the patient determine her treatment options and ways to minimize the risk of reinfection, such as using estrogen if indicated.

CHAPTER 10

Systemic Disorders Affecting Women

A number of disorders affect women more often than men. Certain endocrine, autoimmune, cerebrovascular, cardiovascular, and gastrointestinal disorders, for example, are predominately found in women. Hormonal shifts may place some women at risk for systemic complications, especially when combined with other factors such as smoking or use of oral contraceptives.

Cardiovascular Disease

Cardiovascular diseases may affect women in ways not previously studied. Since 1910 more women in the United States have died of heart disease than of any other disorder. For most of this century, physicians and researchers treated heart disease as a man's problem. When the American Heart Association held its first public conference for women in 1964, it focused on how women could help protect their husband's hearts. Women are more likely than men to die soon after a heart attack; if they survive, they are more likely to have a second heart attack later on, and are more apt to be sidelined by pain and disability.

Coronary heart disease is the number one killer of American women. Of the 540,000 Americans who die each year of this disease, nearly half (250,000) are women. The death rate for coronary heart disease is 19% higher for black women than for white women.

The three major risk factors for cardiovascular disease are high blood pressure, cigarette smoking, and high serum cholesterol and lipid levels. Other risk factors are diabetes, obesity, and physical inactivity. After menopause women are more vulnerable to cardiovascular disease. Women who have had early natural or surgically induced menopause have twice the risk of developing coronary heart disease as do women of the same age who have not entered menopause.

Nearly 58 million Americans have hypertension, and half of them are women. More than half of women over age 55 have hypertension. High blood pressure is common in black women and often more serious than it is in white women. Approximately 25 million American women smoke cigarettes. Although the percentage of women and girls who smoke has declined (from 34% in 1965 to 28% in 1985), those who do smoke are likely to begin at an earlier age and to smoke more heavily than in the past. Among teenagers 17 to 19 years of age, more girls than boys smoke, for the first time in history.

PATHOPHYSIOLOGY

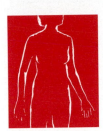

Women who smoke are two to six times as likely to suffer a heart attack as nonsmoking women, and the risk increases with the number of cigarettes smoked per day. Although women have a lower rate of coronary artery disease than men, if a woman smokes heavily, her risk is the same as a man's. Women who smoke heavily tend to reach menopause earlier, which further increases their risk of coronary artery disease.

Women who smoke and have high blood pressure and high serum cholesterol and lipid levels have eight times the risk of developing coronary artery disease than do nonsmoking women with normal blood pressure and serum cholesterol and lipid levels. Women who smoke and also take birth control pills are at especially high risk for cardiovascular disease. Women smokers who use oral contraceptives are about 39 times more likely to have a heart attack than women who neither smoke nor use birth control pills. Low-tar and low-nicotine cigarettes do not lessen the risk of cardiovascular disease, although the risk rapidly declines if the individual stops smoking.

CLINICAL MANIFESTATIONS

A major symptom of cardiac disease is high blood pressure, or hypertension. Birth control pills contribute to hypertension in some women. Hypertension cannot be cured, but it can usually be controlled through antihypertensive medications, a low-sodium diet, regular exercise, and avoiding alcohol.

Women tend to have lower cholesterol levels than men until age 45, at which time their levels exceed those of men. More than one third of American women have elevated cholesterol levels (over 200 mg/dl). The risk of coronary heart disease increases as the cholesterol level rises. Over a period of years, cholesterol plaques deposit on the walls of the coronary arteries and decrease blood supply to the heart muscle. Serum cholesterol levels can be reduced by 10% to 15% with a low-cholesterol diet and cholesterol-lowering drugs.

The classic warning sign of coronary artery disease is chest pain. It can occur as angina (a severe, constricting pain) or myocardial infarction (heart attack). The pain of angina is the result of an imbalance between supply and demand in the coronary blood flow. Anginal pain reflects myocardial ischemia, whereas a heart attack is actual necrosis of the myocardium. Many heart attacks are the result of thrombus formation in the area of coronary artery plaques.

COMPLICATIONS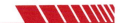

Complications of coronary artery disease include sudden death, cardiac dysrhythmias (ventricular tachycardia or fibrillation), congestive heart failure, and cardiogenic shock.

DIAGNOSTIC STUDIES AND FINDINGS

Diagnostic test	Findings
Electrocardiogram (ECG)	Ischemia appears as elevated ST and then T wave inversion; injury appears as ST elevation; necrosis appears as Q wave or persistent ST wave increase
Right and left coronary angiography (cardiac catheterization)	Decreased perfusion indicates narrowing or occlusion of coronary artery; ejection fraction (EF) is computed to determine heart's pumping ability
Cardiac enzymes: creatine phosphokinase (CPK), lactate dehydrogenase (LDH), and serum glutamate oxaloacetate transaminase (SGOT)	Elevated with cardiac damage
Stress testing (ECG during exercise)	Evaluates cardiovascular response to progressive graded workload
Scintigraphic myocardial imaging	Identifies myocardial infarction and perfusion

MEDICAL MANAGEMENT

Medical therapy is aimed at reducing myocardial oxygen demand. The precipitating factors that bring on an attack of angina are identified and avoided. Risk factors are identified and corrected.

DRUG THERAPY

Drug therapy consists of vasodilators (nitrates), beta-adrenergic blocking agents, and calcium channel blockers.

SURGERY

Surgical intervention does not alter the atherosclerotic process. It does decrease anginal pain and improve the myocardial blood supply.

A coronary artery bypass graft (CABG) improves myocardial blood flow through the use of saphenous vein or internal mammary artery bypass grafts, which detour around the blocked coronary artery. Anywhere from one to four coronary arteries may be grafted. Women who have coronary artery bypass surgery are less likely than men to survive the procedure.

Percutaneous transluminal coronary angioplasty (PTCA) is an alternative to coronary bypass surgery for single-vessel coronary disease. A balloon-tipped catheter is inserted under fluoroscopy and advanced to the area of the coronary obstruction. The balloon is inflated to compress the plaque, widening the clogged coronary artery, and then removed. About 5% to 10% of patients who undergo PTCA have subsequent coronary occlusion, coronary collapse, or coronary spasm. Preparations are made for emergency bypass surgery during all PTCA procedures.

1 ASSESS*

ASSESSMENT	OBSERVATIONS
Chest pain	Location and radiation to other sites; severity of pain on a scale of 1 to 10; quality of pain (squeezing, pressure, or heaviness); onset; duration; precipitating and relieving factors; associated factors, such as diaphoresis, cool skin
Vital signs	Increased B/P caused by anxiety; decreased B/P resulting from cardiogenic shock; increased heart rate resulting from congestive heart failure (CHF); decreased heart rate as a result of dysrhythmias (bradycardia or complete heart block); mild temperature elevation caused by inflammation response to myocardial infarction

*Nursing care should be well documented in the patient's permanent health care record.

2 DIAGNOSE

NURSING DIAGNOSIS	SUBJECTIVE FINDINGS	OBJECTIVE FINDINGS
Pain (acute) related to coronary occlusion	Complains of crushing or squeezing chest pain	Anxiety, pallor, muscle tightness
Anxiety related to threat of death	Expresses fear of dying	Fearful, restless

NURSING DIAGNOSIS	SUBJECTIVE FINDINGS	OBJECTIVE FINDINGS
Altered tissue perfusion related to cardiovascular insufficiency	Reports history of hypertension or angina	Increased B/P

3   PLAN

Patient goals

1. The patient's chest pain will be relieved within 1 hour of arrival at the hospital.
2. The patient will be able to identify factors that increase cardiac workload.
3. The patient will use effective coping mechanisms to decrease anxiety.
4. The patient will understand both the risk factors for cardiac disease and how she must change her lifestyle to reduce those risks.

4   IMPLEMENT

NURSING DIAGNOSIS	NURSING INTERVENTIONS	RATIONALE
Pain (acute) related to coronary occlusion	Assess and document onset, location, and duration of pain.	Medication can be administered to improve cardiac blood flow.
Anxiety related to threat of death	Assess existing coping mechanisms.	Coping with a life-threatening illness can cause feelings of fear, anger, or depression.
Altered tissue perfusion related to cardiovascular insufficiency	Assess and document history of angina and/or hypertension.	Risk factors for cardiovascular disease must be identified.

5   EVALUATE

PATIENT OUTCOME	DATA INDICATING THAT OUTCOME IS REACHED
Patient has no more chest pain.	Myocardial perfusion has been restored.
Patient understands what causes increased cardiac workload.	Patient can describe the factors that increase cardiac workload.
Patient's anxiety has decreased, and she is able to cope effectively.	Patient reports and exhibits effective coping, as evidenced by positive statements.

➜ ❯ ❯

PATIENT OUTCOME	DATA INDICATING THAT OUTCOME IS REACHED
Patient understands risk factors associated with cardiac disease and necessary medical treatment.	Patient can describe the development of cardiovascular disease and the risk factors leading to it; her medication regimen; the rationale for any surgical intervention planned; the need for continued medical follow-up; and life-style changes that will be necessary.

PATIENT TEACHING

1. Review the pathophysiology and treatment associated with cardiac disease.
2. Help the patient and family develop life-style goals that will minimize cardiac problems and promote optimum cardiac function.
3. Refer the patient to rehabilitation and nutritional counselors as needed.

Mitral Stenosis and Mitral Valve Prolapse

Mitral stenosis is a fibrotic thickening and fusion of valve commissures with adhesions and scarring, resulting primarily from rheumatic fever. **Mitral valve prolapse** is the superior systolic displacement of the mitral leaflets.

Mitral stenosis is the most common disease of the mitral valve, and two thirds of all individuals with mitral stenosis are women. Mitral valve prolapse occurs in both sexes and in people of all ages, although it is detected most frequently in women under age 40.

PATHOPHYSIOLOGY

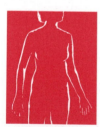

Rheumatic fever can cause thickening of the mitral valve, leading to fibrosis and immobility of the valve. Hypertrophy of the left atrium develops as a compensatory mechanism, since additional force is needed to pass blood through the narrowed valve. Pulmonary hypertension develops as a result of left atrial (LA) enlargement, causing right-sided heart failure and a decrease in cardiac output (CO). Mitral valve prolapse (MVP) is an excessive valvuloventricular disproportion. MVP is

characterized by a connective tissue abnormality of the mitral leaflets, annulus, and chordae tendineae (Figure 10-1).

CLINICAL MANIFESTATIONS

A latency period of about 20 years separates the onset of rheumatic fever and the development of mitral stenosis. The main patient complaint is dyspnea, which results from pulmonary hypertension. Other symptoms include easy fatigability, chest pain, jugular venous distention, and right upper quadrant pain from liver congestion. The symptoms may be preceded by emotional stress, respiratory infection, sexual intercourse, or atrial fibrillation with rapid ventricular response.

The clinical manifestations of MVP depend on the amount of leaflet prolapse in the atrium and whether mitral regurgitation results.

COMPLICATIONS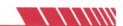

Complications may include ineffective endocarditis, embolism, pulmonary edema, left ventricular (LV) and right ventricular (RV) failure, or ruptured papillary muscles of the chordae tendineae.

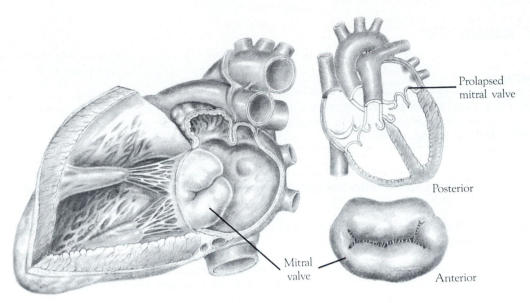

Prolapsed
mitral valve

Posterior

Mitral
valve

Anterior

FIGURE 10-1
Mitral valve prolapse. (From Canobbio.[20])

DIAGNOSTIC STUDIES AND FINDINGS

Diagnostic test	Findings	
	Mitral stenosis	**Mitral valve prolapse**
Electrocardiogram (ECG)	LA enlargement; notched P wave (P mitrale); RV hypertrophy	Normal; may show ST segment and T-wave abnormalities, especially in inferior leads or prominent ∩ waves; dysrhythmias, supraventricular tachyrhythmias, premature atrial or ventricular beats
Chest x-ray	LA and RV enlargement; pulmonary venous congestion; interstitial pulmonary edema	Identifies or confirms presence of skeletal abnormalities
Echocardiogram	Decreased excursion of leaflets; diminished E to F slope	2-D records mild to moderate superior systolic displacement of posterior and/or both mitral leaflets and the coaptation of point of the cusps; records atrial size, chordal rupture; Doppler records degree of mitral regurgitation
Radionuclide studies	To determine resting and exercise ejection fraction (EF)	To determine resting and exercise EF
Cardiac catheterization	Pressure across mitral valve increased; LA pressure increased; increased pulmonary capillary wedge pressure (PCWP); low CO	Normal unless mitral regurgitation present; LV angiogram shows the prolapsed mitral valve

(From Canobbio[20].)

MEDICAL MANAGEMENT

DRUG THERAPY

Pulmonary congestion is treated with diuretics and sodium restriction. Pulmonary hypertension is treated with bed rest in the high Fowler's position. Atrial fibrillation is treated with synchronized cardioversion, digitalis, quinidine, and anticoagulants.

SURGERY

Surgery is indicated for individuals who face activity restrictions despite medical treatment. The following are possible procedures.

Mitral commissurotomy is the incision of the stenotic valve leaflets at their borders. The commissurotomy may be closed or open; the mortality rate is 2%.

Open mitral commissurotomy is performed through a median sternotomy or right anterolateral thoracotomy incision. Cardiopulmonary bypass is used. An incision is made into the left atrium, the mitral valve is inspected, and any atrial thrombi are removed. The valve leaflets are incised and attached to the chordae tendineae.

Closed mitral commissurotomy is done without cardiac bypass through a left posterolateral thoracotomy approach. The fifth rib is removed, and the atrium is palpated for thrombi. If a thrombus is found, the procedure is converted to an open commissurotomy approach. If no thrombus is present, the surgeon inserts a finger into the valve and then uses a dilator to open the valve and relieve the stenosis.

Mitral valve replacement is considered when a valve is too diseased and calcified to be repaired through a commissurotomy. The incision is through a median sternotomy approach, and cardiac bypass is used. The diseased valve is excised, and the artificial valve is sutured to the annulus. The mortality rate for mitral valve replacement is 10%.

1 ASSESS*

ASSESSMENT	OBSERVATIONS
Dyspnea	Dyspnea on exertion, paroxysmal nocturnal dyspnea, orthopnea (these are due to pulmonary hypertension)
Dry cough	Dysphagia, hoarseness (due to bronchial irritation from left atrial enlargement)
Fatigue	Weakness (due to decreased cardiac output)
Diastolic murmur	Auscultation of opening snap (due to forceful opening of mitral valve)

*Nursing care should be well documented in the patient's permanent health record.

2 DIAGNOSE

NURSING DIAGNOSIS	SUBJECTIVE FINDINGS	OBJECTIVE FINDINGS
Decreased cardiac output related to impaired coronary blood flow	Complains of fatigue and weakness	Decreased B/P and cardiac output
Ineffective breathing pattern related to decreased cardiac output	Complains of shortness of breath	Tachypnea, adventitious breath sounds
Anxiety related to threat to health status	Complains of feeling anxious and powerless	Talks about threat to health status

3 PLAN

Patient goals
1. The patient's cardiac output will improve.
2. The patient's breathing pattern will improve.

3. The patient will practice effective coping skills.

4 IMPLEMENT

NURSING DIAGNOSIS	NURSING INTERVENTIONS	RATIONALE
Decreased cardiac output related to impaired coronary blood flow	Assess vital signs q 2 h and prn; intake and output; daily weight measurements.	Decrease in B/P reflects a decreased cardiac output; increase in weight reflects fluid retention from deteriorating cardiac output and impending heart failure
Ineffective breathing pattern related to decreased cardiac output	Monitor respiratory rate and rhythm q 2 h and prn.	Pulmonary hypertension causes changes in the respiratory status, such as dyspnea, loss of lung volume, and increased risk of pneumonia.
Anxiety related to threat to health status	Assess coping mechanisms.	Coping with a life-threatening illness can lead to feelings of fear, anger, or depression.

5 EVALUATE

PATIENT OUTCOME	DATA INDICATING THAT OUTCOME IS REACHED
Patient's cardiac output has improved.	Patient has fewer complaints of fatigue; weight is stable.

→ > >

PATIENT OUTCOME	DATA INDICATING THAT OUTCOME IS REACHED
Patient's breathing pattern has improved.	Patient does not complain of dyspnea.
Patient's anxiety has been alleviated.	Patient exhibits effective coping mechanisms.

PATIENT TEACHING

1. Assess the patient's current knowledge about her condition, and discuss the cause and treatment; discuss contraception and pregnancy issues as appropriate.
2. Have the patient and family repeat the warning signs that require medical intervention.
3. Explain the purpose of antibiotic prophylaxis and ways to prevent infectious endocarditis.
4. Help the patient and family plan a life-style that includes good nutrition, rest, hygiene, dental care, and modified activity.

Migraine Headaches

Migraine headaches comprise a complex symptomatology of severe head pain associated with vertigo, nausea, vomiting, and photophobia. The discomfort often is unilateral, and the headaches recur at random.

Approximately 30 million individuals in the United States seek health care for recurring headaches. *Migraine headaches* are classified as vascular headaches that generally begin in childhood, adolescence, or early adulthood. Approximately 5% of the general population experience migraines.

PATHOPHYSIOLOGY

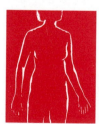

Cephalalgia (headache) is head discomfort resulting from stimulation of pain-sensitive areas in the cranium and/or extracranial tissues. Pain may also occur in the neck and face. The exact pathophysiology of a migraine headache is unknown. It is known that intracranial and extracranial arteries constrict and then dilate several minutes later. The vasoconstriction causes the aura characteristic of a classic migraine, and the vasodilation produces the headache.

Young women are the most susceptible to migraine headaches, especially before or during their menstrual period. Head pain may also be caused by chemical irritation from cosmetic products.

Circumstances and agents thought to bring on migraine headaches include emotional stress, menstruation, too much or too little sleep, and dietary ingredients such as tyramine, nitrate, and glutamate.

CLINICAL MANIFESTATIONS

A migraine headache is characterized by throbbing, unilateral head pain associated with nausea and vomiting. Symptoms of headaches vary according to the cause and type of headache (Table 10-1).

COMPLICATIONS

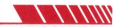

The complications of headaches are chronic pain and depression. Activities of daily living may be interrupted, and accidents may result from distraction caused by the pain.

Table 10-1

CLINICAL MANIFESTATIONS OF HEADACHES

Type	Pain	Location	Onset	Duration	Other
Classic migraine	Throbbing, high intensity	Usually unilateral in temporal area but may occur in any area of the head	Hours	Hours to days	Prodrome/aura: visual disturbances, sensory symptoms, mild paresis, nausea, vomiting
Common migraine	Throbbing intense pain; progresses to generalized nonthrobbing pain	Usually frontal or temporal region	Gradual	Hours to days	No aura; nausea; vomiting
Cluster	Sudden, usually awaking patient at night	Orbitotemporal area, usually unilateral	Sudden	½ to 1 hour; occur in clusters	No prodrome; lacrimation; rhinorrhea; nasal congestion; flushing of face; Horner's sign
Muscle contraction	Aching, tightness, or pressure	Suboccipital, occipital, frontal, temporal, parietal	Gradual	Hours to days (variable)	Muscle tension
Traumatic headaches	Dull, generalized pain	Varies	Gradual	Varies	Intensified by physical exertion; lack of concentration; dizziness
Traction headaches	Deep, dull, steady ache	Varies	Varies	Varies	Varies
Temporal arteritis	Variable intensity; unilateral or bilateral tenderness of painful area	Temporal occipital, frontooccipital areas	Gradual	Hours to days	Visual loss

(From Chipps.[23])

DIAGNOSTIC STUDIES AND FINDINGS

Diagnostic test	Findings
Neurologic history and examination	Identifies precipitating influences, effect on activities of daily living, and neurologic deficits
Cervical and skull x-rays	Detects brain abnormalities
Provocative histamine test	Positive test indicates a vascular component to headache
Cerebral angiogram	Detects vascular abnormality
Computed tomography (CT) and magnetic resonance imaging (MRI) scans	Detect intracranial lesions

MEDICAL MANAGEMENT

GENERAL MANAGEMENT

Nutrition: Diet counseling to eliminate foods that may provoke headaches (vinegar, chocolate, pork, onions, sour cream, alcohol, caffeine, citrus fruits, bananas, yogurt, figs, cheese, lunch meats, chicken livers, broad bean pods, marinated foods, avocados, monosodium glutamate [MSG]).

Application of heat and cold to the affected area.

Counseling: Behavioral modification, stress reduction, and biofeedback.

DRUG THERAPY

Drug therapy for migraine headaches is used for prophylactic treatment (Table 10-2), symptomatic treatment (Table 10-3), or both.

Table 10-2

PROPHYLACTIC MEDICATIONS FOR MIGRAINE HEADACHES

Medication	Dosage
Beta blockers	
Propranolol (Inderal)	40 mg tid-qid
Methysergide maleate (Sansert)	2 mg tid with meals
Tricyclic antidepressants	
Amitriptyline (Elavil)	10-100 mg qhs
Imipramine (Tofranil)	10-75 mg in divided doses
Desipramine (Norpramin)	25-75 mg in divided doses
Nonsteroidal antiinflammatory agents	
Naproxen (Anaprox)	550 mg bid with meals
Calcium channel blockers	
Verapamil (Calan, Isoptin)	80 mg tid-qid
Monoamine oxidase inhibitors	
Phenelzine sulfate (Nardil)	15 mg tid-qid

(From Whitney and Daroff.[107b])

Table 10-3

SYMPTOMATIC MEDICATIONS FOR MIGRAINE HEADACHES

Medication	Dosage

Ergotamine tartrate (Ergostat, Ergomar)	1 tablet sublingual at onset of migraine; may repeat in 20-30 min
	    Maximum dosage: 3 tablets/24 h
	                              6 tablets/wk

Ergotamine tartrate with caffeine (Cafergot)	Tablets: 1-2 PO at onset of headache, may repeat 1 tablet in 30 min
	    Maximum dosage: 6 tablets/24 h
	                              12 tablets/wk
	Suppository: 1 at onset of migraine; may repeat in 1 h
	    Maximum dosage: 2 suppositories/24 h
	                              5 suppositories/wk

Isometheptene/ dichloralphenazone/ acetaminophen (Midrin)	2 capsules at onset of migraine; may repeat 1 capsule in 1 h Maximum dosage: 5 capsules/12 h
Naproxen sodium (Anaprox)	275 mg tablets: 3 tablets at onset, may repeat 2 tablets in 1 h Maximum dosage: 5 tablets/24 h

(From Whitney and Daroff.[107b])

 1 ASSESS*

ASSESSMENT	OBSERVATIONS
History of headaches	Location and type of pain, frequency of attacks, length of headaches, auras, age of onset
Headache pain	Severity on a scale of 1-10, associated symptoms
Neurologic examination	Focal deficits, visual field deficits
Psychosocial	Changes in affect (irritability, apathy, depression)

*Nursing care should be well documented in the patient's permanent health care record.

2 DIAGNOSE

NURSING DIAGNOSIS	SUBJECTIVE FINDINGS	OBJECTIVE FINDINGS
Pain (acute) related to headache	Complains of headache	Increased B/P, heart rate; guarding; rubbing location of pain; photophobia
Ineffective individual coping related to pain	Complains of anxiety	Changes in affect (anxiety, irritability, depression)

3 PLAN

Patient goals

1. The patient will be able to prevent some headaches and will achieve relief of headache pain.

2. The patient will demonstrate effective coping by having normal affect at time of discharge.

4 IMPLEMENT

NURSING DIAGNOSIS	NURSING INTERVENTIONS	RATIONALE
Pain (acute) related to headache	Assess and document onset, location, aura, and duration of pain.	Aura often precedes migraines.
	Instruct patient to report headache pain.	Medication given at beginning of headache may decrease or eliminate headache.
	Provide quiet environment.	Quiet affords comfort, rest, and relaxation.
	Apply cold compress to head and forehead.	Application of cold causes vasoconstriction, which may decrease pain.
	Administer medications as prescribed, and monitor effects.	For effective pain management, medication must be administered as prescribed.
Ineffective individual coping related to pain	Assess existing coping mechanisms.	Coping with a chronic illness may cause feelings of anger, fear, and depression.
	Encourage patient to discuss her feelings and concerns.	To establish a therapeutic relationship.
	Provide support and information.	To reduce negative feelings.

5 EVALUATE

PATIENT OUTCOME	DATA INDICATING THAT OUTCOME IS REACHED
Patient experiences fewer headaches and is able to obtain relief.	Patient has effectively used dietary guidelines, decreased her stress level, and administers prophylactic medications to eliminate headaches.
Patient is able to cope effectively.	Patient expresses and exhibits effective coping, as evidenced by positive comments.

Cerebrovascular Accident

Cerebrovascular accident (CVA or stroke) occurs when a cerebral blood vessel is occluded by an embolism or thrombus or as a result of cerebral hemorrhage, causing ischemia of the brain tissue normally perfused by the damaged blood vessel.

Stroke is the third leading cause of death in the United States. It claims 150,300 lives each year, and 60.6% of these are women.

The risk factors that predispose women to strokes are hypertension, diabetes mellitus, a high serum cholesterol level, obesity, a sedentary life-style, cigarette smoking, stress, and use of oral contraceptives. Women who smoke and use oral contraceptives are 22 times as likely to have a stroke as women who neither smoke nor use oral contraceptives.

PATHOPHYSIOLOGY

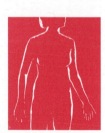

The pathologic mechanisms of stroke are commonly listed as hemorrhagic, thrombotic, and embolic in the most recent vascular literature. Hemorrhage may be subarachnoid, from rupture of the subarachnoid artery, or intraparenchymal, from rupture of an intraparenchymal artery. Embolic occlusion is caused by tumors, valvular cardiac disease and, most commonly, plaques that are released from cerebral vessels and cause infarction. Thrombotic arterial occlusion produces various ischemic or hypoxic insults. Table 10-4 compares seven types of strokes.

CLINICAL MANIFESTATIONS

The classic warning signs of a stroke are minor numbness, temporary speech difficulties, blurred vision, headache, dizziness, loss of consciousness, and/or paralysis.

COMPLICATIONS

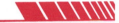

The complications of a stroke are seizures, increased intracranial pressure, contractures, loss of muscle tone, deep vein thrombosis, pulmonary embolism, malnutrition, aspiration, urinary incontinence, bowel incontinence, and depression.

Table 10-4

COMPARISON OF SEVEN TYPES OF STROKES

	Intracerebral hemorrhage	Subarachnoid hemorrhage	Subdural hemorrhage
Onset	Rapid; minutes to 1-2 h	Sudden; varied progression	Insidious; occasionally acute
Duration	Permanent if lesion is large; small lesions are potentially reversible	Variable; complete clearing may occur in days or weeks	Hours to months
Relation to activity	Usually occurs during activity	Most commonly related to head trauma	Usually related to head trauma
Contributing or associated factors	Hypertensive cardiovascular disease; coagulation defects	Intracerebral arterial aneurysm; trauma; vascular malformations	Chronic alcoholism
Sensorium	Coma common	Coma common	Generally clouded
Nuchal (neck) rigidity	Frequently present	Present	Rare
Location of cerebral deficit	Focal; arterial syndrome not common	Diffuse aneurysm may give focal sign before and after	Frontal lobe signs; ipsilateral pupil may dilate
Convulsions	Common	Common	Infrequent
Cerebrospinal fluid	Bloody unless hemorrhage is entirely intracerebral	Grossly bloody; increased pressure	Normal to slightly elevated protein
Skull x-rays	Pineal shift, edema, hemorrhage, or hematoma	Normal or calcified aneurysm	Frequent contralateral shift of pineal gland

(From Thompson.[104])

DIAGNOSTIC STUDIES AND FINDINGS

Diagnostic test	Findings
Computed tomography (CT) scan	Infarct appears as decreased density; shift of midline structures and ventricular system
Magnetic resonance imaging (MRI) study	Infarct appears as area of high density
Brain scan	Infarct shows as area of decreased perfusion
Electroencephalography (EEG)	Focal slowing around area of lesion

Epidural hemorrhage	Focal cerebral ischemia	Cerebral thrombosis	Cerebral embolism
Rapid; minutes to hours	Rapid; seconds to minutes	Minutes to hours	Sudden
Initially fluctuating; then steadily progressive	Seconds to minutes	Permanent if lesion is large; potentially reversible if lesion is small	Rapid improvement may occur, depending on collateral flow
Almost always related to head trauma	Occurs during activity if related to decreased cardiac output	Usually occurs at rest	Unrelated to activity
Any condition that predisposes to trauma	Peripheral and coronary atherosclerosis; hypertension	Peripheral and coronary atherosclerosis; hypertension	Atrial fibrillation; aortic and mitral valve disease; myocardial infarct; atherosclerotic plaque
Rapidly advancing coma	Usually conscious	Usually conscious	Usually conscious
Rare	Absent	Absent	Absent
Temporal lobe signs; ipsilateral pupil may dilate; high intracranial pressure (ICP)	Focal; or arterial syndrome	Focal; or arterial syndrome	Focal; or arterial syndrome
Common	Rare	Rare	Rare
Increased pressure; color and cells usually normal	Usually normal	Usually normal	Usually normal
Frequently fracture across middle meningeal artery groove	May show calcification of intracranial arteries	Possible arterial calcification and pineal shift from edema	Usually normal

MEDICAL MANAGEMENT

GENERAL MANAGEMENT

Cardiac monitoring is conducted, since embolic strokes may have cardiac origin.

Head of bed is kept flat if increased cerebral perfusion is desired (as with thrombotic or embolic stroke); head of bed is elevated if decreased cerebral perfusion is desired (as with hemorrhagic stroke or increased intracranial pressure). Bed rest is desired.

Controlled mechanical ventilation and hyperventilation are used to treat increased intracranial pressure (ICP).

Arterial blood gas analysis is done to monitor respiratory and metabolic functions.

Seizure control is achieved with anticonvulsants and seizure precautions.

Intake and output records are kept, and an indwelling urinary catheter is used as needed to ensure accurate output.

Pulmonary embolism is prevented with anticoagulants, TED hose, and passive range-of-motion exercises.

Ineffective swallowing and decreased level of consciousness may require use of enteral tube feedings.

Impaired communication and muscle control require an organized approach to regulate the bowel and bladder.

SURGERY

Carotid endarterectomy: Surgical removal of atherosclerotic plaques from the internal and external carotid arteries and the common carotid artery.

1 ASSESS*

ASSESSMENT	OBSERVATIONS
Level of consciousness	Varying degrees of consciousness
Communication disorders	Impaired ability to communicate; Wernicke's aphasia (unable to understand speech); Broca's aphasia (able to hear and understand); global aphasia (difficulty communicating); anomia (difficulty finding appropriate words); syntactic aphasia (uses words in wrong syntax or transposes letters); agraphia (unable to write); alexia (unable to read); automatic speech (uses automatic words such as "hello," "ok"); jargon (speaks unintelligible words)
Agnosia	Unable to recognize familiar objects
Apraxia	Unable to perform a task, even though motor and sensory functions are intact
Dysphagia	Difficulty swallowing because of paralysis of tongue and larynx
Short-term memory deficit	Limited day-to-day learning
Motor paralysis	Hemiplegia (paralysis of one side, arm, and leg on side of body opposite brain lesion); monoplegia (paralysis of one extremity, usually the arm); triplegia (paralysis of three extremities, usually both arms and one leg); quadriplegia (paralysis of all four extremities)
Sensory alterations	Hemianesthesia (loss of sensation on side of face, arm and leg of body opposite brain lesion); hyperesthesia/pain (enhanced sensitivity or pain, usually in paralyzed extremity)
Emotional lability	Mood swings, laughs or cries
Impulsiveness/impaired judgment	Acts without considering consequences
Bladder functioning	May have urinary incontinence or retention
Bowel functioning	May have bowel incontinence or constipation

*Nursing care should be well documented in the patient's permanent health care record.

2 DIAGNOSE

NURSING DIAGNOSIS	SUBJECTIVE FINDINGS	OBJECTIVE FINDINGS
Altered cerebral tissue perfusion related to impaired cerebral blood flow, increased ICP, hypoxia, widening pulse pressure, and changes in respiration	Complains of headache	Change in level of consciousness (LOC), seizures, restlessness, lethargy

NURSING DIAGNOSIS	SUBJECTIVE FINDINGS	OBJECTIVE FINDINGS
Impaired physical mobility related to hemiplegia, decreased LOC, sensory deficits	Complains of inability to move extremity or to walk	Hemiplegia; impaired ability to position self
Impaired verbal communication related to aphasia, alexia, agraphia, dysarthria	Complains of difficulty reading, writing, and speaking	Speech unintelligible; unable to read or write
Self-care deficit related to hemiplegia, sensory deficits	Complains of inability to do activities of daily living (ADL)	Impaired ability to bathe, dress, feed, and toilet self
Urinary incontinence related to decreased sensations and impaired mobility, communication, and cognitive functions	Complains of being unable to "get to the bathroom in time"	Urinary incontinence, no communication of need to void

3 PLAN

Patient goals

1. The patient will have improved cerebral tissue perfusion.
2. The patient will be able to ambulate independently or move with assistive devices.
3. The patient will be able to transmit understandable messages.
4. The patient will be able to perform activities of daily living independently.

4 IMPLEMENT

NURSING DIAGNOSIS	NURSING INTERVENTIONS	RATIONALE
Altered cerebral tissue perfusion related to impaired cerebral blood flow, increased ICP, hypoxia, widening pulse pressure, and changes in respiration	Assess neurologic status q 1 h and prn; perform neurologic assessment q 1 h and prn.	LOC reflects neurologic change; neurologic assessment detects changes in cranial nerves.
	Monitor B/P, pulse, and respirations q 1 h and prn.	Changes in vital signs reflect increased ICP.
	Monitor for seizures activity due to cerebral edema or irritation.	Seizure activity may indicate increased intracranial pressure.

→ 〉 〉

NURSING DIAGNOSIS	NURSING INTERVENTIONS	RATIONALE
Impaired physical mobility related to hemiplegia, decreased LOC, sensory deficits	Help patient and family develop plan for maximizing patient mobility; identify resources and services to help with assistance and optimizing self-care.	To promote rehabilitation and self-care.
Impaired verbal communication related to aphasia, alexia, agraphia, dysarthria	Encourage patient to express self and allow time for developing communication skills; obtain supportive services as needed and explore ways to maximize communication, such as nonverbal methods.	To facilitate communication with verbal and nonverbal methods.
Self-care deficit related to hemiplegia, sensory deficits	Assist patient with self-care while encouraging patient involvement; establish levels of tolerance and help patient and family develop progressive activities of self-care.	To provide a plan for improving patient self-care until independent ADLs are established.
Urinary incontinence related to decreased sensations and impaired mobility, communication, and cognitive functions	Maintain routine fluid intake and bladder training; help patient identify way to communicate need to void, or to independently use facilities when needed.	To assist patient in developing toilet routine and self-management of urinary needs.

5 EVALUATE

PATIENT OUTCOME	DATA INDICATING THAT OUTCOME IS REACHED
The patient demonstrates improved cerebral tissue perfusion.	The patient demonstrates improved ability to verbalize, and is free of headaches or seizures.
The patient demonstrates increased mobility.	The patient can turn and position self in bed, and ambulate or independently use assistive devices, such as a wheelchair.
The patient can communicate effectively.	The patient can express her needs with verbal or nonverbal communication techniques.
The patient can perform ADLs.	The patient can perform self-care.

PATIENT TEACHING

1. Assess patient/family knowledge and involve them in planning care.
2. Encourage regular schedules that promote patient's independence.
3. Refer patient to speech therapist and other health care providers, as needed.

Cholelithiasis/Cholecystitis

Cholelithiasis is the formation of stones in the gallbladder. **Cholecystitis** is an inflammation of the gallbladder; it can be acute or chronic and usually is preceded by cholelithiasis.

Cholelithiasis is a common health problem, one that affects 20 million Americans. Gallstones rank fifth as a cause of hospitalization for adults, and removal of the gallbladder is the third most common type of surgery performed. Cholelithiasis is two to three times more common in women than in men.

PATHOPHYSIOLOGY

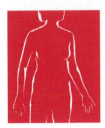

Gallstones are composed primarily of cholesterol, bile salts, and calcium. Three specific factors appear to contribute to the formation of gallstones: metabolic factors, biliary stasis, and inflammation. A combination of elevated serum cholesterol, stasis of bile in the gallbladder, and a heightened inflammatory process caused by gallstone development may lead to cholelithiasis.

CLINICAL MANIFESTATIONS

Cholelithiasis manifests with right upper quadrant pain (which may radiate to right shoulder) that occurs a few hours after the person consumes a high-fat meal. If inflammation is present, the individual may also have fever and chills. If the common bile duct is obstructed, the patient will have clay-colored stools and the urine will contain excess bilirubin. Absorption of vitamin K may be impaired, and the patient will have an elevated prothrombin time.

COMPLICATIONS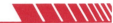

Complications of cholelithiasis/cholecystitis include increased prothrombin time, peritonitis, recurrent attacks, jaundice, obstructed common bile duct, pancreatitis, internal biliary fistulas, and carcinoma.

DIAGNOSTIC STUDIES AND FINDINGS

Diagnostic test	Findings
Serum bilirubin	May be elevated with obstruction of common bile duct
Urine bilirubin	Bilirubin in urine
Alkaline phosphatase	Elevated
Serum prothrombin time	Elevated
Ultrasound of gallbladder	Gallstones
Computed tomography (CT) scan of gallbladder	Gallstones
Cholecystography	Gallstones
Endoscopic retrograde cholangiopancreatography (ERCP)	Gallstones

MEDICAL MANAGEMENT

GENERAL MANAGEMENT

Medical management of cholelithiasis involves keeping the patient NPO, inserting an NG tube for nausea and vomiting, and administering IV fluids, narcotic analgesics (Demerol) for pain, and vitamin K for prolonged prothrombin time.

SURGERY

Obstruction may require surgery.

Gallstone lithotripsy: Lithotripsy involves the use of shock waves to break down gallstones (Figure 10-2). The shock waves are passed through a water medium. Approximately 1,500 small shocks are delivered over 1 to 2 hours. Fragments of the gallstones are excreted through the common bile duct.

Cholecystectomy: Removal of the gallbladder if conservative management is unsuccessful.

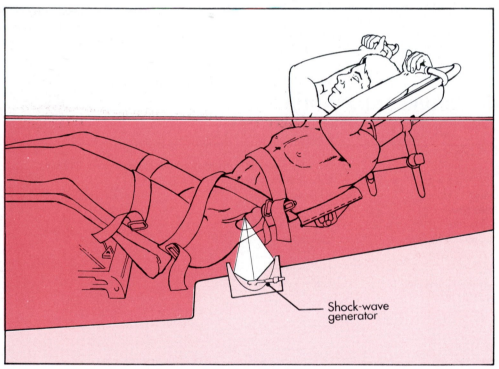

FIGURE 10-2
Patient positioned for shock wave lithotripsy. Area of flank is exposed for efficient shock wave conduction. (From Brundage.[18])

1 ASSESS*

ASSESSMENT	OBSERVATIONS
Pain (acute or chronic)	Location and type of pain, frequency and length of attacks, age of onset, severity of pain on a scale of 1-10, associated symptoms, history of food intake in relation to pain
Abdominal examination	Guarding, tenderness, increased pain on palpation, abdominal distention, nausea, vomiting, clay-colored stools, dark-colored urine

*Nursing care should be well documented in the patient's permanent health care record.

2 DIAGNOSE

NURSING DIAGNOSIS	SUBJECTIVE FINDINGS	OBJECTIVE FINDINGS
Pain (acute) related to gallstones	Complains of pain in upper right side	Increased B/P and heart rate, guarding, tenderness
High risk for injury (bleeding) related to vitamin K impairment	Complains of bruising or bleeding easily	Petechiae, bleeding of gums or from needle sticks
Knowledge deficit related to new illness and diagnosis	Complains of lack of information	Asks questions about workup, medical treatment, and surgery

3 PLAN

Patient goals

1. The patient's abdominal pain will be relieved.
2. The patient will have no bleeding complications.
3. The patient will understand key elements of her illness and surgery.

4 IMPLEMENT

NURSING DIAGNOSIS	NURSING INTERVENTIONS	RATIONALE
Pain (acute) related to gallstones	Assess and document onset, location, and duration of pain.	Right upper quadrant pain associated with meals is diagnostic of gallstones.
High risk for injury (bleeding) related to vitamin K impairment	Assess and document petechiae and bleeding; administer vitamin K.	Impaired absorption of vitamin K leads to bleeding complications.
Knowledge deficit related to new illness and diagnosis	Teach patient about her illness and surgery.	Instruction prepares patient for diagnosis and surgery.

5 EVALUATE

PATIENT OUTCOME	DATA INDICATING THAT OUTCOME IS REACHED
Patient's pain has been relieved.	Patient states that pain is gone.
Patient has no bleeding complications.	Patient shows no signs of bleeding or undetected hemorrhage.
Patient understands her treatment options.	Patient can describe and has selected medical treatment and surgery.

PATIENT TEACHING

1. Help the patient devise pain-relief measures.
2. Discuss with the patient and family medical and surgical options (e.g., laser techniques, dietary management).
3. Refer the patient to dietary counseling if needed.

Endocrine Disorders

The endocrine system consists of the anterior and posterior pituitary, the thyroid, parathyroid, adrenal cortex and medulla, pancreas, gonads, pineal body, and thymus, as well as specialized gastrointestinal cell (Figure 10-3). These ductless glands secrete hormones directly into extracellular spaces, from which they pass into the blood. The hormones, along with the nervous system, act to coordinate body processes to maintain homeostasis via synergistic and inhibitory relationships. Several endocrine disturbances are common to women.

Anterior pituitary disorders that commonly affect women are related to the secretion of prolactin (PRL), follicle-stimulating hormone (FSH), luteinizing hormone (LH), and thyroid-stimulating hormone (TSH). Alterations in normal secretion of these hormones have wide-ranging effects. Menstrual dysfunction, infertility, decreased libido, galactorrhea, and depression are expressions of anterior pituitary dysfunction in women.

Thyroid disorders affect women more often than men, for unknown reasons. The incidence of these disorders is six times greater in women. The ages for diagnosis of thyroid dysfunction are 30 to 40 for Graves' disease, 40 to 50 for subacute thyroiditis, 60 to 70 for toxic multinodular goiters, and 30 to 50 for Hashimoto's thyroiditis.

Parathyroid disorders are twice as common in women than men. The age for diagnosis is anywhere from 30 to 70 years. The peak incidence for parathyroid dysfunction is during the postmenopausal years.

Adrenal disorders such as Cushing's disease are more commonly seen in women than men. Naturally occurring Cushing's disease usually is diagnosed between 30 and 60 years of age. The physical effects are emotionally devastating.

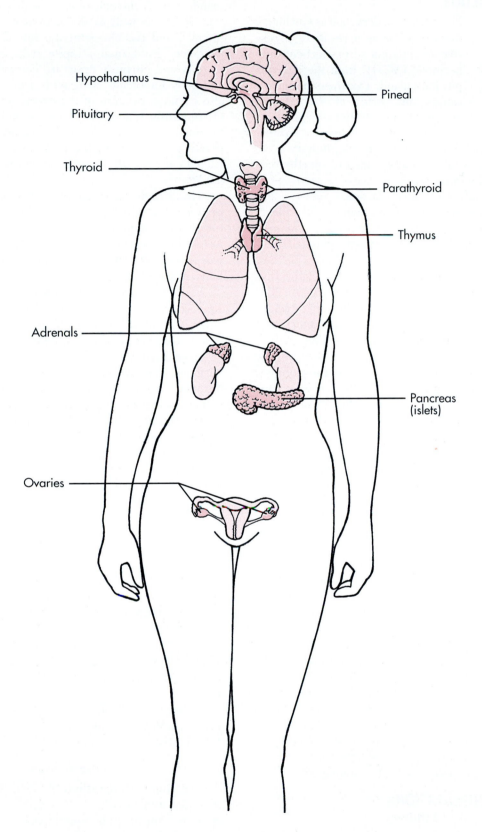

FIGURE 10-3
Endocrine glands and their location in women.

PATHOPHYSIOLOGY

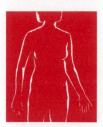

Pituitary disorders such as Cushing's disease occur as a result of excessive secretion of adrenocorticotropic hormone (ACTH) from the anterior pituitary gland. This overstimulation causes the cortex of the adrenal glands to secrete excessive corticosteroids, leading to toxicity. Excessive production of TSH from the anterior pituitary overstimulates the thyroid gland and leads to hyperthyroidism. Pituitary adenomas result in excessive secretion of prolactin, which adversely affects lactation, menses, and fertility. An inadequate level of oxytocin directly affects pregnancy, labor, and lactation. Menopause is a time of excessive secretion of pituitary gonadotropins (LH and FSH).

Thyroid disorders affect the production of the thyroid hormones, thyroxine (T_4) and triiodothyronine (T_3), which regulate metabolism and growth and development. Graves' disease, toxic multinodular goiters, and thyroiditis occur as a result of excessive thyroid hormone secretion. Graves' disease is believed to be due to an autoimmune disorder in which immunoglobulins stimulate the thyroid gland to secrete excessive hormones. Hyperfunctioning in toxic multinodular goiters is due to autonomously functioning thyroid tissue. The mechanism of hyperfunction in subacute thyroiditis is thought to be due to viral infection of the gland, which causes it to release large quantities of preformed hormones. Hashimoto's thyroiditis is an autoimmune disorder in which lymphocytic and antibody infiltration creates hyposecretion of thyroid hormones.

Parathyroid disorders related to primary hyperparathyroidism involve a single parathyroid adenoma. The cause is unknown. Some speculate that radiation of the neck is a possible cause. Parathyroid hyperplasia can be a secondary development in chronic renal disease, vitamin D deficiency, pregnancy, lack of calcium, and hyperphosphatemia.

Adrenal disorders involving hypersecretion of corticosteroids may result from ACTH oversecretion by the pituitary gland, caused by an adenoma. Primary adrenal tumors also cause hypersecretion of the adrenal cortex, since neoplastic tissue produces cortisol independently of ACTH. Thus hypercortisolism (Cushing's syndrome) is either ACTH dependent or ACTH independent. High cortisol levels adversely affect many tissues and physiologic processes, with devastating effects.

CLINICAL MANIFESTATIONS

Pituitary

In **Cushing's disease,** the excessive secretion of ACTH leads to the symptoms of Cushing's syndrome. Clinical manifestations include obesity with a central distribution of fat, as well as dorsocervical fat pads ("buffalo hump"), and the characteristic round "moon face" appearance. Epidermal atrophy with connective tissue fragility and purplish striae are commonly seen. Facial and body hirsutism, along with acne and seborrhea, is also common because of the excess adrenal androgens. Osteoporosis, glucose intolerance, and a predisposition to renal calculi are frequent clinical features. The psychologic impact of the change in appearance often leads to anxiety, depression, irritability, and emotional lability.

Thyrotropin, or thyroid-stimulating hormone, when produced in excess manifests as hyperthyroidism (thyrotoxicosis). Symptoms include weakness, sweating, weight loss, nervousness, heat intolerance, tachycardia, palpations, exophthalmos, tremors, restlessness, irritability, and easy fatigability.

Excessive secretion of **prolactin** leads to hypogonadism, which manifests as anovulation, menstrual irregularity, and infertility, as well as hyperinsulinemia, glucose intolerance, and galactorrhea.

Irregularities in the secretion of the gonadotropin hormones, **luteinizing hormone** and **follicle-stimulating hormone,** manifest as reproductive and menstrual difficulties. Infertility and menstrual irregularities are common. LH and FSH are controlled by pituitary **gonadotropin-releasing hormone (GnRH),** which also may augment secretion of ACTH in Cushing's disease.

Insufficient **oxytocin** during pregnancy may interfere with labor and with postpartum lactation. It is also believed that insufficient oxytocin may act as a diabetogenic factor in late pregnancy.

Thyroid

Graves' disease manifests as thyrotoxicosis, goiter, exophthalmos, and pretibial edema. Symptoms include palpitations, nervousness, irritability, intolerance to heat, hyperkinesia, fatigue, weight loss, and thyroid enlargement.

Symptoms of **toxic multinodular goiter (Marine-Lenhart syndrome)** include tachycardia, dysrhythmia, nervousness, tremors, sweating, and gland enlargement.

Subacute or **Hashimoto's thyroiditis** manifests with early symptoms of malaise; neck pain; dysphagia; an enlarged, tender gland; and periods of thyrotoxicosis.

Parathyroid

Symptoms of **parathyroid** disturbances vary from muscular weakness in the lower extremities, decreased appetite, constipation, somnolence, and short attention span to calcium loss, osteoporosis, bone fragility, kidney stones, and peptic ulcer. Facial muscle contraction when the facial nerve is tapped (Chvostek's sign) and carpal spasm after application of a cuff (Trousseau's phenomenon) are positive signs of hypoparathyroidism. Deep tendon reflexes may be hyperactive. Hyperparathyroidism, commonly found in women, manifests as skeletal pain with progressive kyphosis, polyuria and polydipsia, thirst, anorexia, and nausea and vomiting resulting from hypercalcemia.

Adrenal

Hypercortisolism is manifested as **Cushing's syndrome.** The psychologically devastating symptoms include obesity, with a "moon face" appearance, and a large pad of fatty tissue ("buffalo hump") at the back of the neck. Hirsutism, acne, seborrhea, purple striae, and osteoporosis are also present.

Complications

Disorders of the pituitary gland can result in adrenal insufficiency leading to shock and subsequent death. Mortality from hypertension occurs in Cushing's disease, and severe emotional disturbances often seen in Cushing's syndrome can lead to suicide. Pituitary necrosis (Sheehan's syndrome) can occur from severe postpartum hemorrhage, and an elevated prolactin level is associated with premature osteoporosis, infertility, and galactorrhea.

Overstimulation of the thyroid gland can lead to life-threatening thyroid storm, whereas severe hypothyroidism leads to myxedema coma. Life-threatening complications of parathyroid dysfunction are associated with pathologic fractures and renal failure.

Adrenal complications are associated with excess cortisol. Peptic ulcers, hypertension, hyperglycemia, hypokalemia, and suppressed immunity are serious complications. Psychosis is also a serious complication to be considered.

DIAGNOSTIC TESTS AND FINDINGS

Diagnostic test	Findings
Adrenal disorders	
Cushing's syndrome	
Hemoglobin (Hgb)	High normal
Hematocrit (Hct)	High normal
White blood count (WBC)	Normal
Lymphocytes	Decreased
Esinophils	Decreased
Serum phosphorus	Decreased
Calcium	Increased (40% cases)
Cortisol	Moderate increase
Adrenal androgens	Moderate increase
Adrenocorticotropin (ACTH)	Normal to moderate increase
Urine 17-hydroxycorticosteroids with a 2-day dexamethasone suppression	Increased
Thyroid-stimulating hormone (TSH)	May be abnormal, but cannot be used alone to evaluate pituitary function
Prolactin (PRL)	Varies
Follicle-stimulative and luteinizing hormones (FSH/LH)	Varies but is increased in menopause
Thyroid disorders	
Graves' disease	
Thyroxine (T$_4$)	Decreased
Triiodothyronine (T$_3$)	Increased
TSH	Suppressed
Cholesterol	Increased
Radioactive iodine uptake	Decreased
Thyroid-stimulating immunoglobulins	Present
Electrocardiogram (ECG)	Tachycardia or bradycardia

Continued.

DIAGNOSTIC TESTS AND FINDINGS—cont'd

Diagnostic test	Findings
Toxic multinodular goiter	
TSH	Suppressed
T_3	Increased
T_4	Normal to slightly elevated
Radioactive scan	Multiple, functioning nodules
Subacute thyroiditis (findings vary with disease process)	
TSH	Suppressed, increased (late)
T_3	Increased (early), decreased (late)
T_4	Increased (early) decreased (late)
Erythrocyte sedimentation rate (ESR)	Markedly elevated
Radioactive iodine uptake	Low
Hashimoto's thyroiditis	
T_3	Decreased
T_4	Decreased
TSH	Increased
Thyroglobulin autoantibodies (microsomal)	Strongly positive
Fine needle biopsy	Lymphocytic infiltrate

Parathyroid disorders

Hyperparathyroidism	
Serum calcium	Increased
Serum phosphate	Decreased
Urine calcium	Normal or increased
Urine phosphate	Increased
Radioimmunoassay: immunoradiometric assay (IRMA)	Increased in parathyroid hormones

Adrenal disorders

Hypercortisolism	
Glucose tolerance test	Impaired
Plasma cortisol	High without diurnal variation
Eosinophils	Low
Lymphocytes	Decreased
RBCs	Increased
WBCs	Increased
Serum bicarbonate	Increased
Chloride	Decreased
Potassium	Decreased
Urine 17-hydroxycorticosteroids	Low to high
Free cortisol	High

MEDICAL MANAGEMENT

GENERAL MANAGEMENT

Management of *anterior pituitary disorders* is directed at promoting normal pituitary function and preventing further loss of function. The surgical approach to treat tumors is a transfrontal (transsphenoidal) adenomectomy. Residual tissue may be treated with radiation therapy, but complications involving adjacent tissue occur. Drug therapy involves hormonal replacement using natural or synthetic hormones. Treatment of *prolactin disorders* focuses on decreasing hormone levels to suppress galactorrhea and regulate the menstrual cycle. Bromocriptine is the drug of choice. With *ACTH disorders*, lifelong replacement with cortisone or hydrocortisone (cortisol) is indicated with complete deficiency. Dosage regulation is required before surgery or during periods of stress or illness.

TSH disorders usually involve antithyroid hormones to prevent an increase in thyroid hormone levels. With TSH deficiency, L-thyroxine is used as a replacement, depending on the clinical picture. *FSH-LH disorders* are treated with small doses of estrogen replacement to correct deficiencies. Drug therapy is highly individualized, and small doses are used to avoid thromboembolism and hyperlipidemia.

Treatment of *thyroid disorders* is also highly individualized and depends on the clinical picture. Thyroid hormone antagonists are used to treat thyrotoxicosis to prevent the formation of thyroid hormones. Prophylthiouracil (PTU) is the usual drug of choice. Methimazole is also used, as is adjunctive therapy with propranolol to control cardiac symptoms. Drug therapy must be initiated 2 to 3 months before surgical intervention (subtotal thyroidectomy) or treatment with ^{131}I. Management of *parathyroid* disorders focuses on identification of the underlying cause and surgery if symptoms indicate. Medical management involves calcium regulation with close observation of laboratory values, renal studies, and clinical response. Corticosteroids are sometimes indicated, and unresponsive hypercalcemia involves the administration of phosphorus. Additionally, calcium gluconate and possibly vitamin D replacements are indicated in hypoparathyroidism to control tetany and prevent seizures. Magnesium replacement is indicated in hypomagnesemia-induced hypoparathyroidism.

Disorders of the *adrenal cortex* are treated by unilateral or bilateral adrenalectomy in hyperfunctioning disorders. Radiation is also used to treat hyperplasia or to prevent postoperative progression of ACTH-secreting adenomas. Following treatment, steroid replacement is indicated either temporarily or for life. Drug treatment approaches to hyperfunction include mitotane, cyproheptadine, and bromocriptine. The drug focus for hypofunction is on careful hormonal replacement. Dosage adjustments must be made during periods of infection, stress, or trauma. Abrupt discontinuation of corticosteroids leads to circulatory collapse, shock, and death.

1 ASSESS*

	ASSESSMENT	OBSERVATIONS
Pituitary disorders	Onset and duration of symptoms; family history; medical history; pain; visual disturbances; fatigability; delayed wound healing; skin changes; personality changes; sexuality changes; hair distribution; weight changes; history of postpartum hemorrhage, lactation failure, amenorrhea	Muscle weakness; poor wound healing; paresthesia; joint pain; fatigue; lethargy; dyspnea; sweating; palpitations; tachycardia; bradycardia; abnormal fat distribution; nausea/vomiting; diarrhea/constipation; irritability; hirsutism; milky breast discharge; visual disturbances; skin pigmentation abnormalities; striae

*Nursing care should be well documented in the patient's permanent health care record.

→ › ›

	ASSESSMENT	OBSERVATIONS
Thyroid disorders	Onset and duration of symptoms; family history; medical history; chief complaint; sleep pattern changes; mood swings; irritability; nervousness; palpitations; chest pain; exercise intolerance; weakness; temperature intolerance; skin changes; lethargy; muscle/joint pain; gastrointestinal changes; menstrual irregularities; pregnancy history; past head/neck trauma, surgery, radiation; medications; change in interpersonal relationships	Neck pain; dysphagia; irritability; difficulty concentrating; nervousness; tremor; chest pain; palpitations; exercise intolerance; dry, rough skin; coarse/fine hair; muscle/joint pain; diarrhea/constipation; brittle nails; visual changes; staring appearance; lack of facial expression; thick tongue and lips; facial edema; palpable gland; pretibial edema; altered tendon reflexes
Parathyroid disorders	Onset and duration of symptoms; family history; medical history; chief complaint; muscle fatigability, cramping, tremors; change in energy level; lower extremity weakness; nausea/vomiting; nocturnal leg twitching; joint pain; headaches; emotional lability; memory loss; depression; visual disturbances; medications	Spinal change; tetany; choking sensation; lethargy; decreased reflexes; cardiopulmonary changes; positive Chvostek's/Trousseau's signs; muscle weakness; lack of coordination; hypotonia; disorientation; dry, scaly skin; ridged, brittle nails; alopecia; increased caries and tooth staining; hypertension; visual changes; candidal infections
Adrenal disorders	Onset and duration of symptoms; family history; medical history; medications; muscle weakness; fatigability; bone/joint pain; osteoporosis; depression; confusion; headaches; change in physical appearance; weight gain; fat distribution; masculinization; menstrual changes; renal changes; thirst; anorexia; abdominal pain; dizziness/faintness	Moon face; buffalo hump fat distribution; alopecia; hirsutism; truncal obesity with extremity wasting; bruising; petechiae; facial redness; acne; striae; mucosal changes; edema; paresthesia; cardiovascular changes; abnormal skin pigmentation; emotional lability; fatigue/lethargy; joint pain

2 DIAGNOSE

NURSING DIAGNOSIS	SUBJECTIVE FINDINGS	OBJECTIVE FINDINGS
Body image disturbance related to hormone imbalance and physical changes	Expresses negative feelings about physical changes and focuses on the loss with feelings of hopelessness and helplessness	Social withdrawal, avoidance of self-care, emotional lability, denial, depression
Impaired adjustment related to impact on self-esteem, impaired cognition, and/or incomplete grieving	Reports powerlessness and lack of coping skills with unrealistic expectations and goals, noncompliance, and lack of confidence	Distorted concept of chronic illness and treatment regimen; inability to problem solve; denial; inappropriate goal setting; emotional lability
Knowledge deficit related to limited information, misinterpretation of disease process, treatment, prognosis, and community resources	Reports inaccurate information about illness, medication protocols, treatment regimen, and symptoms of complications	Noncompliant behavior, inaccurate perception of health care plan and potential complications, lack of awareness of community resources

3 PLAN

Patient goals

1. The patient will acknowledge the changes in her body image and will understand the steps toward increasing acceptance.
2. The patient will express her grief, identify her personal strengths, and set realistic goals.
3. The patient will verbalize correct information about the disease process, expected outcomes, medication regimen, and health care resources.

4 IMPLEMENT

NURSING DIAGNOSIS	NURSING INTERVENTIONS	RATIONALE
Body image disturbance related to hormone imbalance and physical changes	Encourage patient to express her feelings; help her identify her strengths, alternate behavior, and a realistic plan of action.	Verbalization decreases anxiety, and identifying an effective coping pattern encourages acceptance and realistic planning.
Impaired adjustment related to impact on self-esteem, impaired cognition, and/or incomplete grieving	Help patient identify strengths and participate in accurate, realistic goal setting and problem solving; incorporate family and community resources.	Allows for progression in the grieving process and movement to clearer cognition with realistic problem-solving skills.
Knowledge deficit related to limited information, misinterpretation of disease process, treatment, prognosis, and community resources	Provide information (verbal and written) about management of the chronic illness; reinforce learning and help patient develop a written health care plan incorporating community resources.	Increased knowledge promotes greater compliance and understanding of the disease process.

5 EVALUATE

PATIENT OUTCOME	DATA INDICATING THAT OUTCOME IS REACHED
Patient shows increased acceptance of body changes.	Patient adopts changes in life-style and habits that demonstrate acceptance of altered body image.
Patient demonstrates improved cognition and problem-solving ability.	Patient demonstrates increased emotional stability and is able to set accurate, realistic goals.
Patient better understands the disorder, treatment regimen, medication side effects, and potential complications.	Patient can verbalize accurate information, exhibits increased compliance, and has formulated a realistic health plan.

PATIENT TEACHING

1. Explain the disease process and treatment regimen.
2. Discuss medication compliance and side effects.
3. Explain the symptoms requiring immediate medical attention.
4. Help the patient explore coping patterns.
5. Explore support systems and community resources.
6. Address the patient's sexuality concerns and problems with self-image.
7. Instruct the patient in methods to promote comfort.
8. Explain the need for increased oral hygiene and dental follow-up.
9. Discuss measures to promote skin integrity.
10. Explain the impact of the disorder on future pregnancies and the need for prepregnancy counseling.

Autoimmune Disorders

Immunity is the body's ability to identify and attack foreign invading substances via the immune system's classic antibody-antigen response. This protective process depends on the immune system's ability to distinguish nonself (antigens) from self (somatic) tissue. **Autoimmunity** is the failure of the immune system to make this important distinction; as a result, the protective cell-mediated immune response becomes self-destructive. Several autoimmune disorders are prevalent in women, such as *systemic lupus erythematosus, rheumatoid arthritis, progressive systemic sclerosis (scleroderma), polymyositis/dermatomyositis, and Sjögren's syndrome.*

Systemic lupus erythematosus (SLE) is a chronic, inflammatory, autoimmune disease with an insidious onset that affects the vascular and connective tissue of the joints, skin, pleura, kidneys, pericardium, and central nervous system. SLE affects women more often than men, and usually develops between the ages of 15 and 64 (the average age of onset is 30). Three times as many black and Asian women are affected as white women.

Rheumatoid arthritis (RA) is an inflammatory autoimmune disease with variable symptoms. It occurs more often in women than men (75% of the 6 million Americans with the disease are women). The peak age of onset is between 35 and 45, although the disorder can occur in juveniles. Because RA is a disabling disease, it is a significant health concern.

Progressive systemic sclerosis (SS) or scleroderma is an autoimmune connective tissue disorder that affects women three times more frequently than men. The ratio increases during the childbearing years to 15:1, and the average age of onset is between 30 and 50 years.

Polymyositis/dermatomyositis is an inflammatory autoimmune disorder that affects striated muscle fibers. Twice as many women are affected as men, and the average age of onset is between 50 and 60 years. This disorder is frequently associated with malignant neoplasms.

Sjögren's syndrome (keratoconjunctivitis sicca) is an autoimmune inflammatory disorder that affects the lacrimal and salivary glands. It is frequently associated with other connective tissue disorders and rheumatoid arthritis. More than 90% of affected individuals are women.

PATHOPHYSIOLOGY

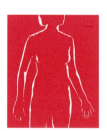

The pathophysiology of autoimmune disorders is believed to be the result of an alteration in normal tissue caused by infections, drugs, or unknown factors, which causes the immune system to recognize the altered tissue as foreign. Also, tissue similarity to specific antigens may initiate an immune response as well as alter the function of suppressor T cells and increase B-cell activation. Changes in the normally protective immune response result in autoantibody formation (antinuclear or ANA antibodies and rheumatoid factor or RF antibodies). The subsequent hypersensitivity reaction results in inflammation, which is common to all autoimmune pathophysiologic mechanisms. Persistent inflammation leads to tissue damage and permanent loss of function; however, recurring remission is common.

In *systemic lupus erythematosus*, both vascular and connective tissues become inflamed through deposition of immune complexes in the kidneys, joints, skin,

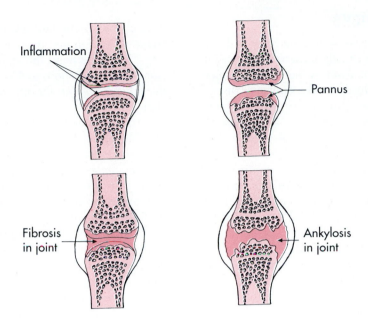

FIGURE 10-4
Pathologic changes in the joint with rheumatoid arthritis. (From Mudge-Grout.[82])

brain, pleura, and peritoneum. The result is a necrotizing vasculitis of small arteries, glomerular capillaries, retinal capillaries, fibrous synovitis, and central nervous system lesions. Scarring can lead to disabling outcomes and death from renal failure.

In *rheumatoid arthritis*, nonsuppurative inflammation within diarthrodial and intraarticular joints occurs, leading to synovial inflammation and vascular congestion (Figure 10-4). As a result, tissue damage occurs through fibrin deposition and cellular infiltration, which release harmful substances and lead to synovial thickening. Both cartilage and supporting joint structures are damaged, and immobility with deformity occurs.

In *scleroderma*, degenerative, fibrotic changes in the skin, skeletal muscles, blood vessels, synovium, and internal organs are caused by a disruption in the immune response. As a result, interstitial fibroblasts appear, which stimulate excessive collagen production, leading to fibrosis. Parenchymal cells of the small arteries of the skin, lungs, kidneys, heart, and esophagus become thickened, giving a characteristic fibrotic rigidity along with subcutaneous atrophy.

In *polymyositis/dermatomyositis*, collagen tissue and striated muscle fibers become inflamed. A diffuse inflammatory myopathy develops, caused by lymphocyte infiltrates. Fibrotic lesions, along with necrosis, lead to painful changes in the skin and muscles.

In *Sjögren's syndrome*, the lacrimal and salivary glands are infiltrated by lymphocytes. The glands be-

---

CONDITIONS ASSOCIATED WITH SJÖGREN'S SYNDROME

Systemic lupus erythematosus (SLE)
Rheumatoid arthritis
Raynaud's syndrome
Primary biliary cirrhosis
Chronic active hepatitis
Autoimmune diseases of the liver
Hyperglobulinemic purpura
Myasthenia gravis
Graft-versus-host disease
Polyarteritis
Hashimoto's thyroiditis
Pemphigus
Systemic sclerosis (scleroderma)
Polymyositis
Cryoglobulinemia
Pancreatitis
Waldenström's macroglobulinemia
Myeloma

(Adapted from Katz, editor; and Andreoli et al, editors.)

---

come inflamed, and the production of tears and saliva decreases, causing dryness and discomfort, with subsequent lesions. Additional pathophysiology usually includes rheumatoid arthritis and autoimmune connective tissue disorders.

CLINICAL MANIFESTATIONS

Systemic lupus erythematosus symptoms vary with the severity of the disease and usually have an insidious onset. Chronic fatigue, slight fever, weight loss, intolerance to sunlight, and a diffuse maculopapular or discoid rash on the extremities are common. The characteristic "butterfly" rash may appear on the face, and migratory polyarthritic symptoms and anemia also are seen. Twenty-five percent of SLE patients have cardiopulmonary symptoms: pericarditis, myocarditis, pleurisy, and painful intermittent attacks of ischemia of the extremities (Raynaud's phenomenon). Kidney involvement in the later stages is the leading cause of death in SLE patients.

Symptoms of *rheumatoid arthritis* include early manifestations of low-grade fever, easy fatigability, and generalized aching (fibrositis) with characteristic morning stiffness. As the disease progresses, symptoms become more localized, involving specific articular inflammation, swelling, pain, redness, warmth, and tenderness. Formation of subcutaneous nodules over bony prominences, bursae, and tendon sheaths is common. Chronic polyarthritis with erosions and deformity occurs, with fusiform of the fingers being common. Involvement usually is bilateral, and the joints most often affected are the hands, wrists, feet, ankles, elbows, and knees. Symptoms of RA may appear as an isolated incident with lifelong remission, or they may be chronic with periods of remission and exacerbation. Overexertion, mental or emotional stress, and physical trauma can lead to exacerbation with increased severity of symptoms.

Scleroderma manifestations range from generalized cutaneous thickening to severe visceral involvement. Less severe symptoms include the CREST syndrome, which manifests as *c*alcinosis, *R*aynaud's phenomenon, *e*sophageal dysfunction, *s*clerodactyly, and *t*elangiectasis. Skin thickening is limited to the fingers and face with characteristic tautness and pursed lips. As the soft tissue of the digits atrophies, flexion contractures occur, giving the hand the appearance of a claw. Progression involves esophageal dysfunction, gastrointestinal disturbances, and fibrotic pulmonary and myocardial changes.

Polymyositis/dermatomyositis is characterized by pain, atrophy, and contractures of proximal muscles. Individuals with this disorder are unable to raise their arms over their head and have a great deal of difficulty getting up from a seated position. Involvement of neck and throat muscles leads to dysphagia. The skin often exhibits dusky red lesions, particularly on the face, neck, shoulders, chest, and upper back. There are periods of exacerbation and remission. This disorder has been shown to have a positive association with malignant neoplasms.

Sjögren's syndrome often manifests along with the symptoms of rheumatoid arthritis and other autoimmune connective tissue disorders (see the box below). Dryness of the eyes, giving them a "gritty" sensation, is a common finding, along with photosensitivity. Dryness of the mouth leads to difficulty chewing and swallowing as well as painful buccal membrane fissures and dental caries. Nasal and respiratory dryness is manifested as a dry cough.

COMPLICATIONS

- Progressive, uncontrolled *systemic lupus erythematosus* usually leads to lupus nephritis, with subsequent renal failure. Dialysis and transplantation are common. High-dose steroidal therapy to control inflammation frequently causes avascular necrosis of the hip and other joints, necessitating surgical replacement. Central nervous system involvement with seizure activity is a contributing cause of death, along with renal failure and infections resulting from depressed immunity from steroid therapy.
- Complications of *rheumatoid arthritis* are related to the disabling joint destruction and deformity that occur. Severe, disabling pain often causes RA individuals to become depressed, since normal activities are severely limited. Surgical intervention to replace diseased joints, fuse joints, and remove and resurface synovial surfaces gives hope to these individuals.
- *Scleroderma* complications involve immobilizing contractures and deformities of the extremities. As the lungs, kidneys, and heart become fibrotic, chest expansion is limited, resulting in diffuse alveolar thickening and dyspnea. Fibrotic changes in the heart can lead to dys-

---

SICCA COMPLEX

The hallmark of Sjögren's syndrome is a nonspecific lymphocytic infiltration of exocrine glands, primarily the lacrimal and salivary glands, which results in a decrease in lacrimal and salivary secretions. The cellular infiltration insidiously destroys glandular tissue, producing the combination of ocular and oral membrane dryness. Persistent dryness is caused by insufficient secretion from the lacrimal, salivary, and mucous glands.

(From Mudge-Grout.[82])

rhythmias, and kidney changes can lead to renal compromise and failure.

Polymyositis/dermatomyositis symptoms vary, with frequent remissions and complete recovery in some individuals. The disease usually progresses to a stationary point, with muscular atrophy and contractures of affected voluntary muscle groups. The myocardium and unstriated muscles usually escape serious damage but when they are affected, cardiac dysrhythmias can occur.

Sjögren's syndrome, if progressive, can involve the visceral organs, lymph nodes, and bone marrow via lymphocytic infiltration. Extraglandular proliferation can lead to lymphoma, and lacrimal involvement can cause severe visual disturbances. Decreased salivation and dysphagia can lead to nutritional complications as well as dental caries and painful mouth lesions.

DIAGNOSIS OF SYSTEMIC LUPUS ERYTHEMATOSUS

Systemic lupus erythematosus (SLE) can be diagnosed only through a comprehensive history and physical examination and in-depth evaluation of laboratory data. No single test is diagnostic for SLE, and clinical manifestations may in some cases make it difficult to differentiate from rheumatoid arthritis. In addition, the onset of the disorder can be insidious and the symptoms vague, which may present an initial diagnostic problem.

Since the symptoms of SLE can affect almost every organ, 11 clinical findings have been developed to assist in the diagnosis. The presence of four or more of these symptoms, either simultaneously or serially, in conjunction with positive laboratory data generally confirms the diagnosis of SLE.

1. **Malar rash:** fixed erythema, flat or raised, over malar eminence, tending to spare nasolabial folds
2. **Discoid rash:** erythematous, raised patches with adherent keratotic scaling and follicular plugging; atrophic scarring
3. **Photosensitivity:** skin rash as a result of unusual reaction to sunlight; based on patient history or observation
4. **Oral or nasopharyngeal ulcers:** usually painless
5. **Arthritis:** nonerosive, minimum two-joint involvement, characterized by tenderness, swelling, or effusion
6. **Serositis:** pleuritis, convincing history of pleuritic pain or rub that is ausculated; evidence of pleural effusion or pericarditis documented by electrocardiogram, rub, or evidence of pericardial effusion
7. **Renal disorders:** persistent proteinuria of 500 mg/day or 3+ if quantitative; no preformed or cellular casts; may be red cell, hemoglobin, granular, tubular, or mixed
8. **Neurologic disorders:** seizures in the absence of offending drugs or known metabolic derangements (e.g., uremia, ketoacidosis, electrolyte imbalance) or psychosis in the absence of offending drugs or known metabolic derangements
9. **Hematologic disorders:** hemolytic anemia with reticulocytosis or leukopenia with a WBC <4,000/μL total on two or more occasions, or thrombocytopenia with a platelet count of <100,000/μL in the absence of offending drugs or lymphopenia
10. **Immunologic disorders:** manifested by positive LE-cell preparation, anti-DNA antibodies directed against the genetic material in host cells, or a false-positive serologic test for syphilis (VDRL). Known to be positive for at least 6 months and confirmed by *Treponema pallidum* immobilization or fluorescent treponemal antibody absorption test
11. **Antinuclear antibody (ANA):** abnormal titer of antinuclear antibody by immunofluorescence or equivalent assay at any point in time in the absence of drugs known to be associated with drug-induced lupus syndrome

(From Mudge-Grout.[82])

DIAGNOSTIC STUDIES AND FINDINGS

Diagnostic test	Findings
Systemic lupus erythematosus	
Erythrocyte sedimentation rate (ESR)	Elevated
Complete blood count (CBC)	Leukopenia, hypochromic anemia, thrombocytopenia
Gamma globulin	Elevated
Lupus erythematosus (LE) factor	Positive in 80% of cases
Antinuclear antigen (ANA)	High positive, but not specific for SLE
Serum complement level	Decreased
Serology (VDRL)	False positive
Serum albumin	Decreased
Urinalysis	Hematuria, proteinuria, casts (with kidney involvement)
See the box on page 191 for further information.	
Rheumatoid arthritis	
CBC	Normal WBC or mild leukocytosis; mild hypochromic anemia in active disease, leukopenia or thrombocytopenia in chronic disease
C-reactive protein (CRP)	Positive in active stage
ESR	Elevated in active stage
Rh factor	Present in 60%-70% of cases; depends on severity
ANA	Positive with a speckled pattern
Scleroderma	
ESR	Mildly elevated
ANA	SLC-70 in diffuse disease; ACA antibody in CREST syndrome
RF	Present
Urinalysis	Hematuria, proteinuria, casts (with kidney involvement)
X-ray	Digital tuft resorption, distal esophageal hypomobility, pulmonary fibrosis
Skin biopsy	Dermal collagen thickening, condensation, or homogenization
Polymyositis/dermatomyositis	
CBC	Leukocytosis
ESR	Elevated in active disease
Creatine phosphokinase (CPK)	Elevated in active disease
Serum glutamate oxaloacetate transaminase (SGOT)	Elevated in active disease
Aldolase	Elevated in active disease
ANA	Positive for PM-1, JO-1 (speckled pattern)
Urine (24 hour)	Abnormal creatine/creatinine ratio
Sjögren's syndrome	
CBC	Leukopenia, anemia
ESR	Elevated
Rh factor	Present
ANA	Positive
Gamma globulins	Excess
Schirmer eye test	Decreased tears
Salivary flow rate	Decreased
Histology	Lymphocytic infiltration of lacrimal and salivary glands

NURSING DIAGNOSIS	SUBJECTIVE FINDINGS	OBJECTIVE FINDINGS
Knowledge deficit related to lack of information about disease process, treatment, prognosis, and available resources	Reports misinformation about disease, treatment regimen, medications, and prognosis; expresses concern about family and financial impact of chronic illness	Inadequate knowledge base regarding disease process and treatment; exhibits anxiety regarding prognosis and financial/family impact

3 PLAN

Patient goals

1. The patient's pain, stiffness, and discomfort from skin, mucous membrane, and ophthalmic discomfort will decrease, and the patient will take measures to avoid exacerbation of symptoms.
2. The patient will increase her activity tolerance, will balance activity and rest, and will improve joint function and range of motion.
3. The patient will discuss her sexual concerns and seek measures to relieve pain and improve sexuality.
4. The patient will become more knowledgeable about the disease process, treatment goals, medication regimen, and community resources.

4 IMPLEMENT

NURSING DIAGNOSIS	NURSING INTERVENTIONS	RATIONALE
Pain related to joint inflammation, headaches, and skin lesions	Administer analgesic/antiinflammatory drugs as indicated; assess pain relief and aggravating factors; promote functional joint alignment, skin and mouth care; apply warmth and splints as indicated.	To provide comfort and maintain function.
Impaired physical mobility related to joint/muscle pain, tenderness, and stiffness	Individualize activities and exercise; maintain a balance between activity and rest; give medications before range-of-motion and therapeutic activities; promote safety as indicated.	To promote improved function and lessen exacerbations, and to prevent deformities and accidental injury.
Altered sexuality patterns related to decreased libido, increased pain and discomfort	Establish rapport to encourage patient to discuss her concerns; ensure confidentiality; promote comfort measures.	To promote open communication and decrease fears by exploring alternatives, and to improve sexuality.
Knowledge deficit related to lack of information about disease process, treatment, prognosis, and available resources	Provide accurate information about the disease, medication/treatment regimen, and available resources; reinforce learning.	To promote compliance and accurate health care goals.

5 EVALUATE

PATIENT OUTCOME	DATA INDICATING THAT OUTCOME IS REACHED
Patient has less pain in joints and muscles, and skin and mucous membrane irritation has been relieved.	Patient appears comfortable during activities and reports increased psychologic comfort.
Patient maintains optimum joint function.	Patient exhibits functional range of motion without deformity, and increased activity tolerance without exacerbation of symptoms.
Patient identifies areas of sexual dysfunction.	Patient shows increased knowledge and coping methods to improve sexual function and sexuality.
Patient can give accurate information about the disease.	Patient sets realistic health care goals based on accurate information.

PATIENT TEACHING

1. Provide written and verbal information about the disease, treatment regimen, and medications.
2. Reinforce learning with a written health care plan containing realistic goals.
3. Assess activity and rest program to prevent exacerbations.
4. Reinforce avoidance of sunlight to prevent photosensitivity reaction or exacerbation (SLE).
5. Teach the patient how to use splints, warmth, and antiinflammatory medications to control exacerbations and prevent deformity.
6. Provide information about support groups, community resources, and health care needs.
7. Emphasize the importance of follow-up visits with health care providers.
8. Instruct the patient in the implications of the disease for pregnancy and the need for prepregnancy counseling.
9. Instruct the patient in the impact of the disease on sexual function and sexuality.

Multiple Sclerosis*

Multiple sclerosis (MS) is a chronic, relapsing neurologic disease of unknown cause or cure. It is characterized by disseminating inflammatory demyelination in the central nervous system (CNS), thought to be caused by a defect in the immunoregulatory system.

Some researchers have suggested that multiple sclerosis (MS) may have an epidemiologic, genetic, or viral cause. Only the epidemiologic theory is discussed here. The incidence of MS in the United States is 40 to 60 cases per 10,000 population. Worldwide the disease is

*Information on multiple sclerosis presented here is adapted from Mudge-Grout CL: *Immunologic disorders*, St. Louis, 1992, Mosby, pages 272-290.[82]

seen more in western Europe, southern Canada, south-ern Australia, and New Zealand. Because the preva-lence of MS is low in warmer climates and higher in colder climates, geographic areas close to the equator have a lower incidence. Local epidemics have also been described, indicating the possibility of a transmissible cause.

Individuals who move from areas of higher MS prevalence to areas of lower prevalence after 15 years of age retain the risk of MS associated with their previous environment. However, individuals younger than 15 years of age acquire the risk of the new environment, indicating a possible epidemiologic cause.

Most people diagnosed with MS are women; the female-to-male ratio is 2 to 3:1. Multiple sclerosis oc-curs in all races but predominates among Caucasians. Clinical onset of the disease occurs between 20 and 40 years of age in 75% of cases. It is rare in childhood, and the incidence decreases significantly after age 55. This distribution in age may suggest that a critical event (e.g., possible viral exposure) occurs during adoles-cence and is a predisposing factor to the onset of MS.

PATHOPHYSIOLOGY

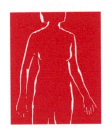

Multiple sclerosis damages the my-elin sheath of the body's central nervous system (Figure 10-5). The myelin sheath is a white, fatty tissue that surrounds most of the axons of the nervous system; it acts as an in-sulator and promotes the conduc-tion of nerve impulses. In MS only the white fibrous tracts of the central nervous system (the brain and the spinal cord) are affected. As the my-elin is damaged, it is replaced first by lymphocytes and then by sclerotic tissue. Initially the myelin sheath con-tinues to transmit impulses. However, as the disease progresses, the myelin sheath is permanently destroyed and replaced with scar tissue, resulting in significant in-terference in neural transmission.

The proposed pathologic features of MS include two processes: the interaction between the immune system and the central nervous system, and the formation of demyelinating lesions.

The immunoregulatory response that occurs in MS is not completely understood. It may be directed to-ward antigens of a virus infection or an unknown auto-antigen of myelin or oligodendroglial cells. When the immune response is triggered, it causes a mild, recur-rent inflammatory reaction. The inflammation causes a vasculitis that breaks down the blood-brain barrier.

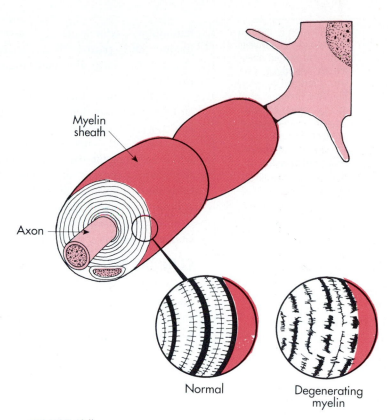

Myelin
sheath

Axon

Normal

Degenerating
myelin

FIGURE 10-5
In multiple sclerosis the myelin sheath is progressively de-stroyed until the myelin is totally disrupted and the axon is nonfunctional. (From Mudge-Grout.[82])

Formation of Lesions

It is unknown whether the lesions of MS are a cause or an effect of the interaction between the central nervous system and the immune system.

The pathology of plaque formation involves a num-ber of processes, including breakdown of the myelin structure, lysis of oligodendrocytes, and activation of astroglial processes.

The plaques, or lesions, of MS involve the white matter of the central nervous system. These neuro-pathologic lesions are primarily confined to the CNS. They are multifocal plaques of demyelination that are distributed randomly within the white matter of the ce-rebrum, cerebellum, brainstem, and spinal cord.

Plaque formation has two stages, the acute (or early) stage and the chronic (or late) stage. The acute stage is the process of perivascular infiltration of T lymphocytes and macrophages. This occurs in conjunction with peri-venular demyelination, primarily around the third and fourth ventricles. A mild lymphocytic meningitis ac-companies these changes. The external surface of the brain appears normal, but the ventricles may be en-larged and brain weight may be diminished. The in-

Demyelination is the process whereby the myelin sheath and myelin sheath cells are destroyed. Demyelination causes four significant changes in the central nervous system: decreased nerve conduction velocity, nerve conduction block, differential rate of transmission of impulses, and complete failure of impulse transmission. These changes predispose the individual with MS to the numerous signs and symptoms of the disease. During a remission, demyelinated areas are healed with fibrotic tissue. If the nerve fiber is destroyed during the demyelination process, the symptoms are permanent.

flammatory edema in and around the plaque and partial demyelination are thought to cause the neurologic symptoms of MS.

In the chronic stage, plaque formation and the process of demyelination are characterized by a proliferation of astrocytic processes and degeneration of axons, which lead to glial scarring. Plasma cells in the plaques secrete oligoclonal IgG antibody into the cerebrospinal fluid and extracellular fluid. Neurologic defects progress over years, with subsequent loss of function and increasing disability.

CLINICAL MANIFESTATIONS

The clinical manifestations of MS vary considerably and are characterized by periods of exacerbation and remission. How they manifest clinically depends on the area of CNS involvement. Initial symptoms generally manifest involvement of the cerebrum, the cerebellum, the brainstem, or the spinal cord. After several years, these patients show symptoms of mixed CNS involvement. Symptoms are caused by plaque formation and myelin loss in the white matter of the brain, usually in the periventricular area, which is thought to prevent conduction of nerve impulses.

Symptoms may develop acutely, with a rapid onset, or chronically, over several years. Acute exacerbations develop over a few days and persist for days or weeks, with eventual recovery. Chronic exacer-

bations develop at varying intervals, with less-than-complete recovery and decreasing function. The frequency of exacerbations varies considerably. Approximately 60% of individuals with MS are fully functional at 10 years; 25% to 30% are functional 30 years after onset.

Increased body temperature, infection, elevated serum calcium levels, and stress are factors that contribute to periods of exacerbation. Increases in body temperature and serum calcium levels cause leakage through the demyelinated neurons, aggravating the symptoms of MS. Infection tends to stimulate the immune system. Stress, both physical and emotional, can increase the symptoms of MS by imposing functional demands that may exceed the conduction capacity of the demyelinated neurons. Increases in body temperature can be external (e.g., hot bath, sunbathing) or internal (fever). Although heat may exacerbate symptoms, it does not contribute to the disease process itself.

COMPLICATIONS

The complications of multiple sclerosis include aspiration, pneumonia, respiratory failure, infection, contractures, psychosis, complications of immobility, and bladder control problems.

DIAGNOSTIC STUDIES AND FINDINGS

Diagnostic test	Findings
Lumbar puncture for cerebrospinal fluid specimen	
Electrophoresis	>90% have oligoclonal IgG bands
IgG antibody	75% have increased levels
Gamma globulin	Elevated
Protein	Normal or elevated
White blood count (WBC)	Elevated
VDRL	Negative
Radioimmunoassay (RIA)	Myelin protein
Serum IgG antibody	Elevated
Serum antibody titers	Titers to many viruses may be elevated (e.g., herpes simplex type 1, parainfluenza, rubella, mumps, measles, Epstein-Barr virus)
Computed tomography (CT) scan	Areas of low attenuation around cerebral ventricles; may show ventricular enlargement and cerebral atrophy
Magnetic resonance imaging (MRI) studies	Visualization of plaques in cerebral white matter and brainstem lesions not detected by CT
Evoked response studies	Decreased conduction velocity in visual, auditory, and somatosensory pathways
Positron emission tomography (PET) studies	May show altered locations and patterns of cerebral glucose metabolism

(From Mudge-Grout.[82])

There is no single diagnostic test for MS. Diagnosis is based on a complete history and physical and a comprehensive neurologic examination, supported by information from the tests listed here.

SIGNS AND SYMPTOMS OF MULTIPLE SCLEROSIS

Motor	Sensory	Cognitive	Psychologic
Muscle weakness (90%)	Numbness	Decreased short-term memory	Depression (30%-40%)
Muscle spasticity	Vertigo	Decreased ability to solve abstract problems	Anxiety
Nystagmus (70%)	Diplopia	Poor judgment	Denial
Ataxia	Blurred vision	Intellectual changes	Frustration
Intention tremor	Eyeball pain	Inability to concentrate	Restlessness
Fatigue (>90%)	Scotomas	Confusion	Anger
Constipation	Impaired color perception	Disorientation	Apathy
Bladder dysfunction (80%-90%) (urgency, hesitancy, incontinence)	Decreased hearing		Irritability
Dysarthria	Paresthesia		Instability, dementia, euphoria
Dysphagia	Loss of sphincter control		
Seizures	Facial sensory deficit		
Women: diminished orgasmic response	Hemisensory loss, sexual dysfunction (90%)		
Men: neurogenic impotence; premature, delayed ejaculation	Decreased libido, impaired genital sensation, sexual dysfunction (70%)		

MEDICAL MANAGEMENT

The goals of medical management are to preserve function and prevent complications.

GENERAL MANAGEMENT

Activity: Promote routine activity with a regular exercise program (consult with exercise physiologist or physical therapist); use braces, splints, cane, walker, or wheelchair when necessary to maintain optimum functioning.

Nutrition: Maintain optimum nutritional intake (consult dietician).

Promote independence: Consult occupational therapist and home nursing service and, when necessary, extended-care facilities.

Cognitive or psychologic support: Consult psychiatrist, assess medications, and refer patient to support groups.

Visual support: Teach use of aids and eye patch; refer patient to support groups for the blind.

Urinary impairment: Monitor for infection; institute bladder training program.

Dysphagia/dysphasia: Refer to speech therapist; with risk of aspiration, institute tube feedings when necessary to maintain nutritional intake.

DRUG THERAPY

Antiinflammatory drugs (used during periods of exacerbation and for maintenance therapy during remissions): corticosteroids: prednisone, 0.5-1 mg/kg/day in divided doses, taper to maintenance dosage; prednisolone, dexamethasone (Decadron), 0.75-9 mg/day, taper to maintenance dosage; methylprednisolone (Solu-Medrol), "pulse therapy" 1-2 mg/kg/day IV in divided doses for 3-7 days; adrenocorticotropic hormone (ACTH, Athcar), 40-50 U bid for 7-10 days.

Immunosuppressive drugs (currently under investigation): cyclophosphamide (Cytoxan), cyclosporine (Sandimmune), azathioprine (Imuran), alpha- and beta-interferons, monoclonal antibodies.

Antispasmodic drugs: Baclofen (Lioresal), 15-25 mg PO tid; diazepam (Valium), 5-10 mg PO qid; dantrolene (Dantrium), 25 mg PO qid, maintenance dosage increased to 400 mg/day; cyclobenzaprine (Flexeril), 10 mg tid.

Tremor-reducing drugs: Beta-adrenergic blocking agents; propranolol (Inderal), 40-240 mg/day PO; primidone (Mysoline), 100 mg qd, increase to 250 mg tid; isoniazid (INH), 5 mg/kg/day, maximum 30 mg qd; trihexyphenidyl (Artane), 1-15 mg qd; hydroxyzine (Vistaril), 50-100 mg qd in divided doses.

Drugs to minimize bladder dysfunction: Hyporeflexia causing urinary retention: cholinergic drugs: bethanechol (Urecholine), 10-50 mg tid. Hyperreflexia causing frequency and urgency: anticholinergics: propantheline (Pro-Banthine), 20-75 mg qd in divided doses; oxybutynin (Ditropan), 1-5 mg qid; imipramine (Tofranil), 50-150 mg qd.

Drugs to decrease fatigue: Amantadine (Symmetrel), 100-200 mg qd; methylphenidate (Ritalin) 20-60 mg qd in divided doses (should not be taken after 6 PM).

Drugs to decrease pain: Carbamazepine (Tegretol), 200 mg bid, increase to 800-1,200 mg qd in divided doses; amitriptyline (Elavil), 25-150 mg qd in divided doses; imipramine (Tofranil), 100-300 mg qd in divided doses; antiinflammatory drugs (acetaminophen, aspirin, ibuprofen).

Antibiotics: To treat infections, particularly urinary tract infections.

ADJUNCTIVE THERAPY

Physical therapy; occupational therapy; hydrotherapy; speech therapy; sexual therapy; plasmapheresis.

SURGERY

Contralateral thalamotomy to relieve pain, tremors, and rigidity; rhizotomy to relieve intractable pain; penile implants for impotence; gastrostomy tube placement for nutritional support.

(From Mudge-Grout.[82])

1 ASSESS*

ASSESSMENT	OBSERVATIONS
History	Emotional or physical stress, recent infection, exposure to heat
Motor	Initial presentation demonstrates weakness in lower extremities; impaired motor function after a hot bath or shower (Uhthoff sign); uncoordinated movements, hyperactive reflexes; intention tremors of upper extremity; ataxia of lower extremities; staggering gait; intermittent spastic weakness of speech muscles; dysphasia and dysphagia; facial palsy; nystagmus; loss of sphincter control (urinary and later bowel incontinence)
Sensory	Numbness and tingling in involved extremity or the face; loss of joint sensation and proprioception; loss of sensation of position, shape, texture, and vibration (50%); eye pain and diplopia; vertigo; decreased libido
Psychologic/ cognitive	Emotional lability, irritability, depression, changes in memory

*Nursing care should be well documented in the patient's permanent health care record.

2 DIAGNOSE

NURSING DIAGNOSIS	SUBJECTIVE FINDINGS	OBJECTIVE FINDINGS
Impaired physical mobility related to muscle weakness and fatigue	Complains of difficulty walking and controlling movements; reports inability to perform activities of daily living (ADLs), fatigue, and tremors with exertion	Spasticity and tremors; focal motor deficits; intention tremor with purposeful movements; progressive muscle atrophy, psychomotor incoordination, listlessness
Altered patterns of urinary elimination (functional, stress, and urge incontinence, and retention) related to altered nerve impulse transmission	Complains of urgency and intermittent urinary incontinence; reports urinary frequency, dysuria	Urinary incontinence, decreased bladder sensation, >150 ml residual urine after voiding; *urinalysis:* bacteriuria; elevated WBC; microhematuria; cloudy, turbid urine; fever; serum WBC >10,000
Altered thought processes and impaired verbal communication related to altered nerve innervation	Reports forgetfulness and memory loss; complains of inability to express self and articulate words	Slowness in thinking and problem solving, altered judgment, short-term memory loss; slurred, jerky speech pattern; slow speech with decreased fluency; tremors of lips, tongue, and jaw; faint voice with fluctuations in volume
Sensory-perceptual alterations (visual) related to optic nerve demyelination	Reports decreased vision in one eye; complains of seeing double (diplopia) and having blurred vision	Diplopia, nystagmus, optic neuritis; able to identify only large objects
High risk for ineffective individual coping related to multiple stressors	Reports feelings of uselessness and lack of control over life	Lack of social support systems and adequate resources

→ › ›

NURSING DIAGNOSIS	SUBJECTIVE FINDINGS	OBJECTIVE FINDINGS
Self-care deficit in all ADLs related to progressive dysfunction, mental changes, and neurologic impairment	Reports inability to care for self	Remains in bed much of the day; decreased participation in self-care activities; has neglected appearance

Other related nursing diagnoses: Altered family processes related to role changes; **Social isolation** related to deteriorating function; **Impaired swallowing** related to progressive dysphagia; **Altered nutrition** related to dysphagia and fatigue; **Body image disturbance** related to incontinence and ataxia; **Powerlessness** related to progressive debilitation and perceived lack of control over disease outcome and health care management; **Bowel incontinence** related to progressive neuromuscular impairment; **Chronic pain** related to altered nerve transmission; **Sexual dysfunction** related to altered nerve innervation.

3 PLAN

Patient goals

1. The patient will remain mobile without weakness or fatigue.
2. Urinary incontinence and retention will be resolved, or the patient will develop strategies for management.
3. The effects of altered thought and speech processes will have a minimal effect on the patient's life.
4. The patient will demonstrate restored visual acuity or will develop strategies for coping with visual impairments.
5. The patient will develop methods of coping with multiple stressors.
6. The patient will increase her ability to complete ADLs or develop strategies and explore resources to assist in coping with self-care and routine activities.

4 IMPLEMENT

NURSING DIAGNOSIS	NURSING INTERVENTIONS	RATIONALE
Impaired physical mobility related to muscle weakness and fatigue	Assess range of motion (ROM) and level of mobility.	To establish baseline and guide therapeutic interventions.
	Consult with patient, exercise physiologist, physical therapist, and occupational therapist to develop daily exercise program.	Professional health team members provide an important service in complex care; a routine exercise program will assist in maintaining a maximum level of mobility.
	Problem solve with patient to determine strategies for decreasing fatigue (e.g., fatigue occurs most often in the afternoon, so the most demanding activities should be performed in the morning).	To identify ways to conserve energy, thereby decreasing fatigue and weakness.
	Help patient reposition herself q 2 h; perform ROM exercises, hydrotherapy with tepid water, and splint use as needed. Administer antispasmodic medications as ordered, and monitor patient's response; administer Ritalin or Symmetrel as ordered, and monitor patient's response.	To prevent complications of immobility and contractures; to temporarily relieve spasticity; to decrease fatigue; and to promote optimal movements that otherwise might be impossible.

NURSING DIAGNOSIS	NURSING INTERVENTIONS	RATIONALE
Altered patterns of urinary elimination (functional, stress, and urge incontinence, and retention) related to altered nerve impulse transmission	Assess current voiding pattern and factors associated with incontinence episodes or urinary retention.	To assist in guiding therapeutic interventions.
	Implement techniques to ensure complete bladder emptying (e.g., tapping or stroking bladder, Credé's maneuver [bladder massage], coughing, listening to running water, pouring lukewarm water over perineal area, stimulating anus digitally).	To ensure complete bladder emptying, prevent urinary incontinence, and decrease risk of infection from residual urine.
	Instruct patient to control fluid intake and balance intake with *voiding schedule;* patient should receive 2,000-2,500 ml/day.	To assist in scheduling voiding times, to prevent incontinence and possible infection, and to ensure renal perfusion.
	Teach patient to use urinary control devices as needed.	To control urinary leakage between toilet trips.
	If bladder regimen fails, institute clean intermittent catheterization and instruct patient and family in procedure and associated perineal skin and hygiene measures.	To restore urinary continence; intermittent straight catheterization decreases the risk of infection compared to a permanent, indwelling catheter; to prevent irritation and breakdown of perineal skin.
	Administer drugs to minimize bladder dysfunction (e.g., Pro-Banthine) as ordered, and monitor patient response.	To promote urinary continence and prevent bladder spasms.
	Teach patient perineal (Kegel) exercises.	To improve muscle tone of urinary sphincter.
Altered thought processes and impaired verbal communication related to altered nerve innervation	Assess cognitive, emotional, and neurologic processes.	To establish baseline functioning and guide therapeutic interventions.
	Encourage patient to have familiar people and objects in her environment; reorient as indicated to new events (e.g., provide clocks, calendars, newspaper).	To provide tangible reminders as an aid to memory and to maintain orientation.
	Encourage patient to make a list or write things down.	To prevent or control forgetfulness.
	Develop an outline of daily activities, and structure time.	To provide a familiar routine and control forgetfulness.
	Encourage patient to speak slowly and to concentrate and stay focused on content of communication.	Slowed speech will improve diction and decrease slurring of words.
	Allow patient adequate time to express herself.	To decrease frustration and promote communication.
	Provide alternative methods of communication (e.g., picture books, magnetic slate); consult speech therapist.	To provide a means for patient to communicate.

➜ ❯ ❯

NURSING DIAGNOSIS	NURSING INTERVENTIONS	RATIONALE
Sensory-perceptual alterations (visual) related to optic nerve demyelination	Assess degree of visual impairment.	To establish baseline and guide therapeutic interventions.
	Alternate patching patient's eyes q 2 h as ordered and monitor patient response.	To relieve diplopia; double vision stems from weakness in one or more eye muscles.
	Refer patient with decreased visual acuity to the Association for the Blind or the National MS Society.	These organizations may send a representative to the home to teach the patient and family adaptive strategies.
	Administer tremor-reducing medications (e.g., Inderal) as ordered.	To decrease eye tremors.
High risk for ineffective individual coping related to multiple stressors	Encourage patient to identify stressors and to verbalize feelings; help patient set realistic goals for coping with stress.	To help patient develop an awareness of emotional reactions to stress and facilitate coping.
	Help patient identify past behaviors that were effective in coping with stress.	To facilitate patient involvement in problem solving.
Self-care deficit in all ADLs related to progressive dysfunction, mental changes, and neurologic impairment	Assess patient's ability to perform ADLs; assess effort involved to complete task.	To establish baseline functioning and guide therapeutic intervention.
	Refer patient to occupational therapist for assistive devices and home maintenance equipment.	To encourage independence and self-care.
	Teach significant other to assist with or provide ADLs.	To maintain care at home for as long as possible.

5 EVALUATE

PATIENT OUTCOME	DATA INDICATING THAT OUTCOME IS REACHED
Patient maintains muscular functioning.	Patient participates in routine exercise program; satisfactory ROM is maintained; muscle mass without atrophy is maintained; and unaffected muscle groups have been strengthened.
Urinary continence or retention has been restored, and patient has developed management strategies.	Regular, complete bladder emptying has been achieved; perineal skin is intact; there is no urinary leakage or dribbling; and patient demonstrates strategies for urinary continence (e.g., double voiding, voiding schedule, fluid control, access to toilet). Less than 150 ml of residual urine is present after voiding; patient demonstrates double-voiding technique and can perform intermittent catheterization.
Effects of altered thought processes on patient's life and routine activities are minimized.	Patient can participate and complete ADLs without evidence of frustration and depression and can communicate her feelings and needs without excess frustration.

PATIENT OUTCOME	DATA INDICATING THAT OUTCOME IS REACHED
Patient's visual capacity has increased, or patient has developed strategies with decreased vision.	No injury ensues related to impaired vision; patient can perform routine activities; and nystagmus is controlled.
Patient can cope with and respond to stressful events.	Patient recognizes source of stress and demonstrates effective skills for coping with stress; patient uses resources for help in coping with stress.
Patient can independently perform ADLs or uses modified equipment, strategies, and resources for assistance.	Patient can perform routine ADLs without fatigue; she uses assistive devices to facilitate ADLs (e.g., specialized eating utensils); and she uses community resources to assist with ADLs (e.g., transportation services).

PATIENT TEACHING

1. Instruct the patient and family about the disease, diagnostic procedures, treatments, supportive functional activities, and medications.
2. Teach the patient and family about medications: purpose, dosage, route and time of administration, and side effects.
3. Encourage the patient to keep a diary of her illness (i.e., symptoms, medications, and treatments used).
4. Stress the importance of paced and structured routine activities.
5. Teach the patient to adhere to her activity and rest schedule to prevent overwhelming fatigue.
6. Instruct the patient and family in passive and active ROM exercises.
7. Teach the patient to monitor her response to activity and to alter her activity when the signs and symptoms of excessive fatigue develop.
8. Emphasize the importance of diversional activities to reduce stress and fatigue.
9. Instruct the patient and family in visualization and stress-reducing exercises to prevent overwhelming fatigue and potential periods of exacerbation.
10. Teach the patient and family to clean toileting device regularly; white vinegar may be used to clean and deodorize the receptacle.
11. Teach the patient and family the Credé method of bladder emptying (apply pressure on the lower abdominal wall, manually compressing the bladder and allowing expulsion of urine).
12. Instruct the patient and family in intermittent catheterization and how to use clean technique at home.
13. Stress the importance of speech therapy to assist with communication.
14. Teach the patient and family forms of communication other than speaking (e.g., pictures, magnet drawing board, using objects to point to, signaling with eye movements).
15. Instruct the family to provide a safe environment to prevent injuries caused by visual impairment.
16. Teach the patient about factors that may cause an exacerbation of symptoms: overexertion, hot baths, excessive sun exposure, fever, emotional or physical stress, high humidity, extreme hot or cold weather, and pregnancy.
17. Instruct the patient in community resources and services and how to use these programs.
18. Instruct the patient in strategies for simplifying ADLs (e.g., allow for periods of rest, develop a routine and schedule, use assistive devices, maximize resources).
19. Refer the patient and family to the MS Society.

Eating Disorders: Obesity, Bulimia, and Anorexia

Obesity is a body weight more than 20% higher than the desirable weight for adults of a given sex and height. **Bulimia** is a binge-and-purge disorder. **Anorexia** is the intense fear of being obese and the intentional limitation of food intake.

Eating disorders such as anorexia nervosa and bulimia nervosa have been known since ancient times, when they were described as "nervous consumption" and "anorexia hysteria." Currently obesity is the most common type of malnutrition in the United States. Compulsive overeating leading to obesity is also a known eating disorder. In the United States more women than men suffer from eating disorders. Eighty percent of children of two overweight parents will also be overweight. The incidence of eating disorders, especially anorexia and bulimia, is high in certain subgroups such as models, ballet dancers, and flight attendants. It is estimated that 5% to 15% of adolescent girls meet the criteria for bulimia.

PATHOPHYSIOLOGY

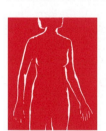

A person's desirable weight is obtained from standard height/weight tables that contain arbitrary figures derived from pooled life insurance data. The greater the obesity, the greater the health risk. Massive, or morbid, obesity is defined as being 100 pounds over desirable weight and is extremely hazardous to health. Patients with bulimia can eat as much as 25,000 calories at one sitting. Not only are bulimics addicted to food, they also have a morbid fear of getting fat. They usually induce vomiting or take laxatives, or both, to purge themselves of unwanted calories.

Some researchers think that compulsive overeating, obesity, and bulimia begin early in life, when a girl learns to numb emotional pain by overeating. In time food becomes a narcotic, or a "fix," that temporarily alleviates psychologic discomfort. As with many drugs, more and more food is soon required to produce an anesthetizing effect. Before long the bulimic is hooked on huge quantities of food, particularly junk food.

CLINICAL MANIFESTATIONS

In general the signs and symptoms of eating disorders are amenorrhea; behavioral changes, which include agitation, disorganized thinking, and hyperactivity; sleep disturbances; gastrointestinal complaints; and weight fluctuations. Individuals diagnosed with anorexia experience weight loss that is at least 15% less than their ideal body weight. Anorexics are terrified of being obese and feel very overweight even when they are emaciated. Bulimics tend to be overachievers at work, yet have a poor opinion of themselves. The disorder tends to appear in families that have a high incidence of severe depression, drug abuse, and alcoholism. Individuals may have a weight loss or gain of 10 pounds a week. Constipation may result from chronic laxative abuse. Swollen parotid glands and ulcerated gums or eroded tooth enamel may result from vomiting.

COMPLICATIONS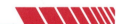

Complications of obesity include atherosclerosis, hypertension, gallstones, diabetes mellitus, osteoarthritis, and respiratory insufficiency. Complications of anorexia include amenorrhea, hypoglycemia, malnutrition, and cardiac dysrhythmias. Complications of bulimia include amenorrhea, loss of tooth enamel, constipation or diarrhea, GI bleeding, gastritis and esophagitis, and malnutrition.

DIAGNOSTIC STUDIES AND FINDINGS

Diagnostic test	Findings
Increased blood urea nitrogen (BUN), low creatinine, albumin, total protein	Low levels suggest malnutrition
Upper gastrointestinal x-ray	May show evidence of gastritis, esophagitis, or GI bleeding
Clinical history	Positive for manifestations of eating disorders

MEDICAL MANAGEMENT

GENERAL MANAGEMENT

Medical management centers around nutritional management in the form of IV therapy, hyperalimentation, or tube feedings. Supplemental vitamins are given. Psychotherapy is used for behavior modification.

SURGERY

Gastric resections for GI bleeding or obesity management may be performed if medical management is unsuccessful.

1 ASSESS*

ASSESSMENT	OBSERVATIONS
Description of typical eating pattern	Weight compared to ideal body weight (IBW), percentage above or below IBW
History of binging or purging	Evidence of tooth enamel loss, mouth ulcerations
Laxative use	Constipation or diarrhea
Family history	Positive family history of alcoholism, drug addiction, or depression
GI disturbances	Abnormal upper GI x-ray

*Nursing care should be well documented in the patient's permanent health care record.

2 DIAGNOSE

NURSING DIAGNOSIS	SUBJECTIVE FINDINGS	OBJECTIVE FINDINGS
Ineffective individual coping related to undereating or overeating	Complains of being overweight	*Obesity:* weight >20% IBW; *bulimia:* weight at IBW; *anorexia:* weight 15% less than IBW
Altered nutrition: less than body requirements related to eating disorder	Describes food history	Abnormal laboratory chemistries: increased BUN, low creatinine, albumin, and total protein

→ > >

3 PLAN

Patient goals

1. The patient will be able to describe an adequate and nutritional diet in 3 days and will understand the elements of her eating disorder in 1 day.
2. The patient will demonstrate effective coping skills.
3. The patient will practice adequate nutrition.

4 IMPLEMENT

NURSING DIAGNOSIS	NURSING INTERVENTIONS	RATIONALE
Ineffective individual coping related to undereating or overeating	Assess existing coping mechanism.	Ineffective coping with stress leads to eating disorders.
Altered nutrition: less than body requirements related to eating disorder	Monitor IV fluids, hyperalimentation, or tube feedings.	Nutritional support must be maintained until a normal eating pattern is restored.
	Monitor laboratory values.	Quantitative measurement of laboratory values provides information on patient's intake.

5 EVALUATE

PATIENT OUTCOME	DATA INDICATING THAT OUTCOME IS REACHED
Patient understands her eating disorder and what constitutes adequate nutrition.	Patient can describe an adequate and nutritional diet and the elements of her eating disorder.
Patient demonstrates effective coping skills.	Patient can cope without manifesting signs of her eating disorder such as binging or purging or avoiding food.
Patient practices adequate nutrition.	Patient's laboratory values are within normal range.

PATIENT TEACHING

1. Help the patient identify her eating disorder and underlying misconceptions of self.
2. Help the patient devise a plan for problem solving and correcting potentially harmful eating patterns.
3. Refer the patient and family to nutritional and psychologic counseling as needed.
4. Encourage follow-up visits to reassess progress and plan additional therapeutic steps as needed.
5. Discuss medical and surgical options to assist with eating disorder if needed.

CHAPTER 11

Fertility, Infertility, and Contraception

Fertility is the ability to conceive and bear children. **Infertility** is the *inability* (1) to conceive within at least 12 months of unprotected intercourse, or (2) to carry a pregnancy to viability. *Primary infertility* is infertility in a couple who has never had a pregnancy; *secondary infertility* is infertility in a couple who has had a child but cannot conceive again in a reasonable time frame. **Contraception** is the regulation or prevention of fertilization and/or implantation of a fertilized ovum in the uterus.

Disorders of pregnancy are not addressed in this chapter, but the process of fertilization and the factors that influence it are discussed to provide a basis for understanding diagnostic procedures, therapy, and techniques used in both supporting fertility and achieving contraception.

Fertility and Infertility

As a girl matures and achieves menarche, the assumption is made that she is fertile, or capable of conceiving and bearing a child. Efforts to prevent conception often begin when the young woman becomes sexually active, supporting this assumption of fertility.

In the United States approximately 17.3 million couples desire children, but 2.4 million (approximately 15%) have a problem with conception. Infertility is a unique medical problem in that it occurs between two individuals. It can involve just male, just female, or both male and female causative factors. In general, male factors are responsible for about 40% of cases of infertility. Major female factors include tubal disease (20%) and hormonal factors (20%). Cervical problems, including immobilization of the sperm, account for approximately 5% of cases of infertility. In about 20% to 30% of cases, both partners are subfertile. Infertility is unexplained in 5% to 10% of affected couples.

PATHOPHYSIOLOGY

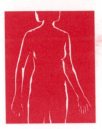 Both the female and the male reproductive systems play important roles in the process of fertilization. The female system (1) provides for the development and release of ova, (2) provides an environment in which fertilization can occur, and (3) provides an environment in which the fertilized ovum can develop and mature (see Figure 1-11). The male system (1) provides an adequate number of viable sperm, and (2) facilitates the transport of sperm to the female for fertilization. For pregnancy to occur, the woman must ovulate a normal, fertilizable ovum that can reach the oviduct. The man must be able to produce a sufficient number of normal, mature, motile sperm that can be ejaculated into the woman's vagina. The spermatozoa must be able to pass through the cervical mucus and through a patent cervical os, ascend the uterus, pass into the oviduct at the appropriate stage of the menstrual cycle, and penetrate the ovum. After fertilization the ovum must implant in a prepared endometrium in the uterus and develop normally. Interference in any of these mechanisms may result in infertility.

Factors that may influence fertility include the age of the man or woman; the frequency of intercourse; infection; abnormalities of the genital tract, endocrine system, or immunologic system; diabetes; thyroid dysfunction; and environmental and life-style factors (see the box on page 213 for a summary of factors that influence fertility).

In women, fertility is low at very young ages, peaks in the mid twenties, and begins to decline after age 30 until menopause, which usually occurs in the early fifties. In men, fertility peaks a little later than in women and declines after age 40, although pregnancies have been reported involving men who were 80 and 90 years old. The frequency of intercourse with ejaculation appears to influence the quality and motility of sperm. The optimum frequency appears to be four or more times per week; about 80% of couples conceive within 12 months with this frequency.

CLINICAL MANIFESTATIONS

The clinical manifestations of infertility are inability to conceive after 12 months of regular sexual intercourse without use of contraception; inability to carry a pregnancy to live birth; and inability to conceive after delivery of a viable infant (secondary infertility).

COMPLICATIONS

The emotional response to infertility can be devastating. The inability to have children may become a life crisis for the couple, who often feel frustration, anger, loss, guilt, and depression. Also, there are often sociocultural pressures, as well as personal ones, for bearing children that the couple may not be able to meet. These pressures can cause severe emotional stress for one or both members of the couple.

DIAGNOSING INFERTILITY

Evaluations for infertility should begin with the simplest and least invasive laboratory tests. These include semen analysis (Table 11-2), basal body temperature (BBT) charts for women (Figures 11-1 and 11-2), and endocrine studies for both men and women. Diagnosis generally is divided into the categories of female factors (ovulatory, tubal, peritoneal, uterine, and cervical) and male factors (semen/sperm adequacy, sperm penetrability, and antibody compatibility). A summary of the main reproductive organ problems to be evaluated and the tests performed is presented under Diagnostic Studies and Findings: Female and Male. Additional information on BBT charts, LH surge tests, and cervical mucus tests is given in the contraceptive section beginning on page 221.

Diagnostic studies themselves are stressful and time consuming. They may continue for years, and for 5% to 10% of couples, no physical reason for the infertility will be identified. Although many of the physical reasons for infertility can be treated, the treatments are not without risk. Treatment can include surgery with all of its attendant risks of bleeding, infection, adhesions, and anesthesia. Medications such as hormone stimulation for ovulation induction may result in hyperstimulation, increasing the risk of multiple pregnancies and hypovolemic shock. Minor complications include nausea, flushing, headache, vaginal dryness, and depression.

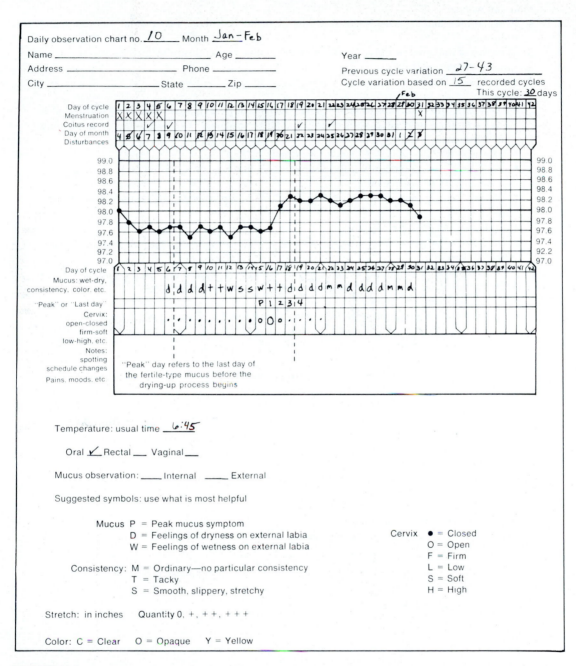

FIGURE 11-1

Example of a completed sympto-thermal contraceptive method chart. (From Bobak and Jensen.[13])

EVALUATING FERTILITY: SEXUAL HISTORY

The most important diagnostic tool in a fertility evaluation is a complete and comprehensive patient history. This should include the following:

Man and woman

1. Personal information: (name, age, sex, education, marital status, occupation, environmental exposures)
2. Duration of impaired fertility, length of contraceptive and noncontraceptive exposure
3. Prior marriages or children
4. Past physical health

Woman

- Menarche, interval, and duration for last menstrual period, regularity of menstrual periods, symptoms associated with cycle (i.e., Mittelschmerz, cramping, signs of impending menstruation)
- Infectious diseases of pelvis, cervix, or vagina
- Obstetric history, number of pregnancies and/or abortions, time to initiate each pregnancy, complications of pregnancies
- Previous tests performed for infertility (medication, laparoscopy, abdominal or pelvic surgery)
- Chronic and hereditary diseases
- Drug use or exposure (i.e., diethylstilbestrol [DES], ibuprofen, alcohol, nicotine, recreational drugs)
- Psychosomatic evaluation (general and specific to infertility)
- Environmental exposure (metals, dyes, drugs, radiation, anesthetic gases)
- Stress (physical and emotional)
- Sexual practices and knowledge (frequency of intercourse, duration of exposure, use of lubricants; positions used; postcoital activities [douching]; areas of concern about sexual relationship; awareness of optimal sexual practices for conception)

Man

- Urogenital history (age, duration of infertility, history of prior paternity, testicular trauma, mumps, torsion, cryptorchidism, surgery)
- Sexual practices and knowledge (frequency of intercourse, normal erectile and ejaculatory function; positions used; areas of concern about sexual relationship; awareness of optimal sexual practices for conception)
- Systemic illnesses and/or medications
- Drug use or exposure (i.e., alcohol, recreational drugs)
- Environmental exposure (metals, dyes, drugs, radiation, anesthetic gases, Agent Orange, occupational toxic chemicals)

5. Psychosocial status (stressors related to infertility)
   - Why do they each want children?
   - How has infertility affected their relationship?
   - Are their expectations realistic?

DIFFERENTIAL DIAGNOSIS

Reproductive disorder; e.g., congenital defect, hormonal imbalance, endometriosis versus systemic disorder; e.g., endocrine condition.

Table 11-1

MALE SERUM HORMONAL PROFILE IN INFERTILITY EVALUATION

T	FSH	LH	Diagnosis
Low	High	High	Primary hypogonadism
Low	Low	Low	Secondary hypogonadism
Normal	Normal	Normal	Germ cell aplasia
High	High	High	Androgen insensitivity
Normal	Normal	Normal	Nonendocrine cause

T = testosterone
FSH = follicle stimulating hormone
LH = luteinizing hormone

EXAMINATION OF THE MALE

As with the female partner, an infertility evaluation of the male begins with a comprehensive history to determine factors that may have affected his fertility. Physical assessment should include a review of systems with focus on those areas that might indicate an infertility diagnosis, i.e., endocrine disorders, testicular abnormalities, epididymal disorders, varicocele, and prostate or seminal vesicle disorders. The infertility workup may include a physical exam, with special attention to habitus and fat and hair distribution.

Genital tract inspection and exam should include the penis and urethra; scrotal size; position, size, and consistency of testes, epididymis, and vasa deferentia, serum hormonal profile (Table 11-1), semen analysis (Table 11-2), and testicular biopsy, among others. Presence of a varicocele will provide further information upon which to make a diagnosis.

PHASES OF FERTILITY EVALUATION

The series of tests usually conducted to evaluate fertility proceeds in three phases:

PHASE 1   The physician performs a postcoital test, examining the environment of the vagina and cervix; the cervical mucus, the motility of the man's sperm, and the woman's hormone levels are evaluated.

PHASE 2   The uterine cavity and fallopian tubes are evaluated; a hysterosalpingogram is performed to visualize these organs and detect any abnormalities. Hormone response within the uterus may be evaluated through an endometrial biopsy.

PHASE 3   Surgical procedures are performed to visualize the uterus, abdominal cavity, ovaries, and fallopian tubes to rule out endometriosis and adhesions. Procedures of choice include laparoscopy and hysteroscopy.

MALE ENDOCRINE DISORDERS THAT INFLUENCE FERTILITY

Hypothalamic disorders

Kallmann's syndrome

Pituitary disorders

Panhypopituitary syndrome (result of trauma surgery or irradiation)
Hypogonadism (low serum follicle-stimulating hormone [FSH], luteinizing hormone [LH], or testosterone levels)
Growth hormone (GH) insufficiency

Testicular disorders

Hypergonadotropic hypogonadism (elevated serum FSH and LH with suppressed testosterone levels)
Idiopathic hypogonadism

Hyperprolactinemia

Adrenal disorders

Adrenal insufficiency
Adrenogenital syndrome
Congenital adrenal hyperplasia

Hypothyroidism (rare)

Table 11-2

NORMAL SEMEN ANALYSIS PARAMETERS

Ejaculate volume	1.5-5 ml
Semen liquefication	Within 30 minutes
Semen pH	7.2-7.8
Sperm concentration	>20 million/ml
Motility	>60% of sperm are moving
Morphology (normal forms)	>60% of sperm are mature and normally formed (without significant WBCs, RBCs, agglutination, or hyperviscosity)
Viscosity	Can be poured from pipette in droplets rather than a thick strand

DIAGNOSTIC STUDIES AND FINDINGS

Diagnostic test	Findings
Female	
Endocrine evaluation	
Follicle-stimulating hormone (FSH)	Elevated with ovarian failure, suppressed with pituitary or hypothalamic disorder *Normal values:* follicular phase 5-20 IU/d; mid-cycle 15-60 IU/d; luteal phase 5-15 IU/d; menopausal 50-100 IU/d
Luteinizing hormone (LH)	Elevated with ovarian failure, suppressed with pituitary or hypothalamic disorder, suppressed with hyperprolactinemia *Normal values:* pre- or post-ovulatory 5-22 mU/ml; mid-cycle peak 30-250 mU/ml
Prolactin	Elevated with hyperprolactinemia; marked elevation may indicate tumor *Normal values:* 20-24, >40-90 if lactating
Serum progesterone level	Collected day 6-8 after ovulation, provides evidence of ovulation *Normal values:* preovulation: 20-150 ng/dl; mid-cycle: 300-2400 ng/dl; pregnancy: >2400 ng/dl
Estradiol (E₂)	Suppressed with endocrine disorder
Basal body temperature (BBT)	Indirect evidence of luteinization noted in biphasal body temperature surge of 0.5° to 0.8° during last 2 weeks of cycle (not definitively diagnostic)
Endometrial biopsy	Obtained within 1 to 2 days of LH surge; detects inadequate progestin production and ovulation, and presence of endometriosis
Serial ultrasonography of pelvis	Dominant follicle; ovulation detected by disappearance of preovulatory follicle (more specific than BBT)
Postcoital (Sims-Huhner) test	Fewer than five highly motile spermatozoa in the upper cervix, inadequate spinnbarkeit, and arborization suggest secretory defect
Evaluation of cervical mucus	Thickening of cervical mucus with tacky character and loss of crystalline fern pattern on drying within 24 hours of ovulation
In vitro SCMI test	Character of cervical mucus using donor sperm and donor mucus; numbers of sperm, assessment of sperm—sperm, cervical mucus interaction (SCMI)
Hysterosalpingogram	Scheduled after menstruation and before ovulation to detect anatomic defects of the uterus and tubes, as well as polyps, tumors, or proximal or distal tubular stenosis (An oil- or water-based dye is infused into the uterine cavity through the cervix. The choice of dye depends on the goals of the examination; the oil-based contrast results in higher subsequent pregnancy rates with generally better imaging, whereas water-based contrast offers greater comfort, better imaging of rugae, and diminished retention when a granuloma is present.)

DIAGNOSTIC STUDIES AND FINDINGS—cont'd

Diagnostic test	Findings
Diagnostic laparoscopy	(See Diagnostic Procedures, Chapter 3) Evidence of pelvic organs, tubal patency, infection, endometriosis, uterine mobility; presence of synechiae or compromising myoma; peritubal adhesions, and/or anomalous growth (congenital abnormality, fibroids, polyps, Asherman's syndrome)
Immunologic compatibility evaluation	Antigen-antibody response between ovum, vagina, and sperm

Male

Testicular biopsy	To distinguish ductal obstruction from parenchymal dysfunction
Vasography (typically combined with testicular biopsy)	Ductal obstruction causing oligospermia or aspermia
Sperm penetration assay (SPA)	To determine fertilization potential for assisted in vitro fertilization procedures; quantifies potential for ovum penetration with or without zona stripping
Mucus migration test	Objective comparison of sperm movement in an in vitro setting; quantifies motility
Venography	Testicular venous reflux, indicating "subclinical" varicocele
Transrectal ultrasound	Abnormal anatomy of accessory sex organs (seminal vesicles, vas deferens); spermatocele or obstruction
Immunologic compatibility evaluation	Antigen-antibody response between ovum, vagina, and sperm

(From Gray.[39])

MEDICAL MANAGEMENT

Management of infertility is provided by different medical specialists; a gynecologist may treat the woman's problems, and a urologist oversees treatment of the man. Reproductive endocrinologists specialize in hormone disorders. They are especially valuable in evaluating and treating infertility and often have the most current methods and information available. Successful management requires that the caregiver establish a rapport with the couple seeking evaluation. The couple should be evaluated together.

The technology involved in treating infertility has escalated in the past 10 years. Various medical protocols and surgical procedures have been developed to correct conditions affecting fertility or to bypass the problem that is preventing conception.

GENERAL MANAGEMENT AND DRUG THERAPY

Dosage regimens are not exact for all women. Dosage regimens must be determined on the basis of expected and actual response to treatment; close monitoring is imperative.

Marked elevation of FSH that is resistant to pharmacotherapy warrants a guarded diagnosis (adoption and other alternatives should be discussed).

Embryo or egg donation.

Clomiphene citrate (Clomid, Serophene) therapy—*Major indication:* Ovulation induction to stimulate production of follicle-stimulating hormone (FSH). Clomiphene citrate stimulates ovulation in as many as 95% of anovulatory women. *Usual adult dosage:* 50 to 100 mg po daily, beginning on cycle days 3 to 7 or 5 to 9. Some patients may be given higher doses to induce ovulation, but incidence of side effects increases as dose increases.

Supplementation of clomiphene citrate with estrogen, corticosteroids, and human chorionic gonadotropin (hCG)—*Major indication:* For ovulation induction to stimulate the luteinizing hormone surge in women who do not respond to clomiphene by itself; hCG is administered at mid-cycle. *Usual adult dosage:* 2,500 to 5,000 IU IM; for infertility patients, 10,000 IU IM may be given at mid-cycle.

MEDICAL MANAGEMENT—cont'd

Therapy with human menopausal gonadotropin (HMG) (Perganol) in combination with hCG—*Major indication*: For women who fail to respond to oral clomiphene therapy; for women who respond with ovulation but fail to conceive; or for women with pituitary or hypothalamic insufficiency. *Usual adult dosage*: 150 IU IM on cycle days 3 to 7, followed by daily dosages. Ultrasonography is used to time the dosage of hCG accurately based on the number of maturing follicles and serum estradiol (E_2) levels.

Progestin injections—*Major indication*: Used in women with amenorrhea. *Usual adult dosage*: A normal endometrium and estrogenic stimulation can be demonstrated with a positive response to one intramuscular injection of 100-200 mg of progesterone or oral Provera, 10 mg daily for 5 days.

Antiinfective medications for pelvic inflammatory disease

Therapy with danazol (Danocrine) for endometriosis—*Major indication*: For endometriosis. *Usual adult dosage*: 200 to 400 mg orally, twice a day, usually for 3 to 6 months.

Therapy with gonadotropin-releasing hormone (GnRH) (Factrel) or its analogs—*Major indication*: Simulates the luteinizing hormone surge in ovulation induction. Helps prepare the endometrium to become more receptive for implantation of ova. *Usual adult dosage*: 20 to 40 µg subcutaneous (by infusion pump) at 2-hour intervals, starting on day 3 of menses.

Intrauterine insemination

In vitro fertilization (IVF) with embryo transfer

Ovum transfer

Gamete intrafallopian transfer (GIFT)

Surrogate motherhood

SURGERY

Corrective surgeries include reversal of tubal ligation or reconstruction of obstructed fallopian tube and surgical or laser resection of endometrial lesions.

Among the most effective surgical procedures are in vitro fertilization (IVF), gamete intrafallopian transfer (GIFT), zygote intrafallopian transfer (ZIFT), cryopreservation, and surrogate motherhood.

IVF, GIFT, and ZIFT address specific problems through follicular stimulation to encourage the development of multiple follicles and resulting ova. The ova are retrieved through laparoscopy-guided aspiration or by transvaginal, transurethral, or percutaneous-transvesicular aspiration using ultrasonic guidance.

With **IVF,** the egg and sperm are combined in a petri dish, where fertilization can occur. They are incubated for 48 to 72 hours, and if conception occurs, the embryo is transferred through a catheter to the uterus. Hopefully the embryo implants in the uterus and continues on to a successful pregnancy.

In **GIFT,** after ova retrieval the ova and sperm are placed in the same catheter and then are injected directly into the fallopian tube. If conception occurs, the embryo travels down through the fallopian tube to the uterus for implantation. **ZIFT** combines the techniques used in IVF and GIFT. The ova are retrieved and placed in a petri dish with sperm. If conception occurs, the zygote is injected into the fallopian tube, travels through the tube to the uterus, and implants in the uterus.

MEDICAL MANAGEMENT—cont'd

OTHER OPTIONS

Cryopreservation is a technique developed to preserve a zygote for future transfer. Physicians are hesitant to return more than four embryos at one time, but often more ova are retrieved. Some couples elect to have the remaining embryos cryopreserved for later transfer. This negates the need for hormonal stimulation and an additional surgical procedure to retrieve eggs in the next attempt.

Surrogate motherhood is used in instances when the woman cannot physically support a pregnancy. Another woman carries the fertilized ovum retrieved from the female partner and fertilized by the male partner's sperm. Other scenarios include any combination of a donated sperm and/or donated ovum, carried to viability by a third person (surrogate mother). The resulting infant must be adopted legally by the couple even if their sperm and/or ovum are used for conception.

1 ASSESS*

ASSESSMENT	OBSERVATIONS
Ovulatory patterns	Frequency of ovulatory/menstrual cycles; occurrence of oligomenorrhea and amenorrhea; use of oral contraceptives
Endocrine abnormalities	Precocious or delayed puberty; abnormal female body habitus; evidence of masculinization; anovulation; polycystic ovaries; chromosomal abnormalities; adrenal or pituitary tumors; hypothyroidism
Pelvic abnormalities	Abnormal vaginal mucosa; evidence of cervical obstruction; uterine/vaginal/fallopian tube obstructions; evidence of congenital uterine/vaginal structural abnormalities
Endometriosis	Pelvic or lower back pain exacerbated during premenstrual period and alleviated by menses; pelvic or lower back pain with positive culture results for pathogens
Pelvic infection	Inflammation and pelvic pain with positive culture results for pathogens

*Nursing care should be well documented in the patient's permanent health care record.

2 DIAGNOSE

NURSING DIAGNOSIS	SUBJECTIVE FINDINGS	OBJECTIVE FINDINGS
Sexual dysfunction related to female factor infertility	Individual or couple reports inability to conceive a child after a reasonable period of anticipatory (unprotected) sexual intercourse	Conception has not been achieved after 1 year of anticipatory (unprotected) intercourse

NURSING DIAGNOSIS	SUBJECTIVE FINDINGS	OBJECTIVE FINDINGS
Knowledge deficit related to optimum techniques for attaining pregnancy	Couple expresses uncertainty about techniques for maximizing likelihood of conception	Couple uses ineffective or suboptimum techniques to promote conception
Low self-esteem, situational, related to infertility	Couple expresses feelings of uncertainty about sexual compatibility or the stability of their relationship	Stated feelings or behaviors reveal feelings of self-degradation or worthlessness related to infertility

3 PLAN

Patient goals

1. Conception will be achieved.
2. The couple will learn effective techniques to maximize the likelihood of conception.
3. The couple will regain their feelings of self-worth.
4. The marital relationship will remain intact and positive.

(From Gray.[39])

4 IMPLEMENT

NURSING DIAGNOSIS	NURSING INTERVENTIONS	RATIONALE
Sexual dysfunction related to female factor infertility	Consult the physician about the fertility potential for the woman with a markedly elevated FSH level; help the couple obtain information about adoption, surrogate pregnancy, and embryo or egg donation.	A significantly elevated serum FSH indicates ovarian failure, with a poor prognosis for fertility.
	Teach the patient to take clomiphene as directed.	Clomiphene stimulates ovulation in as many as 95% of anovulatory women.
	Advise the patient taking clomiphene that follow-up evaluation and care are necessary.	The dosage often must be titrated to stimulate ovulation; combination therapy may be indicated.
	Administer hCG with clomiphene as directed.	HCG may be administered with clomiphene to stimulate ovulation in individuals who do not respond to clomiphene alone; hCG is administered at midcycle, and ultrasonography typically is indicated to time the dosage of the drug accurately.
	Administer HMG as directed.	HMG is administered to women who fail to respond to oral clomiphene therapy, to those who respond with ovulation but fail to conceive, and to women with pituitary or hypothalamic insufficiency; therapy usually is combined with hCG and clomiphene.

NURSING DIAGNOSIS	NURSING INTERVENTIONS	RATIONALE
	Help the woman who is significantly obese or has other life-style factors leading to anovulation to change these habits or reduce body weight as indicated.	Life-style factors or significant obesity can predispose a woman to anovulation; eliminating these factors can significantly increase fertility potential.
	Administer GnRH or an analog as directed.	GnRH or an analog is used to restore ovulation in a woman who does not respond to nonpharmacologic measures to restore ovulation.
	If the patient has hyperprolactinemia in association with pituitary enlargement or hyperthyroidism, arrange for her to consult an endocrinologist.	Hyperprolactinemia can be caused by excessive thyroid secretion or pituitary adenoma; optimum care is delivered by a qualified expert.
	Administer or teach the patient to self-administer bromocriptine as directed.	Bromocriptine reduces idiopathic hyperprolactinemia and increases fertility potential.
	Administer or teach the patient to self-administer progestins as directed.	Progestins are administered as intramuscular injections or suppositories or in micronized capsule forms; progestins may enhance fertility potential in women with inadequate luteal phase function.
	Help the woman with endometriosis to obtain care from a gynecologist as indicated.	Approximately 11% to 20% of women with endometriosis experience anovulation, and the disorder is found in 30% to 40% of infertile women, compared to 15% of fertile women; management of the condition by a qualified specialist may reverse anovulation and improve fertility potential.
	Prepare the patient for myomectomy as directed.	Surgical myomectomy may be used for women with recurrent abortions.
	Prepare the patient for in vitro fertilization (IVF) and related procedures as directed.	IVF is used when more conservative measures to manage infertility prove unsuccessful.
	Prepare the patient for gamete intrafallopian tube transfer (GIFT) as directed.	GIFT is used when more conservative infertility treatment strategies prove unsuccessful.
	Prepare the patient for surgical reconstruction of the fallopian tubes.	Obstruction of the tubes may respond to tubal reanastomosis; reanastomosis is most commonly performed to reverse tubal ligation.

NURSING DIAGNOSIS	NURSING INTERVENTIONS	RATIONALE
Knowledge deficit related to optimum techniques for attaining pregnancy	Teach the couple the basic principles of reproduction, including the woman's menstrual cycle, events that accompany ovulation, and optimum frequency for intercourse.	The timing and frequency of intercourse may exacerbate or produce infertility in certain cases.
	Help the couple seek cultural solutions for culturally related habits that influence the frequency and timing of intercourse.	Typically, cultural remedies for infertility problems can be identified to resolve frequency and timing issues that reduce fertility potential.
Low self-esteem, situational, related to infertility	Encourage both partners to express their feelings about infertility, individually and together; reassure them that these concerns are common and neither negative nor positive.	Expressing feelings allows the couple to identify issues related to low self-esteem and to cope with these feelings rather than blindly respond to them.
	Help the couple obtain medical care for infertility issues as indicated.	Seeking medical care for issues related to infertility provides an opportunity to aggressively and jointly pursue a positive solution to a legitimate health problem.
	Refer the couple with significant self-esteem disorders to a qualified counselor.	Significant self-esteem problems affecting the individual and couple are best managed by a specialist.

5 EVALUATE

PATIENT OUTCOME	DATA INDICATING THAT OUTCOME IS REACHED
Conception has been achieved.	Pregnancy has been attained and sustained, producing a viable infant.
The couple can describe effective techniques to maximize the likelihood of conception.	The couple accurately relates the events of the woman's menstrual cycle and the timing of ovulation; they can accurately state the basic principles of timing and frequency of intercourse.
The couple has regained their feelings of self-worth.	Individually and together, the couple expresses feelings of positive self-evaluation and identifies specific actions to resolve infertility problems.
The marital relationship has remained intact and positive.	Individually and together, the couple expresses a resolve to remain within the relationship and to resolve infertility problems together.

PATIENT TEACHING ▪▪▪▪▪▪▪▪▪▪▪▪▪▪▪▪▪▪▪▪▪▪▪▪▪▪▪▪▪▪▪▪▪▪▪▪

1. Teach the couple the basic principles of conception, including the menstrual cycle and the significance of ovulation.
2. Teach the patient the names, indications, actions, dosage, and scheduling of all medications.
3. Emphasize the significance of and provide written instructions for the dosage and scheduling of endo-crine medications or clomiphene. Help the woman determine her ovulatory cycle as indicated.
4. Teach the woman who measures her basal body temperature about the biphasic temperature rise she can expect, the method to determine body temperature, and the significance of assessing the timing of ovulation.

Contraception

Contraception is the regulation or prevention of fertilization and/or implantation of a fertilized ovum in the uterus.

Regulating or preventing fertilization has been a challenge to the medical community for decades. Moral, legal, and ethical issues of birth control have been debated and remain unsettled. Related health care controversies, including sexual activity, the risk of sexually transmitted diseases, and abortion as a birth control measure, continue to challenge our society. This section reviews contraceptive options without addressing the above issues. Approximately 90% of women between the ages of 15 and 45 are using some form of contraception to prevent pregnancy. Success rates are constantly changing because of periodic noncompliance, use of different lubricants, and use of combination procedures such as barrier methods with spermicides. Tables 11-3 and 11-4 present information on the effectiveness of various types of contraception. Table 11-5 presents contraceptive choices for women over 40.

METHODS OF CONTRACEPTION

Natural, physiologic, or **rhythm methods** are methods of birth control that use knowledge of the menstrual cycle or fertility awareness to schedule periodic abstinence from intercourse. These methods include *basal body temperature* (BBT) records, *calendar methods,* and *cervical mucus testing* (Billings or ovulation method) to estimate the time of ovulation. *Symptothermal techniques* combine BBT with cervical mucus methods. A *fertility awareness method* combines the

symptothermal approach with barrier contraception. Generally, abstinence is recommended for ovulatory days 12 through 16 of the menstrual cycle, plus days 11, 17, and 18 to account for the 48 hours that sperm may live.

Another method, the *predictor test of LH surge*, generally used by couples with infertility problems, has been fairly reliable in identifying the LH surge that usually occurs 12 to 24 hours before ovulation. It is available in a home testing kit, does not seem to be influenced by illness or daily habits, and has proved effective as a means of contraception.

The *basal body temperature (BBT)*, the lowest body temperature of a healthy person while awake, varies during the menstrual cycle and has been used for decades in infertility evaluations to determine the time of ovulation. The BBT falls slightly during menses and for the following 5 to 7 days. If ovulation does not occur, the BBT is maintained at 36.2° to 36.3° C (97.2° to 97.4° F). It drops slightly (0.1° F) 24 to 36 hours before ovulation and rises 24 to 72 hours after ovulation. *Abstinence* is practiced from the end of menses until the BBT has remained elevated for 4 days. The BBT remains elevated until 2 to 4 days before menses.

The monthly thermal shift is most apparent if the temperatures are recorded daily for several months. A biphasic pattern indicates normal ovulation and can be used by infertility patients to time intercourse to improve the chance of pregnancy, or as natural birth control by patients attempting to regulate pregnancy. A monophasic pattern is abnormal and requires additional evaluation. The BBT usually is taken with an oral thermometer before the woman arises in the morning, since the BBT is lowest at that time. The BBT can vary

(text continues on page 226)

Table 11-3

CONTRACEPTIVE CHOICES: EFFECTIVENESS RATES

Method	Theoretical effectiveness (%)	Effectiveness for typical user (%)
Natural, physiologic, or rhythm methods		
No method (chance)	15	15
Abstinence	100	Unknown
Fertility awareness (BBT, calendar, cervical mucus tests, rhythm methods, symptothermal methods)	90-98	65-85
Coitus interruptus	85	75-80
Chemical/barrier methods		
Condoms and spermicides	99	95
Condoms		
Men	98	80-90
Women	98+	85
Diaphragm and spermicide	97-98	80-90
Cervical cap	94	82
Spermicide	97-98	75-85
Contraceptive sponge	90	75-85
Hormonal		
Combined oral pills	99	97-98
Progestin-only pill	99	96-97
Postcoital pill	Unknown	Unknown
Contraceptive implant	99+	99+
Intrauterine device	99	95-97
(IUD)		
Tubal sterilization	99+	99+

Adapted from Hatcher R et al, editors[49]; Thompson J[104]; Payne WA, Hahn DB.[86]

Table 11-4

SUMMARY OF METHODS OF CONTROLLING CONCEPTION

Method	Action	Safety/effectiveness	Effects	Contraindications
Oral contraceptive Combination pill: each pill contains progestin and estrogen; schedule: one pill daily for 21 days, then discontinue for 7 days; placebo may be advised for last 7 days; pill cycle started and repeated on fifth day after onset of menstrual flow	Inhibits ovulation by suppressing pituitary gonadotropin Produces cervical mucus that is hostile to sperm Modifies tubal transport of ovum May have effect on endometrium to make implantation unlikely	Failure results from failure to take pill regularly If woman forgets to take pill one day, she can "make up" by taking two pills next day Chances of pregnancy increased if pill is missed for even 1 day Highly acceptable to users; easy to take Linked with mortality caused by thromboembolus phenomena Does not alter fertility	Useful for relief of dysmenorrhea in 60% to 90% of cases; relief of premenstrual tension; regulation of menstrual cycles; relief of acne in 80% to 90% of cases; improved feeling of well-being Minor side effects (usually decrease after third cycle): weight gain, breast tenderness, headaches, corneal edema, nausea, breakthrough bleeding, hypertension Major side effects: thromboembolytic disorders; may decrease lactation in breast-feeding women	Undiagnosed vaginal bleeding, breast or pelvic cancer, liver disease Use with caution with history of epilepsy, multiple sclerosis, porphyria, otosclerosis, asthma, cardiovascular disease, renal disease, thyroid disease, diabetes, uterine fibroid tumors, smoker, age >40

Intrauterine contraceptive device (IUD or IUCD)
Small objects of various shapes made of plastic, nylon, or steel inserted into uterus; medicated with copper or a progestational agent; most have nylon string attached that protrudes from cervix into vagina; inserted using aseptic technique; follow-up visits in 1 month, then individualized
EXAMPLES
ParaGard (Copper T380A)
Progestesert
	Unknown
	
	Copper may interfere with sperm transport; progestational agent causes progestin effects on cervical mucus and endometrial maturation
		Easily inserted
		Can be inserted any time during cycle; presence of menstrual flow rules out early pregnancy
		Can be inserted immediately postpartum, but expulsion rate is higher
		Can be left in place indefinitely
		Effectiveness highly dependent on ensuring that IUD remains in place; women need to be taught to feel for string after each period
		Spontaneous expulsion occurs most often during menstruation (expulsion rates: 10% to 20%)
		Failure rate (pregnancy) 1.5% to 3% during first year of use; rate declines thereafter
		Does not alter fertility
			Uterine cramping, heavy menstrual flow, irregular menses (NOTE: Usually disappear in 2 to 3 months)
			Problems
			  Infection: usually minor and occurs soon after insertion
			  Perforation of uterus: varies with types of device; highest rates in first 6 weeks postpartum; usually occurs at time of insertion
				Current infection of reproductive tract, uterine fibroids, undiagnosed vaginal bleeding, nulligravida, multiple sex partners

Continued.

Table 11-4

SUMMARY OF METHODS OF CONTROLLING CONCEPTION—cont'd

Method	Action	Safety/effectiveness	Effects	Contraindications
Diaphragm (with spermicidal foam, cream, jelly)				
Rubber dome attached to flexible metal ring; inserted into vagina to cover cervix; available in various sizes (requires careful fitting); self-inserted by user; surfaces and rim of diaphragm coated with spermicide before insertion; inserted no more than 2 hours before intercourse and left in place at least 6 hours after intercourse	Provides mechanical barrier to sperm; spermicidal preparation destroys large number of sperm	Highly effective if fitted properly and used correctly Requires sustained motivation for repeated insertion and removal Refitting necessary after childbirth, surgery of cervix and vagina, or weight change of 10 pounds or more	Difficulty in placing or removing diaphragm	Severe uterine prolapse
Cervical cap				
Flexible, natural rubber device available in various sizes (requires careful fitting); inserted by user; inserted any time between 40 hours to 30 minutes before intercourse and left in place at least 8 hours (but no longer than 48 hours) after intercourse	Provides mechanical barrier to sperm	Highly effective if fitted properly and used correctly Requires 30-90 minutes' education time to learn insertion procedure Requires sustained motivation for repeated insertion and removal	Potential for Pap test conversion from normal to abnormal at 3 months' follow-up (use of cervical cap is discontinued if this occurs)	Cervical dysplasia with abnormal Pap smear; history of toxic shock syndrome; concurrent vaginal or cervical infection
Condom				
Thin, flexible latex worn over penis; available without prescription; does not require medical supervision	Provides mechanical barrier to prevent sperm from entering vagina; prevents spread of venereal diseases	Effectiveness increased with use of diaphragm by woman Effectiveness decreased by tearing or slipping of condom during intercourse and by use of condoms without a reservoir end Failure rate: 10% to 15%	None	None
Natural family planning (ovulation, symptothermal, Billings method)				
Periodic abstinence from intercourse during fertile periods of menstrual cycle; days 12 to 16 before expected date of menstruation are possible ovulating days; because sperm can survive up to 48 hours, days 11, 17, and 18 added to fertile period	Sexual abstinence around time of ovulation	Safe Fertile period varies; precise time of ovulation not known Effectiveness increased with calculation of fertile period, high motivation to prevent pregnancy, determination of basal body temperature, and observation of mucous secretions' consistency	Frustration; lack of sexual gratification during period of abstinence	Irregular menstrual cycles; medical contraindications to pregnancy

Table 11-4

SUMMARY OF METHODS OF CONCEPTION CONTROL—cont'd

Method	Action	Safety-Effectiveness	Effects	Contraindications
Chemical contraceptive (jellies, creams, foams, suppositories) Applied inside vagina by means of plunger-type applicator or aerosol spray	Contains spermicidal ingredients; partial barrier to entrance of sperm into cervix	Effectiveness increased when used with diaphragm or condom Easily available without prescription Effectiveness depends on dispersion of substance within vagina	Irritation to skin or mucous membrane	None
Levenorgestrel subdermal implant (Norplant) Six Silastic capsules are implanted in the patient's arm; each capsule contains 36 mg of crystalline levonorgestrel	Inhibits ovulation by suppression of pituitary gonadotropin Produces thick cervical mucus that is hostile to sperm	Contraceptive failure rarely occurs	Irregular bleeding, spotting, or amenorrhea may occur in the first year	Hypertension; history of thromboembolism, valvular heart disease; should not be inserted within the first 6 weeks postpartum; same as for oral contraceptives
Injectable medroxyprogesterone (Depo-Provera) Intramuscular injection of long-acting progestogen of 150 mg every 3 months	Inhibits ovulation	Efficacy similar to surgical sterilization	Amenorrhea may occur in women after 1 year of use	Should be used by women only for long-term deferral of pregnancy; takes average of 22 weeks to ovulate after injection
Vaginal sponge Sponge is inserted adjacent to cervix and releases spermicide	Water activates sponge and facilitates insertion; spermicide is released for 24 hours	At least 6 hours should elapse after last intercourse before removal of sponge Sponge must be discarded after use and is not reusable	Irritation and allergic reactions in 2% to 3%; some increased risk of candidiasis; difficult removal reported in 6% of users	None
Vaginal sheath (female condom) Sheath is made of natural latex rubber with flexible rings at both ends; device is a combination of a diaphragm and condom; closed end of pouch is anchored around cervix, and open ring covers labia	Provides mechanical barrier to prevent sperm from entering vagina and cervix Spermicide jelly, foam, or cream should be added before intercourse	Effectiveness in excess of condom and diaphragm May provide more protection than condoms against sexually transmitted diseases	Relatively loose sheath provides heightened sensation for the man	None

Table 11-5 _____

BIRTH CONTROL CHOICES FOR WOMEN OVER 40

	Birth control method	Birth control effectiveness*
Protection from STDs	**Barrier/chemical methods**	
	Diaphragm plus spermicide	82%-98%
	Cervical cap plus spermicide	82%-98%
	Sponge containing spermicide	72%-90%
	Condom	82%-90%
No protection from STDs	**Intrauterine devices (IUDs)**	
	With copper or progestin hormone	94%-99%
	Oral hormonal methods	
	Birth control pill, low-dose estrogen plus progestin hormones	99%
	Long-acting hormonal methods	
	Progestin hormone implant or injection	99%
	Permanent methods	
	Sterilization (tubal ligation)	99%
	Natural methods	
	Periodic abstinence	81%-86%

*Effectiveness when used as directed.

as a result of fatigue, jet lag, stress, trauma, infection, alcohol consumption, and sleeping in a heated bed or under a ceiling fan (Figure 11-2).

Using the *calendar method* is more risky in that ovulation may vary, and using past data to predict future ovulation is not always accurate. This method is most successful when a record of a woman's menstrual cycle has been kept for 1 year before the method is used for contraception. To determine the beginning of the fertile time, 18 days are subtracted from the length of the shortest cycle of the year. The end of the fertile period is calculated by subtracting 11 days from the longest cycle. Intercourse should be avoided from day 5 to day 20 of the woman's menstrual cycle. Because ovulation occurs around day 14, plus or minus 2 days, this method identifies a relative range of safety. However, ovulatory activity is particularly variable during the first few weeks postpartum, during lactation, and during the time near menarche and menopause.

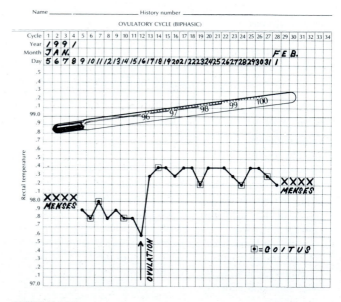

FIGURE 11-2
Special thermometer for recording BBT, marked in tenths to enable a person to read it more easily. Basal temperature shows drop and sharp rise at time of ovulation. Biphasic curve indicates ovulatory cycle.

Table 11-6 _____

CERVICAL MUCUS CHARACTERISTICS ACCORDING TO MUCUS TYPE AND TIME OF CYCLE

Mucus type and time of cycle	Amount	Viscosity	Color	Spinnbarkeit (cm/in)
Dry days—postmenstruation	Moderate	Thick	Cloudy, yellow, or white	<2.5 (1 in)
Onset of mucus symptoms and cloudy or sticky secretion—nearing ovulation	Increasing	Somewhat thick to thin	Mixed cloudy and clear	2.5-3.75 (1-1½ in)
Peak symptoms—ovulation	Maximum	Very thin and slippery	Clear	15-20 (6-8 in)
Postovulation (about 3 days)	Decreasing	Thin	Mixed cloudy and clear	10-15 (4-6 in)
Tacky mucus—nearing menstruation	Minimal	Thick	Cloudy	<2.5-3.75 (1-1½ in)

From Stenchever.[101]

CALENDAR METHOD CALCULATIONS

BEGINNING OF FERTILE TIME	END OF FERTILE TIME
Shortest cycle	Longest cycle
23 days	31 days
−18	−11
5th day	20th day

Example shows that abstinence should be practiced from day 5 until after day 20 of the cycle.

The *cervical mucus (Billings or ovulation) method* involves an evaluation of cervical mucus from the vaginal introitus to predict ovulation. Before ovulation, the cervical mucus is thin, clear, and watery. During or just preceding ovulation, the mucus becomes thicker, more abundant, and "stretchy" and can be pulled like taffy 5 cm or more (spinnbarkeit). Sperm survives well in this mucosal environment. A woman should analyze her mucus several times a day and keep an accurate record of monthly changes before using the characteristics of cervical mucus to predict ovulation. The fertile time begins with the appearance of slippery mucus and lasts for approximately 72 hours. The characteristics of the cervical mucus can be changed by sperm, water-soluble lubricants, contraceptive foams or jellies, and vaginal infections such as yeast infection or candidiasis (Table 11-6).

Chemical/barrier methods involve the use of spermicides to kill sperm and mechanical barriers to obstruct the passage of sperm through the cervical os. These methods may be used alone, or they may be combined for greater effectiveness.

Chemical methods involve the use of spermicidal *foams, creams, jellies,* and *suppositories* to kill sperm. The woman inserts her choice of chemical deep into her vagina with an applicator before she has sex. There are some concerns about the efficacy of chemical barriers: their efficacy may be decreased if foam cans are not shaken well, or if intercourse occurs too soon (within 10 to 30 minutes) or too late (1 hour) after insertion; and reapplication is needed if coitus is repeated. Unfortunately, local irritation or allergic reactions may occur, and the risk of monilial infection (yeast infection or candidiasis) increases. Over-the-counter spermicides and sponges usually contain excellent brochures that describe insertion guidelines and removal procedures, if needed. Some spermicides are inserted with tampon-type devices.

Mechanical barrier methods include *diaphragms, cervical caps,* and *male* and *female condoms (vaginal sheaths).* All these devices are used to block sperm from passing through the cervical os to fertilize an ovum, and all work best when used with spermicidal foams, creams, or jellies.

The *diaphragm* is a latex, dome-shaped cap that covers the cervical area. It must be fitted to the individual woman, and insertion requires teaching and practice. A diaphragm should be inserted no more than 2 hours before intercourse and should be left in place for at least 6 hours after intercourse.

The *cervical cap* is smaller and thicker than a dia-

CONDOM USE EFFECTIVENESS

Condom use efficacy increases when these precautions are taken:

Avoid storing condoms in extreme conditions, such as heat or direct sunlight.

Open and handle condoms gently, and avoid tearing them with sharp objects (jewelry) or fingernails.

Keep sand, dirt, or abrasive substances away from the condoms.

Use prelubricated condoms when possible, since they are usually less likely to tear and break.

Safe **lubricants that don't cause damage to latex condoms include:**

K-Y Jelly	H-R Lubricating Jelly	Probe
Duragel	Lubafax	Personal Lubricant
Astro-Glide	Ortho-Gynol	Koromex Gel
Carbowax	Transi-Lube	Glycerin U.S.P.
Intercept	Silicones DC 360	Norform Insert
Semicid	Condom-Mate	Lubrin Insert

Substances that cause *damage* to condom latex in less than 1 hour include:

Mineral oil	Baby oil	Petroleum jelly
Suntan oils	Palm oil	Insect repellants
Burn ointments	Hemorrhoidal ointments	Rubbing alcohol
Olive oil	Peanut oil	Corn oil
Margarine	Sunflower oil	Coconut oil
Dairy butter	Fish oils (cod, shark)	Monistat vaginal cream
Vagisil ointment	Estrace vaginal cream	Femstat vaginal cream
Rendell's Cone vaginal spermicide	Pharmatex Ovule vaginal spermicide	Premarin vaginal cream
		Sexual lubricants: Elbow and Hot Elbow Grease; Shaft

Adapted from material available from Planned Parenthood, Inc.

---

phragm. It comes in four sizes and must also be fitted. It may be difficult to insert. Like diaphragms, cervical caps, once inserted, provide an immediate barrier. The cervical cap may be inserted 40 hours to 30 minutes before intercourse. It should be left in place for at least 8 hours after intercourse but should be removed within 48 hours. The spermicidal sponge usually contains non-oxynol-9, which kills sperm. The sponge also blocks and absorbs sperm. The sponge is effective immediately and continues to provide protection for 24 hours.

Condoms seem to have an added benefit—protection against the spread of sexually transmitted diseases (STDs). They may also help reduce the occurrence of premalignant changes of the cervix. Condoms are best used in conjunction with a spermicide. The *male condom,* or penile sheath, has been used for hundreds of years. It covers an erect penis, leaving room at the end, or tip, for ejaculated fluid. The newer *female condom (vaginal sheath)* combines the features of a diaphragm and a sheath condom. After coitus, care should be taken while removing the condom to prevent leak-

age of semen. See the box above for effectiveness of condoms.

Intrauterine devices (IUDs) are mechanical barriers, usually made of plastic, that are inserted into the uterus. Although considered mechanical barriers, they work by irritating the uterine wall, preventing implantation of the fertilized ovum. Insertion usually is done during menses, when the cervix is partly open. A string or beads hang from the cervix into the vagina to provide a means of checking that the IUD remains in place. These devices also may contain copper or progesterone to prevent implantation.

Hormonal methods of contraception are used primarily to prevent ovulation by altering the fluctuation of hormones required for maturation of the ovum and ovulation. Estrogen and/or progesterone steroids suppress the hypothalamus and the anterior pituitary, causing changes in the production of gonadotropin-releasing hormone (GnRH), follicle-stimulating hormone (FSH), and luteinizing hormone (LH). Without the usual fluctuation of estrogen and progesterone, not enough FSH and LH are secreted to cause follicle maturation and ovulation. Hormonal methods also change the motility of the tubes and uterus, which impairs transport of the egg and sperm.

Hormonal contraceptives also may alter the endometrium and prevent implantation. Withdrawal of these steroids at monthly intervals causes the uterine lining to be shed with menses. "The pill" typically contains both estrogen and progestin. "Mini pills" contain only progestin. Lower dose contraceptives produce fewer side effects. Menstrual problems such as premenstrual syndrome (PMS), dysmenorrhea, menorrhagia, iron-deficiency anemia, and irregular or prolonged periods appear to decrease with hormonal regulation. A decrease may also be seen in endometrial adenocarcinoma, breast disorders, ovarian cysts, gonorrheal pelvic inflammatory disease (PID), and osteoporosis.

The *oral contraceptive*, commonly known as "the pill," is a popular form of birth control. Taking one pill a day is less disruptive than using natural, chemical, or mechanical methods of contraception. It is also convenient to know when menstruation will occur.

Every body system appears to be affected by oral contraceptives. Of women taking oral contraceptives, 1% to 15% develop hypertension and must stop taking them. Oral contraceptives should also be discontinued if headaches are associated with their use. Cerebrovascular accident (CVA, or stroke) has been associated with women who smoke and use oral contraceptives.

Other contraindications for taking steroidal birth control medications are a history of cigarette use and age over 35, nonsmokers over age 45, vascular disorders, hypercholesterolemia, breast cancer, sickle cell disease, diabetes, hypertension, and renal, liver, or gallbladder disease. The correlation between neoplastic disease and the use of oral contraceptives has not been established. There may be an association between the use of hormonal steroids and infertility, and VACTERL syndrome (vertebral, anal, cardiac, tracheal, esophageal, renal, and limb anomalies).

Women taking the "mini-pill," or *oral progestins*, report more irregular bleeding. *Implantable progestins* may also cause irregular bleeding. Subcutaneous implants of time-released progestogen may produce fibrosis or encapsulation at the tissue site. Other side effects reported are prolonged amenorrhea, uterine bleeding, and vascular or thrombolytic disorders. Chloasma (brown patches on the skin), permanent facial pigmentation, weight gain, nausea, and depression are possible side effects of hormonal contraception.

Another hormonal method of contraception uses several different *injectables* that can be instilled monthly, every 2 to 3 months, or every 6 months. These may be more convenient and reliable than oral

contraceptives or barrier methods, but once injected, the dose cannot be easily reversed or controlled. Another method involves the use of *subdermal implants* containing time-released biodegradable pellets inserted under the skin, much like a subdermal injection. These implants require a minor surgical incision to remove. *Contraceptive vaginal rings* (CVRs) have also been used. These are donut-shaped, soft, pliable plastic devices that contain steroids. They are inserted and removed by the woman, resulting in easy reversibility. Increased vaginal discharge, pressure sensations, and accidental expulsion may occur with CVRs.

Postcoital contraception, or the "morning-after pill," decreases the risk of pregnancy when taken within 72 hours of midcycle coitus. These high-dose estrogens (e.g., ethinyl estradiol plus norgestrel [Ovral] and diethylstilbestrol [DES]) probably prevent the blastocyst from implanting into the endometrium. High-dose progestins may have a similar action. Menses may also be induced with RU 486, if the drug is taken later in the menstrual cycle. It may prevent implantation or cause the fertilized zygote to be expelled and reportedly has fewer side effects than other postcoital contraceptives.

Estrogen agents (DES) and the "morning-after pill" have teratogenic effects if the pregnancy is not terminated. Severe nausea; abdominal, chest, and leg pain; headaches; dizziness and weakness; and vision and speech problems may occur. Postcoital pills may aggravate pathologic conditions of the liver and breast.

Surgical contraceptive techniques interrupt the route of the egg or sperm. These techniques usually are considered permanent sterilization. *Tubal ligation* is one of the most common methods. A portion of the fallopian tubes is separated or cut. The surgery can be performed as a laparoscopic procedure in a same-day surgery or ambulatory surgical setting, or shortly after childbirth in the hospital setting. The failure rate (pregnancy) is about 1 in 300 women after tubal ligation. Even though tubal ligation is considered a permanent means of sterilization, reversal of the procedure may have a success rate as high as 70%. *Hysterectomy* is another permanent, surgical method of sterilization in which the uterus and cervix are removed. The ovaries usually are not removed unless a pathologic condition exists.

Abortion is a controversial method of birth control. First trimester abortion typically is done by aspirating intrauterine contents, by either dilation and curettage (D & C) or vacuum aspiration. Second trimester abortion may require drug instillation or hysterotomy. Hypertonic saline solutions and prostaglandins are used to facilitate expulsion. The complications of surgical procedures include hemorrhage, infection, and risks associated with anesthesia.

1 ASSESS*

ASSESSMENT	OBSERVATIONS
History	Age, reproductive data, previously used contraception, current birth control measures, if applicable; life-style information; body image concept
Physical examination	Any systemic disorder or disease that may influence contraceptive choice; breast and gynecologic health
Psychosocial	Anxiety or concern associated with knowledge deficit about contraception

*Nursing care should be well documented in the patient's permanent health care record.

2 DIAGNOSE

NURSING DIAGNOSIS	SUBJECTIVE FINDINGS	OBJECTIVE FINDINGS
Knowledge deficit related to fertility and fertility control	Verbalizes myths or asks for information about menstrual cycle, fertility, and/or fertility control	Patient or couple states misinformation or ineffective contraceptive methods
Anxiety related to risks of pregnancy and/or contraceptive methods	Reports fear of pregnancy or anxiety over possible side effects of contraceptive choice	Withdrawn expression, perspiration, elevated vital signs
High risk for body image disturbance related to contraceptive choices	Reports negative feelings about self associated with birth control techniques	Poor eye contact, folded arms, or withdrawn movements
Decisional conflict related to choice of birth control method	Expresses uncertainty about contraceptive use and desire to change method or switch to a more convenient, reliable technique	Statements reveal concern over selecting birth control method

3 PLAN

Patient goals

1. The patient and couple will understand the woman's menstrual cycle, concepts of fertility, and contraception.
2. The patient will acknowledge her fears and learn about contraceptive choices that minimize her risks.
3. The patient will have a positive body image and self-confidence related to contraceptive use.
4. The patient/couple will choose a contraceptive method appropriate to their needs, or accept and plan for a pregnancy.

4 IMPLEMENT

NURSING DIAGNOSIS	NURSING INTERVENTIONS	RATIONALE
Knowledge deficit related to fertility and fertility control	Help patient and couple identify myths and dispel misinformation.	To clarify what is known and what needs to be learned about reproduction and contraception.
Anxiety related to risks of pregnancy and/or contraceptive methods	Describe the menstrual cycle, and explain the risk of pregnancy during the fertile time.	To provide physiologic information.
	Discuss contraceptive choices, and describe the risks of the methods identified as possible choices for the patient and couple.	To provide information about the advantages and disadvantages of contraceptive choices.
High risk for body image disturbance related to contraceptive choices	Encourage discussion of self-concept as it relates to contraception.	To identify and correct ineffective body image or self-concept.
Decisional conflict related to choice of birth control method	Encourage and answer questions; allow time for the patient and couple to select a choice.	To help relieve tension or anxiety associated with decision making.

5 EVALUATE

PATIENT OUTCOME	DATA INDICATING THAT OUTCOME IS REACHED
Patient and couple understand fertility and fertility control.	Patient can determine the probable fertile period in her menstrual cycle and discuss how hormonal control devices decrease the chance of fertility.
Patient's fears about pregnancy and contraception have been alleviated.	Patient reports no anxiety about pregnancy or contraception.
Patient has self-esteem with regard to her sexuality and birth control technique.	Patient shows self-confidence with regard to her body and choice of contraception.
Patient's anxiety about selecting a contraceptive method has been alleviated.	Patient and couple select and implement contraceptive choice.

PATIENT TEACHING ■ ■ ■ ■ ■ ■ ■ ■ ■ ■ ■ ■ ■ ■ ■ ■ ■

Natural, physiologic, or rhythm methods

1. Describe basal body temperature (BBT), and explain how to take and graph morning temperatures; explain thermometer calibrations.
2. Have the woman demonstrate how to take and record her temperature.
3. Using a raw egg white, demonstrate mucus stretching; provide a chart that describes the monthly changes in vaginal mucus; explain that the fertile period lasts 72 hours after a positive spinnbarkeit result; teach the patient good handwashing techniques to prevent infection.
4. Have the woman describe and report monthly changes in mucus, especially the appearance of slippery, fertile mucus.
5. Describe the calendar method, and have the woman keep a monthly record; recommend that this record be kept for at least 1 year, and schedule frequent visits to address questions and review the record kept by the patient and couple.

Chemical/mechanical barrier methods

1. Describe the different chemical/barrier methods; encourage the woman to read all package inserts.
2. Have the patient describe the effectiveness range for spermicidals (i.e., wait 10 to 30 minutes after insertion before intercourse, but no longer than 1 hour).
3. When appropriate discuss how barriers, especially condoms, may decrease the risk of sexually transmitted diseases.

Hormonal methods

1. Discuss warning signs and side effects (e.g., mid-cycle bleeding and headaches).
2. Discuss the importance of routine screening examinations.
3. Encourage the patient to ask questions; describe long-term risks and help the patient and couple assess future family planning needs.

CHAPTER 12

Therapeutic and Elective Procedures and Surgeries

Surgical interventions for women usually are directed toward three goals: diagnosing or removing abnormal tissue; restoring or improving anatomic structures; and relieving unpleasant symptoms. Procedures may involve relatively minor excisions, such as removal of a Bartholin's gland cyst, or more complex surgery, such as a mastectomy, repair of prolapse, or sphincter reconstruction. Diagnostic and therapeutic options may overlap in function. For example, a dilation and curettage (D & C) may reveal the cause of, as well as correct, dysfunctional bleeding. Elective procedures usually are aimed at improving anatomic structures and body image.

BREAST REDUCTION

Breast reduction involves removing breast tissue (Figure 12-1). It may be done for therapeutic or cosmetic reasons.

The first known procedure was performed in 1923 in Germany to remove the lower half of the breasts and raise the nipples and areolae of a woman with breast hypertrophy. In 1931 the skin excision and wide lateral undermining of breast tissue resulted in recorded complications of decreased skin and nipple vascularity. The modern age of breast reduction began in 1956 with pre-operative marking and keyhole patterns, which were used to ensure contour. These techniques are still used, as are nipple removal and replacement (free graft) after superfluous breast tissue and skin have been removed. A *mastopexy* may be done to remove stretched skin without removing breast tissue. Sagging breasts may be elevated, and excess nipple-areolar tissue may be removed and realigned.

Women with kyphosis or other postural problems, muscle distortion that causes ulnar paresthesia, respiratory difficulties, or disturbed body image are candidates for therapeutic breast reduction or mastopexy.

233

Breast reduction

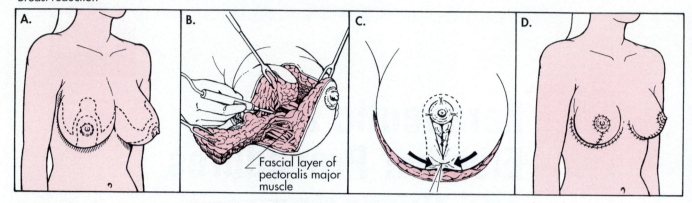

FIGURE 12-1
Breast reduction. **A,** Preoperative markings. **B,** Excess breast tissue is excised. **C,** Skin flaps are thinned and approximated at the inferior margin. **D,** A smaller breast size and improved contour are achieved.

Women wishing to breast-feed may not be candidates for free nipple grafts (complete removal and reattachment of the nipple). If malignancy is present, a mastectomy rather than reduction usually is recommended. Breast reduction does not seem to reduce the risk of breast cancer.

In rare cases hematoma, infection, fat necrosis, and nipple or skin necrosis occur after breast reduction surgery. Other possible complications are asymmetry, scarring, loss of nipple sensation, or thealgia (pain) when the nipple is touched.

NURSING CARE

See pages 238 to 240.

BREAST REMOVAL PROCEDURES FOR CANCER

The surgical treatment for breast cancer is determined by the size of the tumor, whether it has spread, the woman's age and physical condition, and her preference of treatment.

A *lumpectomy,* or *partial mastectomy,* is the removal of a tumor with a wide excision, or margin of healthy tissue (Figure 12-2). A *quadrantectomy* is the removal of a tumor with about one fourth of the breast tissue. Partial breast tissue removal resembles wedge-resection techniques. A *subcutaneous mastectomy* (adenomammectomy) involves removing the breast tissue but leaving the skin and nipple-areola complex intact. In a *simple mastectomy,* the breast tissue and nipple are removed but the skin, underlying chest muscles,

and axillary lymph nodes are not. In a *modified radical mastectomy,* the breast tissue and nipple are removed, but some soft tissue, axillary lymph nodes, and overlying skin are left. A *radical (Halsted) mastectomy* is the total removal of subcutaneous tissue, breast tissue, nipple, skin, muscles, fat, fascia, and lymph nodes. In an *extended radical (supraradical) mastectomy,* the structures involved in a radical mastectomy are removed plus the parasternal lymph nodes.

A lumpectomy with radiation therapy may be an option if the malignant lesion is less than 5 cm or is classified stage II or lower. A modified radical procedure may be indicated if the lesion is localized and small. Prophylactic mastectomies involving total removal of subcutaneous breast tissue have been performed in women with a strong family history of breast cancer in an attempt to eliminate the chance of the disease developing. This practice is very controversial among cancer specialists.

Radical and prophylactic mastectomies may be contraindicated if the woman has severe body image concerns, if she has low risk factors, and if the cancer has been detected early. However, conservative procedures are not recommended for women with risk factors such as a family history of breast cancer, previous benign breast disease or atypical hyperplasia, previous malignancy, or exposure to radiation.

Complications include hemorrhage, infection, tissue necrosis, contractures, deformity, and loss of sensation. Severe muscular and nerve complications are rare but may occur.

NURSING CARE

See pages 238 to 240.

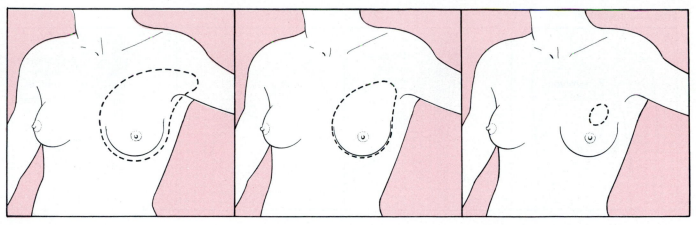

Radical mastectomy   Modified radical mastectomy   Lumpectomy

FIGURE 12-2
Shown above are the areas of tissue removed in a radical mastectomy, a modified radical mastectomy, and a lumpectomy. In a simple mastectomy (not shown), the breast and some nodes are removed. (From Belcher.[9a])

BREAST RECONSTRUCTION

Breast reconstruction is the placement of a soft prosthetic device under the skin, with transplanted tissue often used to form a nipplelike structure. Today reconstruction is more common than in years past. This cosmetic surgery produces a more natural (although not perfect) breast formation after a mastectomy or in cases of congenital absence of breast tissue.

Reconstruction may be an option at the time of mastectomy, although it may be delayed if axillary lymph nodes test positive for cancer. Some women prefer reconstruction over an external prosthesis, which may dislodge. Other indications for reconstruction are congenital or acquired (e.g., through trauma) deformity resulting in the absence of the breast and/or nipple complex, the women's expressed dissatisfaction with her breasts, poor body image, and dysfunctional sexuality.

If the woman has had a mastectomy for cancer, the cosmetic result usually is better if reconstruction and augmentation are performed after chemotherapy and radiation treatments. With some mastectomy procedures there may not be enough tissue or structural support to allow reconstruction.

Several complications may occur. Previously used silicone implants apparently cause long-term immunologic side effects. A number of operations may be required to achieve satisfactory reconstruction. Skin and fat necrosis and hernias may occur, and previous cancer treatments or skin graft complications may result in poor skin and tissue healing.

NURSING CARE
See pages 238 to 240.

BREAST AUGMENTATION

Breast augmentation, or *mammoplasty,* is a procedure to enlarge the breasts. A bilateral augmentation mammoplasty (BAM) may be an outpatient or a same-day surgery procedure. Historically many procedures have been attempted for enlarging the breasts. Prostheses are placed above or beneath the pectoralis major muscle (Figures 12-3 and 12-4). Breast examinations and mammograms are more accurate when prostheses are placed under the muscle.

Breast augmentation is a very common procedure in the United States. The typical woman requesting a bilateral augmentation mammoplasty is married, has children, and is in her thirties. The main indicator for elective breast surgery is the woman's expressed dissatisfaction with her appearance. Physical deformities such as congenital defects (breast hypoplasia or microplasia and agenesis) may cause body image deficiencies.

Some women may have unrealistic expectations of how augmentation will change their body image, personality, or life-style. Counseling may be needed to supplement cosmetic treatment.

As with all surgical procedures, there are risks of

Breast augmentation

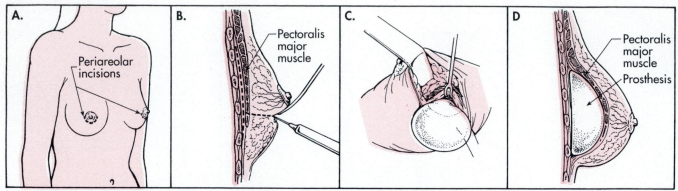

FIGURE 12-3
Breast augmentation. **A,** A periareolar incision allows the scar to be concealed at the border of the pigmented areolar skin. **B,** The incision is made through the breast parenchyma. **C,** A pocket is created below the pectoralis major muscle, and the saline prosthesis is inserted. **D,** Cross-section showing the prosthesis in place.

> For color plates of complications of breast implants, see Color Plates 1, 2, and 3 on page x.

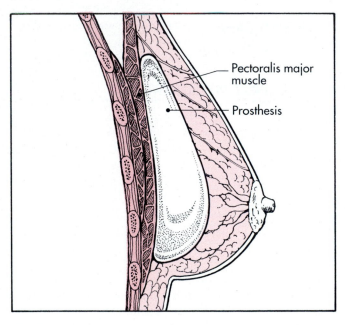

FIGURE 12-4
Breast implant anterior to pectoralis major muscle.

hemorrhage, hematoma, infection, and complications from anesthesia. Mammoplasties may be performed using a local anesthetic, which avoids the risks of general anesthesia. However, with a local anesthetic, the patient may feel some discomfort when the muscle is cut and separated. Surgical alteration of the nipple and breast tissue may impair breast-feeding. Nipple discomfort and numbness may develop if a circumareolar incision is performed. Capsular contractures occur more frequently when the implants are outside the subpectoral area. Silicone leakage may result in severe complications.

NURSING CARE

See pages 238 to 240.

HISTORY OF BREAST AUGMENTATION

Date	Material/procedure	Complications
1890	Liquid paraffin (injection)	Several hard pieces of paraffin dislodged in breast; cysts and sinuses formed; skin necrosis developed; breast condition masked other breast disorders
1895	Breast replaced with lipoma from woman's back	Transplanted benign fat tumor was reabsorbed, leaving a flat breast
1900s	Liquid silicone (injection)	Hard irregularities and deformities developed, similar to paraffin complications; breast condition masked development of other breast disorders
1950s	Polyvinyl, Ivalon sponges	Open-cell sponges caused fibrous growth, hardness, irregularities, and infection
1962	First use of teardrop-shaped, thin-walled, gel-filled sac (position held by tissue ingrowth to posterior wall of fixation patch)	Fixation patch caused capsule contraction; thin-walled sac permitted leakage of gel ("gel bleed")
1964	Gel-filled silicone bag of heat-stable, inert rubber (dimethylsiloxane)	Capsular contractures develop around prosthesis
1965 to 1970s (increased use of silicone for nearly 30 years)	Introduction of single-lumen saline; inflatable implant	Produces less capsular contracture than gel-filled bag; saline is reabsorbed, leaving flat breast
Early 1970s	Beginning use of silicone gel implants with thin layer of polyurethane	"Host" reactions develop, such as inflammation
1980s	Double-lumen adjustable implant with gel-filled inside and outer saline lumen	Capsular contracture rate was similar to that for single-lumen implant
1900s to present	Suction-assisted lipectomy (fat from abdomen and hips is transplanted into breast)	Fat often reabsorbs, leaving large cystic cavities and calcifications that mimic pathologic conditions

COMPLICATIONS OF BREAST IMPLANTS

Approximately 100,000 women a year have cosmetic breast surgery, adding to the 2 million women who already have breast implants. About 40% of these women develop complications, such as rupture or leakage, painful breast hardening, infection, allergic or immunologic reactions, and malignant tumors. Additional surgery often is required.

For many years silicone was considered harmless and biologically inert. Silicone injections and implants were used for breast augmentation in women and transsexual males, and for breast reconstruction after a mastectomy. It is now known that individuals with silicone breast implants may develop a systemic immunologic disease (implants filled with saline do *not* cause systemic reactions). The symptoms associated with this immunologic disease are: foreign body granulomas in the breast and liver; abnormal liver function tests and elevated blood sedimentation rate; biliary cirrhosis; scleroderma; Sjögren's syndrome; general lymphadenopathy; spleen and lymph node enlargement; cervical lymphadenopathy; histologic findings of hyperplastic lymph nodes and granulomas; laboratory results showing antinuclear antibodies and increased lymphocytes, histiocytes, and multinucleated giant cells; nervous system involvement (weakness, attention span deficit, fatigue, insomnia); weight loss; multiple chemical sensitivities syndrome; joint and synovial tissue discomfort; arthritic (polyarthritic) symptoms, including joint and finger edema; connective tissue disease; symptoms similar to those of systemic lupus erythematosus; histopathologic results showing giant cell and vacuole macrophages in removed breast implants.

Gel leakage may result in flat, distorted, or asymmetric breasts. If the implants are successfully removed, the above symptoms may regress or subside. It appears that some people develop an allergic-immunologic reaction to polyurethane and silicone.

1 ASSESS*

	OBSERVATIONS			
ASSESSMENT	**BREAST REDUCTION**	**BREAST REMOVAL**	**BREAST RECONSTRUCTION**	**BREAST AUGMENTATION**
History and preoperative physical manifestations	Large or sagging breasts; postural problems or muscle distortion from heavy breasts	Malignancy present; mastectomy needed	Postmastectomy with adequate tissue for reconstruction	Small breast size or absent breast tissue
Postoperative physical manifestations	Smaller breasts with possible change in nipple location	Absent unilateral or bilateral breasts with possible skin and nipple removal	Breast enlargement with possible tissue transplantation to reconstruct a nipplelike complex	Augmented breasts with possible nipple relocation
Psychosocial	Anxiety associated with knowledge deficit of preoperative and postoperative procedures, and body image disturbance.			

*Nursing care should be well documented in the patient's permanent health care record.

2 DIAGNOSE

NURSING DIAGNOSIS	SUBJECTIVE FINDINGS	OBJECTIVE FINDINGS
Body image disturbance related to breast changes	Reports feelings of disfigurement or altered attractiveness; dissatisfied with outcome	Body language withdrawal; covering of or protective motions over breast(s)
Pain (discomfort) related to breast surgery	Describes breast pain, tingling, tenderness, and factors that may increase or decrease discomfort	Facial expressions of pain; tense muscle tone; guarding or protecting chest area; elevated vital signs or diaphoresis; dilated pupils
High risk for impaired skin integrity related to breast surgery	Reports discomfort, drainage, itching, or pain at incision site	Inflammation, redness, drainage, edema, excoriated incision site

3 PLAN

Patient goals

1. The patient will accept the change in her breasts and her new body image.
2. The patient will have no pain or discomfort.

3. The patient's skin will heal well without infection.

4 IMPLEMENT

NURSING DIAGNOSIS	NURSING INTERVENTIONS	RATIONALE
Body image disturbance related to breast changes	Discuss with patient her expectations of the breast surgery outcome.	To help patient clarify expectations and accept surgical outcome.
Pain (discomfort) related to breast surgery	Explain methods for relieving pain (e.g., relaxation, chest support, changing position).	To decrease need for analgesics.
	Assist with analgesic administration if needed.	To relieve severe pain.
High risk for impaired skin integrity related to breast surgery	Provide, teach, and encourage hygienic measures; apply sterile dressings and antibiotic ointments as needed.	To reduce risk of infection.

5 EVALUATE

PATIENT OUTCOME	DATA INDICATING THAT OUTCOME IS REACHED
Patient has accepted the change in her breasts and body image.	Patient verbalizes acceptance of breast condition.
Patient is comfortable and has no pain or discomfort.	Patient reports no pain and shows no guarding or facial expressions of discomfort.
Patient's skin has healed and shows no signs of infection.	Skin color and turgor are normal; skin shows no signs of infection or unusual deformity.

PATIENT TEACHING

General Guidelines

1. Provide preoperative teaching, as appropriate for any surgery.
2. Review the patient's expectations before and after surgery; show her before and after pictures of other patients; locate support groups as appropriate.
3. Discuss common side effects of breast surgery, such as the potential for impaired breast-feeding.
4. Encourage the patient to ask questions, since unrealistic expectations may surface and provide an opportunity for teaching and psychologic preparation for the surgical outcome.

Breast Reduction

Discuss ways to improve side effects of having large breasts (e.g., practice good posture), and suggest exercises to improve diminished muscle tone.

Breast Removal

Discuss various removal procedures (lumpectomy, partial and radical mastectomy); explain why invasive carcinoma requires more aggressive treatment.

PATIENT TEACHING

Breast Reconstruction

Explain why a reconstructed breast will not look "normal," but that it may appear more natural than a loose prosthesis.

Breast Augmentation

Explain, as appropriate, that enlarged breasts will not necessarily improve body image or sexual relations.

SURGERIES OF THE VULVA AND PERINEUM

A **perineoplasty** is performed to restore normal anatomic structure to the perineum. Surgery is indicated for a congenital defect or an acquired tissue malformation (e.g., episiotomy) that results in either narrowing of the vaginal introitus, causing dyspareunia, or enlargement of the introitus, causing fecal contamination or dissatisfaction with coitus. A narrow or widened introitus may be surgically corrected by incising the midline and loosening or tightening the perineal skin with sutures.

A **hymenotomy** is performed to correct an imperforate hymen or rigid hymenal ring that interferes with menstrual flow or coitus. It is a minor procedure that uses incision techniques to remove hymenal tissue and collected blood and debris. Suturing is usually not needed.

An **anterior colporrhaphy** is performed to repair cystoceles, urethroceles, and/or urinary incontinence.

An incision is made on the midline near the cervix to the urethral meatus. Vaginal epithelium is trimmed and repaired. Complications include urinary retention, urethral stricture, incontinence, fistulas, and cystitis.

A **posterior colporrhaphy** is performed to correct rectoceles and perineal body deficiencies. Surgery involves retracting the vaginal wall, excising the fourchette, and dissecting the underlying fascia. The rectovaginal septum and perineal body are reconstructed. Complications include urinary retention, urethral stricture, incontinence, fistulas, and cystitis.

Urethral and anal sphincter reconstruction may be needed after trauma, particularly childbirth. Rectal surgery is performed by making an H-shaped incision and repairing the fascia and epithelium.

Surgical repair of **genuine stress incontinence (GSI)** may involve vaginal or abdominal procedures and the use of artificial sphincters, slings, or Teflon injections.

Total vulvectomy

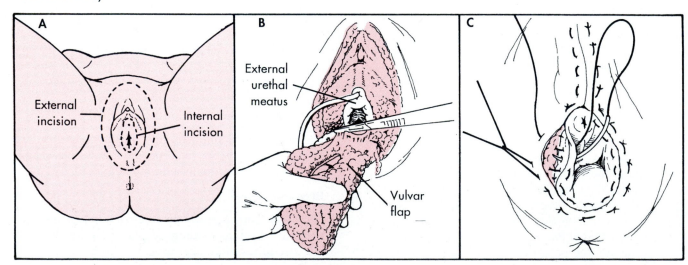

A	B	C
Location of circumscribing lateral and medial vulvar incisions	Posterior dissection involves excision of an appropriate portion of fat	Vulvar wound is closed

FIGURE 12-5
Total vulvectomy. **A,** Location of circumscribing lateral and medial vulvar incisions. **B,** Posterior dissection involves excision of an appropriate portion of fat. **C,** Vulvar wound is closed.

Prolapse repairs may be associated with urethral and anal sphincter reconstruction.

Vaginal vault suspension is performed to correct vaginal vault prolapse, which sometimes is a complication of a hysterectomy. Surgery involves attaching the right sacrospinous or uterosacral ligaments to the vaginal vault.

A **vaginectomy** is performed to treat vaginal intraepithelial neoplasia (VAIN). During surgery cancerous epithelium is removed and the remaining healthy tissue is sutured, or split-thickness skin grafts are used to repair the vagina. Congenital absence of the vagina usually is aided by dilators to lengthen existing tissue. A vaginectomy may not be needed if laser treatment and use of topical 5-fluorouracil succeed in treating VAIN. The risk of surgery increases if general anesthesia is used or with a more extensive reconstruction. Underlying contraindications, such as disease or a pathologic condition, require assessment.

Surgical complications may occur with any of the procedures discussed above. Deformity, infection, and discomfort may result when large amounts of tissue are removed or reconstructed.

A **vulvectomy** is the removal of the vulva (Figure 12-5) to eradicate carcinoma. In a **simple vulvectomy**, the vulva and underlying fatty tissues are removed, but the clitoris is kept intact if possible. In a **radical vulvectomy**, the vulva and groin areas are removed in an attempt to eradicate all invasive carcinoma. Possible surgical complications of a radical vulvectomy include necrosis, edema, hemorrhage, thrombosis, dyspareunia, and introital stenosis.

NURSING CARE

See pages 244 to 247.

VULVAR CYST AND ABSCESS REMOVAL

A **Word catheter** (similar to a Foley catheter) may be used to aid in the treatment of Bartholin's duct abscesses. This procedure may be done using a topical anesthetic or a pudendal block to prevent needle spread of infection. The cystic lesion is punctured, often resulting in a gush of pus or mucoid substance. A culture is done to identify the need for antibiotics. A Word catheter is inserted and left in place for about 2 weeks, so that a new epithelium may develop along the fistulous tract. A topical steroid antibacterial cream may need to be applied for several days before the catheter is removed. The **marsupialization** technique involves suturing the lining of the cyst to the epithelium of the introitus to create a neostoma that does not promote reformation of the cyst or abscess. If cellulitis is present, antibiotics are given.

Catheter drainage procedures and marsupialization may be done to relieve Bartholin's gland abscesses. Bartholin's glands develop cysts or abscesses from infection, tumors, or fluid accumulation. Bartholin's gland cysts are the most common vulvar cysts, and they usually occur unilaterally. Skene's glands may become infected, resulting in enlargement, discomfort, and pus-filled cysts. Epidermal, sebaceous, and sweat gland cysts may also occur in the vulva. These cysts may require incision and drainage.

Repeat surgical intervention may be needed to achieve an epithelialized sinus tract. Acute bartholinitis may result in scar formation or fibrotic tissue.

Cysts and abscesses may cause inflammation, pain, and vulvar deformity. Incision and drainage of a cyst may alleviate the pain only temporarily. Incision and drainage procedures may result in a permanent neostoma. Removal of Bartholin's gland may cause hemorrhage, hematoma, tenderness, restricted activity, and vulvar distortion.

NURSING CARE

See pages 244 to 247.

SURGERIES OF THE UTERUS AND ADNEXA

Women in the United States have approximately twice as many hysterectomies performed as women in Denmark or the United Kingdom. That means that one in every three American women receives a hysterectomy. About 90% of hysterectomies are performed for benign conditions. As many as half of these women have complications, such as infection or urinary problems, and 15% require additional corrective surgery. Approximately 30% of hysterectomies are performed for uterine fibroids, a condition that may not require any treatment. However, hysterectomies performed for cancer treatment or as emergencies to correct hemorrhage may be necessary. Whenever possible, additional tests and medical opinions should be obtained.

A **total hysterectomy** involves the removal of the uterus through the vaginal or abdominal wall (Figure 12-6). A **partial hysterectomy** is the removal of the corpus but not the cervix. A **radical hysterectomy** involves the removal of the uterus, tubes, upper third of the vagina, and possibly the ovaries. A **myomectomy** is the removal of a uterine leiomyoma (benign neoplasm) or a cervical or submucosal myoma. **Uterine septum division** often is done by hysteroscopy to divide the uterine septum within the uterine cavity. **Reconstructive tubal procedures** usually are done by microsurgical techniques during laparoscopic surgery. A **salpingectomy** is the unilateral or bilateral removal of the uterine (fallo-

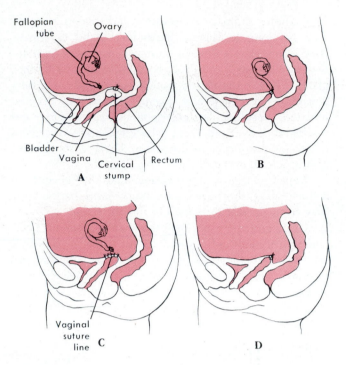

Fallopian tube
Ovary
Bladder
Vagina
Cervical stump
Rectum
A
B
Vaginal suture line
C
D

FIGURE 12-6
A, Subtotal hysterectomy. Note that the cervical stump, fallopian tubes, and ovaries remain. **B,** Total hysterectomy. Fallopian tubes and ovaries remain. **C,** Vaginal hysterectomy. Fallopian tubes and ovaries remain. **D,** Total hysterectomy, salpingectomy, and oophorectomy. Note that the uterus, fallopian tubes, and ovaries are completely removed. (From Phipps.[88])

pian) tubes. An **ovarian cystectomy** is the removal of benign cystic tumors. An **oophorectomy** is the removal of the entire ovary. An **ovarian wedge resection** is the removal of about one third of the ovary.

A radical hysterectomy often is performed when invasive carcinoma is present. Conservative hysterectomy procedures may be commonly indicated for dysfunctional bleeding and endometriosis. Uterine septal and fallopian tube procedures often are performed to improve fertility. A salpingectomy is performed to remove a tubal (ectopic) pregnancy, or it may be indicated for chronic infection (salpingitis) or hydrosalpinx (collection of serous fluid within tube). A bilateral salpingo-oophorectomy (complete removal of both tubes and ovaries) is most often associated with a malignant neoplastic disease or chronic, severe endometriosis. Ovarian surgeries are performed to remove benign cystic tumors or to correct polycystic ovarian syndrome (PCOS).

Radical procedures should be avoided in women wishing to have children, or if malignancy is not present or invasive. Other options should be discussed before invasive procedures are recommended.

Hysterectomy complications may include hemorrhage, infection, inadvertent ligation of the ureter, bladder or bowel transection, or the development of fistulas. Bleeding and infection may occur after myomectomies. Unwanted sterilization may be a consequence for some women who need hysterectomies.

NURSING CARE

See pages 244 to 247.

MINILAPAROTOMY AND STERILIZATION

Tubal ligation is **sterilization** by cutting and tying the uterine tubes. A **minilaparotomy** (laparoscopic, paraumbilical, or belly-button technique) usually is performed as a same-day or outpatient procedure. The procedure takes about 30 to 60 minutes. The patient is placed in the lithotomy position, and a paracervical block usually is given. A local anesthetic is used so that a small incision may be made in the subcutaneous tissue, rectus fascia, muscle, and peritoneum. Trendelenburg's position displaces abdominal contents out of the field of vision and may be used with the lithotomy position. The uterine (fallopian) tube is clearly located and injected with lidocaine, since it usually is sensitive. The **Pomeroy** technique may be used, in which the tube is cut above the clamp, and a piece of the tube is removed for pathologic testing. The ligation is performed bilaterally.

Tubal ligation is available for women who want permanent sterilization. Minilaparotomy techniques are recommended for women post partum.

A minilaparotomy is not usually an option for obese women or women with a history of pelvic disease (such as pelvic inflammatory disease) or previous pelvic surgery. More extensive surgery may be needed to achieve tubal ligation if an underlying pathologic condition exists.

Wound infection and hematomas are rare complications. Inadvertent bladder perforation may occur. Adhesions may develop, especially if the patient has had previous pelvic infections.

NURSING CARE

See pages 244 to 247.

DILATION AND CURETTAGE (D & C)

Metal dilators of increasing size are inserted into the vaginal canal and then the cervical canal. After the cervix has been dilated, curettes are used to scrape or remove endometrial tissue. Curettes have sharp surfaces and can usually empty the entire uterine cavity. Most

D & C procedures can be done as same-day surgery or in an ambulatory outpatient facility.

Dilation and curettage may be needed for a number of diagnostic and therapeutic reasons. For example, scraped endometrial cells may be tested for the presence of cancer or for hormonal imbalances that may be associated with infertility. Tissue may be removed that was causing dysfunctional bleeding. Lost or misplaced intrauterine devices (IUDs) may be retrieved by use of a Randall curette. Incomplete and elective abortions are performed with D & C (or vacuum curettage) procedures.

If pregnancy is suspected and desired, a D & C should be avoided until the status of the pregnancy can be determined. A D & C may be contraindicated if infection is present, since the procedure could spread the organisms.

Hemorrhage or uterine perforation may occur, especially during pregnancy, since the uterus is softer. Infection may occur, resulting in hematuria or a foul vaginal discharge.

NURSING CARE

See pages 244 to 247.

CRYOSURGERY

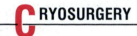

Cryosurgery is a procedure that uses temperature variations to freeze or destroy cells.

The procedure requires a machine that circulates a freezing agent (e.g., nitrous oxide, liquid nitrogen, carbon dioxide snow, liquid oxygen, or Freon) through a pencil or probe. The pencil or probe may be dipped in a transfer agent, such as a lubricating jelly, before it is applied to a small tissue area with moderate pressure for 20 to 30 seconds. The refrigerant solution circulates within the metal probe, and a tingling sensation or mild discomfort may occur. A local anesthetic occasionally is used for the procedure, especially if numerous lesions are present. Analgesics may be used if discomfort occurs during tissue thawing. Tissue necrosis usually occurs within 24 hours of cryosurgery. Crusts develop and drop off within 4 weeks. Scars may develop, since melanocytes are sensitive to freezing.

Cryosurgery has been used successfully to remove such tissue as warts (hyperkeratolytic growths), bunions, cysts, hemorrhoids, and cervical intraepithelial neoplasia (CIN). Conization of the cervix or cryosurgery

may remove atypical cervical tissue and also can rule out invasive cancer that could not be excluded by colposcopy.

Scarring and hyperpigmentation are more likely to occur with overfreezing. Liquid nitrogen may be more painful than other agents. Invasive cancer may resemble cervicitis, and cryosurgery may not remove all of the malignant cells.

Cryosurgery may not remove all of the tissue, and repeat applications may be needed, especially for condylomata. Cervical stenosis may result after cryosurgery to that area. Vaginal discharge may occur following cervical cryosurgery.

NURSING CARE

See pages 244 to 247.

LASERS AND ELECTROSURGERY

Lasers are light amplification from electromagnetic radiation. Waves of infrared light are controlled by the discharge of carbon dioxide, nitrogen, or helium gas. A microscope, carbon dioxide laser probe, and suction device to remove tissue fumes are used. A **loop electrosurgical excision procedure (LEEP)** is done with a triangular wire loop electrode. Other electrosurgical techniques, such as electrodesiccation, are used to remove tissue and control bleeding for dermatologic conditions. A local anesthetic is often required. **Electrolysis** (epilation) is removal of hair through high-frequency alternating electrical currents that destroy the hair follicle.

A laser is more likely to be used to destroy large or deep lesions. Lasers also may be able to destroy lesions that have not been successfully treated with cryosurgery, such as chemical-resistant condylomata. LEEP is used to biopsy ectocervical tissue, to excise endocervical areas, and to remove intraepithelial neoplasia of the genital tract. Electrolysis often is performed by lay people, and hand-held galvanic epilators remove hair without severe pain or scarring.

Bleeding, pain, and scarring occur more frequently with laser treatments than with cryosurgery. Cancer may spread after laser procedures or cryosurgery. Laser treatments are more expensive than cryosurgical procedures.

NURSING CARE

See pages 244 to 247.

SUMMARY OF INITIAL POSTOPERATIVE NURSING INTERVENTIONS FOR MOST ABDOMINAL AND MAJOR GYNECOLOGIC SURGERIES

To evaluate major organ functions and to promote tissue perfusion

Monitor, record, and report vital signs and bowel sounds

Observe surgical site or sites and note and report drainage, hemorrhage, or signs of infection

Observe for signs of potential complications such as paralytic ileus, ligation of ureter from surgical procedure, and thrombophlebitis

Avoid high sitting positions or leg pressure from pillows, bending, or crossing the legs

Encourage use of antiembolic stockings

Encourage movement and ambulation, but prevent orthostatic hypotension

To monitor and promote fluids and nutrition

Administer parenteral fluids as needed

Monitor swallowing reflex and bowel sounds, and progress from NPO to fluids and then to foods as appropriate and tolerated; encourage a high-fiber, high-protein diet, when tolerated, to promote tissue healing

Keep accurate intake and output records, and report and treat inadequate fluid balance, output, or hydration

For indwelling catheters, provide hygienic care and monitor output

Monitor for signs of urinary retention or distended bladder

Promote urination, especially immediately after removal of an indwelling catheter; explain that recatheterization (straight/in and out) may be needed

Use rectal tubes or Harris flush to alleviate flatus, and stool softeners and laxatives as needed to prevent constipation and tissue damage

To promote comfort and prevent associated complications

Monitor breath sounds and encourage coughing, deep breathing, and gradual increases in activity to prevent respiratory complications

Assist with hygienic measures to promote comfort and rest and to decrease the risk of infection

Provide analgesics, if needed, to promote movement and to facilitate comfort so that other pain-relieving techniques may be encouraged

---

1 ASSESS*

OBSERVATIONS

ASSESSMENT	CRYOSURGERY, LASER TREATMENT, AND ELECTROSURGERY	SURGERIES OF THE VULVA AND PERINEUM	SURGERIES OF THE UTERUS AND ADNEXA	MINILAPAROTOMY, STERILIZATION, AND D & C
Physical and psychosocial manifestations	Hyperkeratolytic growths, superficial lesions, excessive or inappropriate hair growth	Anatomic malformation, organ prolapse, sphincter relaxation, cancer	Endometriosis, cancer, tumors and cysts, infertility, configuration problems	Reproductive choice, hemorrhage, pain, discharge, misplaced IUD
Psychosocial	Anxiety associated with knowledge deficit of preoperative and postoperative procedures, and body image disturbance.			

*Nursing care should be well documented in the patient's permanent health care record.

2 DIAGNOSE

NURSING DIAGNOSIS	SUBJECTIVE FINDINGS	OBJECTIVE FINDINGS
Body image disturbance related to perceived unattractiveness	Reports feelings of disfigurement or unattractiveness	Body language withdrawal; covering or protecting of disfigurement or hair growth
Pain (discomfort) related to gynecologic or cosmetic surgery	Describes pelvic and/or back pain and factors that increase or decrease discomfort	Facial expressions of pain; tense muscle tone; guarding or protecting behavior; elevated vital signs or diaphoresis; dilated pupils
High risk for impaired skin integrity related to gynecologic or cosmetic surgery	Reports discomfort, drainage, itching, or pain at incision site	Inflammation, redness, drainage, edema, excoriated incision site

3 PLAN

Patient goals

1. The patient will accept her new body image and gynecologic choices.
2. The patient will have no pain or discomfort.

3. The patient's skin will heal well without infection.

4 IMPLEMENT

NURSING DIAGNOSIS	NURSING INTERVENTIONS	RATIONALE
Body image disturbance related to perceived unattractiveness	Discuss with patient her expectations of the surgical outcome.	To help patient clarify expectations and accept the surgical outcome.
Pain (discomfort) related to gynecologic or cosmetic surgery	Explain methods for relieving pain (e.g., relaxation, chest support, changing position).	To decrease need for analgesics.
	Assist with analgesic administration if needed.	To relieve severe pain.
High risk for impaired skin integrity related to gynecologic or cosmetic surgery	Provide, teach, and encourage hygienic measures; apply sterile dressings and antibiotic ointments as needed.	To reduce risk of infection.

➔ ❯ ❯

5 EVALUATE

PATIENT OUTCOME	DATA INDICATING THAT OUTCOME IS REACHED
Patient has a positive self-concept and body image.	Patient verbalizes acceptance of gynecologic or cosmetic outcome.
Patient is comfortable and has no pain or discomfort.	Patient reports no pain and shows no guarding or facial expressions of discomfort.
Patient's skin has healed and shows no signs of infection.	Skin color and turgor appear normal; skin shows no signs of infection or unusual deformity.

PATIENT TEACHING

General Guidelines

1. Provide preoperative teaching, as appropriate for any surgery.
2. Review the patient's expectations before and after surgery; show her before and after pictures of other patients as appropriate; locate support groups as appropriate.
3. Discuss common side effects of gynecologic and cosmetic surgery, such as the potential for scarring.
4. Encourage the patient to ask questions, since unrealistic expectations may surface and provide an opportunity for teaching and psychologic preparation for the surgical outcome.
5. Discuss the patient's questions about resuming her daily activities, including coitus.

Surgeries of the Vulva and Perineum

1. For surgeries related to or near the bowel, encourage the patient to use stool softeners for 2 to 3 weeks after surgery to aid in defecation, decrease straining, and promote healing.
2. After laser vaporization of vulvar lesions, and as directed following surgery, discuss (if indicated) the use of sitz baths and drying the vulva with a cool blow dryer.
3. After anatomic repairs, discuss the symptoms of complications (e.g., urinary retention, cystitis, and-

fistulas), and emphasize the importance of seeking medical attention.
4. Describe catheterization procedures that may be needed.

Surgery of the Uterus and Adnexa

1. Describe the extent of the surgical intervention (e.g., partial versus total hysterectomy), and explore the need for supplemental estrogen therapy.
2. Discuss the usual need for abstinence and douching for 4 to 6 weeks after a vaginal cuff repair.
3. Discuss the need for frequent walks and avoiding prolonged sitting during recovery from a hysterectomy.
4. Encourage the patient and family to ask questions about options, such as oophorectomy versus ovarian wedge resection.
5. Discuss the use of gonadotropin-releasing hormone (GnRH) analogs before a myomectomy as appropriate.

Minilaparotomy, Sterilization, and D & C

1. Before a tubal ligation, explain that the procedure is considered a permanent sterilization, and assess the patient's understanding of the procedure and its outcome.
2. Describe the spotting and cramping symptoms that may occur after the procedure that are not problem-

atic; also describe the signs of hemorrhage or infection that should receive immediate attention.

3. Explain that coitus and douching may be discouraged for 2 to 3 weeks after cervical dilation.

Cryosurgery, Laser Treatment, and Electrosurgery

1. Discuss the risks of scarring and hyperpigmentation, and help the patient and family explore options.
2. Describe possible blister formation (immediately after carbon dioxide procedure or 5 to 10 hours after liquid nitrogen use).
3. Teach the patient and family about infection control with hygienic measures, by not picking at scabs or puncturing blisters, and by recognizing early signs of infection and seeking medical attention immediately.
4. Discuss methods for avoiding trauma and sunlight after laser treatments.

LIPOSUCTION TECHNIQUES

Liposuction is the removal of fat deposits with suctioning equipment. Suction-assisted lipectomy (SAL) was first used in the 1970s and is now a common cosmetic procedure.

Liposuction is recommended for removing genetically determined fat that cannot be lost through exercise and dieting. Around the age of 40, fat deposits in the face, chest, abdominal area, hips, and legs appear to be most responsive to liposuction techniques. Women generally have the most excess fat accumulation in their hips and thighs, or trochanter areas. Liposuction may be done to obtain symmetry after therapeutic surgery, such as unilateral removal of a malignancy and surrounding tissue from the hip area. Liposuction has been used to decrease insulin requirements for some diabetics.

Obese individuals usually are not candidates for liposuction. Weight loss is recommended before SAL, so that body contour and fat deformities are more pronounced and the risks associated with obesity, such as cardiac and digestive disorders, can be limited.

Liposuction carries operative risks often associated with surgical techniques, such as infection, bleeding, or even death. Breast enlargement from fat transplantation may fail because of local reactions or reabsorption. Postoperative pulmonary complications occur more frequently in smokers.

NURSING CARE

The patient undergoing liposuction requires specific nursing care related to the surgery, and individualized care related to the alteration in body image. Preoperative teaching includes discussion of the liposuction procedure and any other procedures to be performed. It should prepare the patient for the surgical procedure, normal postoperative care and expectations, and any possible complications.

The patient's activity should be limited for about 48 hours after surgery. Discomfort usually can be relieved with a nonaspirin analgesic. The patient's immediate postoperative appearance may distress her. She should be informed that initially the site may appear hard or dimpled, but that it will become smoother and softer. Often the area of liposuction is wrapped with an elastic bandage for 1 to 2 weeks.

Liposuction is performed for individuals seeking a change in body image. This is a variation of the alteration in body image experienced with the loss of a body part. Similar nursing care is warranted. The nurse must be sensitive to the patient's nonverbal responses to the procedure. The nursing care plan should include supporting the patient's decision and assisting her in accepting the new image.

TRANSGENDERED INDIVIDUALS

Health care professionals working with the general population will encounter individuals who have accepted an alternative gender. Nurses must be understanding of the needs of these individuals and professional in their interactions. Nurses must be able to interact in a professional manner, permitting the patient to reveal her/his sexual orientation or gender identification without fear of condemnation or ridicule.

Individuals who have accepted an alternative gender (from the one assigned at birth) are considered transgendered. They consider themselves "trapped" in the wrong gender. This is not a simple choice of gender to them. They feel that they have no real choice but to seek gender reassignment. Transgendered individuals seeking gender reassignment must first undergo extensive psychologic counseling and pass a "true life" test, living the role of the "corrected" gender for a specified length of time. (The male-to-female transsexual is considered here, since this is the individual who will seek health care as a woman. When dressed as a woman, the transgendered person is a **she;** when dressed as a man—a **he.**)

Each individual must decide what degree of medical and/or surgical intervention he/she requires to be able to live in the "correct" gender. Many seek surgical correction of genitalia, whereas some assume the "corrected" gender full-time and have hormonal therapy but no surgical intervention. The goal of the transsexual is to make whatever transition is needed for a happy, productive life-style as easily and as economically as possible. Transsexuals seek to make their outward appearance match their inner view of themselves. The process is very expensive—financially and emotionally.

The preoperative (preop) transsexual and the nonoperative (nonop) transsexual will appear to be the same. The nonop transsexual has gone through the "true life" test and has decided to continue to live in the "correct" gender and not undergo the danger and expense of surgery.

After the "true life" test has been passed, hormonal therapy can be instituted to initiate breast development and increase muscle mass. Other treatments are extensive and conducted over a period of time. Treatment may include electrolysis, tracheal shave, rhinoplasty, removal of the testicles and/or penis, and various other plastic surgical procedures to assist in sexual reconstruction. Sexual reassignment surgery for the male-to-female transsexual may include construction of a vagina, shifting of the urethra, and construction of the labia.

Complications may occur at any stage of the gender reassignment process—during counseling or during any stage of the medical or surgical procedures. If unable to pass the "true life" test, the individual is not considered a good candidate for intervention. Medically, estrogen side-effects may develop (i.e., nausea and skin pigmentation). The surgical risks are similar to those of any major surgical procedure.

Both the postop and nonop transsexual live full-time in their new gender, are undergoing hormone therapy, and usually have had their names changed. Their employers (and perhaps even their families) may or may not know of their change.

NURSING CARE

Nurses must be able to interact with these patients in a professional manner, permitting the patient to reveal her/his sexual orientation or gender identification without fear of condemnation or ridicule. Understanding the psychosocial aspects of the decisions and processes the transsexual individual must undergo will assist the nurse in planning for the health care of this population.

The major nursing concern is to assist the transsexual patient in dealing with the distress associated with changing the outward expression of his/her sexual identity. Nursing interventions include making sure that the patient knows the options available; referring patients to support groups and counseling services; exploring the patient's expectations with him/her; preparing patients for medical and surgical procedures once decisions about the extent of intervention have been made; and supporting patients through the series of procedures required for gender/sexual reassignment (see Chapter 14, Health Promotion for Women, for additional information).

*Adapted from Frye[35b] and Rothblatt.[93a]

CHAPTER 13

Life Cycle Changes

THE PROCESS OF FEMALE MATURATION

Women's health care generally is focused on the nonpregnant adult woman. However, childhood, menarche, pregnancy, menopause, and the postmenopausal years are defined by anatomic and physiologic parameters that are different from those for an adult nonpregnant woman. Changes in the breasts and genitalia throughout the life cycle are contrasted in the following boxes. Breast changes are illustrated in Figure 13-1.

Puberty

Pubescence is the prepubertal growth that usually occurs in spurts during the 2 years preceding puberty. **Puberty** is the age of sexual maturity. *Postpubescence* is the 1 to 2 years after the first menses, when the reproductive cycle becomes established and regular and skeletal growth ends. *Adolescence* is a more general term referring to the period that begins with the growth of secondary sex characteristics and ends when this somatic growth stops. Adolescence is the stage in which psychologic and social maturation occurs. The box on page 252 summarizes the physical and psychosocial development of the maturing young woman.

Many variables can influence sexual maturity, such as nutrition, genetics, physical activity, sanitation and hygiene, climate, environmental light, and congenital or pathologic conditions. The age of menarche has decreased over the past three or four decades, for reasons not fully understood. Puberty in girls occurs between the ages of 8 and 14 years. This developmental stage generally concludes within 3 years. During puberty *thelarche* (breast development) occurs, usually followed in 2 to 6 months by *adrenarche*, or the development of axillary and pubic hair.

Menarche (first menses) usually begins 2 to 2½ years after puberty or at the appearance of secondary sex characteristics (those characteristics that distinguish the sexes without being directly involved in reproduction). Menarche is also known to occur approximately 1 year after peak height velocity, or 6 months after peak

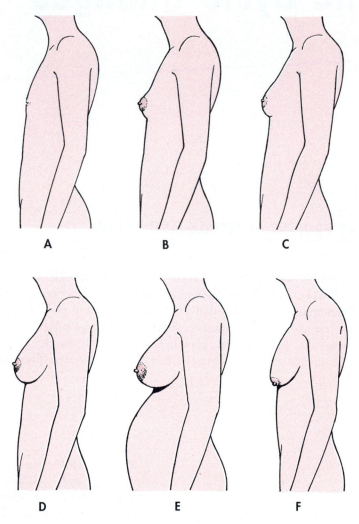

FIGURE 13-1
Appearance of the female breast in various life stages. **A,** Appearance before age 10. **B and C,** appearance between ages 10 and 14. **D,** Appearance of the nulliparous adult breast. **E,** Appearance of the breast during pregnancy. **F,** Appearance of the breast after menopause.

BREAST VARIATIONS THROUGHOUT THE FEMALE LIFE CYCLE

Infant	Child	Adolescent	Pregnant woman	Older woman
Newborns' breasts may be enlarged from estrogen exposure in utero Enlargement of 1-1.5 cm; usually disappears in 2 weeks "Witch's milk" (nipple discharge) may occur	Nipples of girls and boys are similar Chest is smooth, even, and symmetric	Breasts may be tender to touch when developing Initially buds appear Breasts are small and firm; one side may grow slightly faster Areola diameter increases Nipples are more erect, should point symmetrically Breasts grow to protruding, full shape in early adulthood Nipples and areolae become pinker or darker	Breasts may enlarge two to three times during pregnancy Tenderness may occur Breasts have lobular, generalized coarse consistency Superficial veins become prominent Vascular spiders may appear Striae (silver-white or pale lines) may appear Nipples may enlarge and become more erect Areolae darken and broaden Yellowish colostrum is expelled from nipple Lactating deviations include engorgement, skin warmth, pain, inflammation, nipple fissures, and clogged milk ducts	Breasts become stringy, irregular, pendulous, and nodular Borders are less well delineated Breasts may shrink, become flatter, elongated, and less elastic Ligaments weaken Nipples are positioned lower

weight velocity. The average age of menarche in North America is 12½ years.

The mechanism that causes puberty is not fully known. Apparently a central nervous system (CNS) inhibitory factor in the hypothalamus keeps the *hypothalamic-pituitary gonadotropins* dormant during childhood. Hormonal changes appear to begin with the hypothalamus, which stimulates the anterior pituitary gland (adenohypophysis) to release gonadotropins (Figure 13-2). When the gonads are stimulated by gonadotropins, estrogen and progesterone (sex hormones) are secreted from the ovaries. Ovulation generally is established 12 to 24 months after menarche. Puberty appears to correlate with bone age. The first visible sign of puberty in girls usually is the appearance of breast buds. Peak height velocity generally precedes menarche, although growth usually slows after menarche.

The pineal gland (in the middle of the forehead within the brain) produces melatonin, which suppresses gonadal (ovarian) development. In the past the pineal gland was referred to as "the seat of the soul" or "the third eye." It may not be the center of the "soul," as previously thought, but it does seem to be associated with bodily functions. For example, the production of melatonin apparently fluctuates with circadian rhythms. Environmental factors such as photosynthesis change the body's circadian rhythms, which in turn suppress pineal gland production, thus suppressing gonadal and pubertal development.

Normal development of the pubic and axillary hair is caused by increased production of adrenal 17-ketosteroids, dehydroepiandrosterone (DHEA), and DHEA-sulfate (or DHEAS).

PHYSICAL AND PSYCHOSOCIAL DEVELOPMENT OF THE MATURING FEMALE

8-14 years (puberty)	14-20 years (late adolescence)	20 years and older (postadolescence)
Growth: Rapid growth peaks; secondary sex characteristics appear	*Growth:* Growth slows; adult height is attained; structure and reproductive growth are complete	*Growth:* Physical growth is complete; sexual maturity has been reached
Cognition: Has limited concrete and inductive thinking	*Cognition:* Thinking processes include deductive and abstract reasoning; can perceive future implications of behavior	*Cognition:* Can perform complex problem solving; separates fantasy from fact
Identity: Tries various roles; is susceptible to peer pressure; conforms to group norms	*Identity:* Has narcissistic-idealistic fantasies	*Identity:* Body image and gender role definition are secure; self-esteem, physical growth, and social roles have been defined
Superordinate relationships	*Superordinate relationships*	*Superordinate relationships*
Parents: Parents control dependence and independence boundaries	*Parents:* Major parent-child conflicts over independence arise	*Parents:* Has resolved physical and emotional separation from parents
Peers: Conflicts arise in friendships of both sexes	*Peers:* Behavior standards are set by peer group; can be sexually attractive and attracted	*Peers:* Relationship is characterized by giving and sharing; can form lasting alliances
Sexuality: Tries self-exploration; may engage in limited dating and intimacy	*Sexuality:* Has many relationships on various levels; makes decisive declaration of sexual preferences	*Sexuality:* Desires intimacy and commitment rather than exploration and romanticism
Emotionality: Has wide mood swings with outwardly expressed anger	*Emotionality:* Introspective; may withdraw when upset; has difficulty asking for help	*Emotionality:* Has developed emotional constancy; anger is often repressed

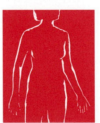

FIGURE 13-2
Hormonal interaction between hypothalamus, pituitary, and gonads. (From Whaley and Wong.[107c])

PATHOPHYSIOLOGY

Pathophysiologic conditions associated with puberty may be related to an exaggeration of physical conditions normally seen during this time. For example, acne may be severe and cause body image disturbance, or it may lead to secondary skin infections. Tallness from a genetically determined growth pattern may occur, causing problems for some girls.

A pathologic condition of the hypothalamus, gonads, or pituitary gland may interfere with puberty. Congenital and pathologic conditions may be more apparent at puberty. For example, Turner's syndrome (caused by the absence of an X chromosome) results in shortness, amenorrhea, and undeveloped secondary sex characteristics.

Primary amenorrhea secondary to inadequate release of gonadotropin-releasing hormone (GnRH) and anosmia (loss of smell) is known as Kallmann's syndrome. Primary amenorrhea with or without breast development and an absent uterus and/or vagina occurs in XY genotypes (phenotypically female with large breasts, immature nipples, and no pubic or axillary hair) and müllerian agenesis (normal breasts, nipples,

VARIATIONS IN GENITALIA THROUGHOUT THE FEMALE LIFE CYCLE

Infant

Vagina: small, narrow tube; few epithelial layers
Clitoris: small
Uterus: 35 mm long
Cervix: two thirds the length of the uterus
Ovaries: small, nonfunctioning, almond shaped, 2-4 mm wide and 10 mm long; contain 700,000 to 2 million ova
Labia majora: hairless
Labia minora: thin, avascular, pale
Hymen: thin tissue inside introitus

Child

Genitalia grow at varying rates
Clitoris remains unchanged until hormonal changes at puberty
Oocytes decrease to 400,000
Ovarian ligaments form outer ovarian layer of connective tissue

Adolescent

Vagina lengthens, epithelial layers thicken
Vaginal secretions become more acidic
Clitoris is more erectile
Uterus, ovaries, and tubes grow
Uterine musculature and vasculature networks increase
Endometrial lining thickens
Uterus reaches true pelvis at puberty
External genitalia assume adult proportions
Labia minora become more vascular
Labia majora and mons pubis develop hair, usually during breast development
Hymen about 1 cm if intact
Adult hypothalamic-pituitary rhythmic cycle established
Ovulation occurs monthly
Adipose tissue develops over hips
Pelvic bones widen
Axillary hair develops

Pregnant woman

Uterus enlarges (due to estrogen and progesterone, then growing fetus)
First trimester: uterine fundus pushes on bladder
Muscular walls become more elastic and stronger
Uterus rises out of pelvis into abdominal cavity
Pelvic ligaments become softer and stronger
Uterine blood and lymph flow increases, causing congestion
Uterus, cervix, and isthmus soften
Cervix turns bluish
Vagina becomes violet in color, walls thicken
Smooth muscle cells hypertrophy
Vaginal secretions become more acidic
Vagina may appear gaping

Older woman

Ovarian function decreases
Menstruation stops at 40-55 years of age (may still be fertile, or ovulation may stop 1-2 years before menopause)
Menopause is completed 1 year after menses stops
Uterine size decreases, endometrium thins
Ovarian size decreases to 1-2 cm
Follicles disappear, surface convolutes
Labia and clitoris become smaller (decreased estrogen)
Labia majora become flatter
Pubic hair becomes sparse and gray
Genital skin becomes shinier, dryer
Vaginal introitus constricts
Vagina narrows, shortens, loses rugation, and becomes pale
Mucosa becomes thinner, dry
Vaginal walls may lose structural integrity
Cervix becomes small, pale
Rectovaginal septum becomes smoother, thinner, pliable
Ligaments and connective tissue may lose tone and elasticity
Pelvic support may weaken

and hair). About 40% of müllerian agenesis is related to renal anomalies. Rare enzyme defects such as 17-alpha-hydroxylase deficiency and 17-20-desmolase deficiency may result in amenorrhea. Pituitary causes of amenorrhea may result from damaged cells (e.g., anoxic damage) or lack of secretion of luteinizing hormone (LH) and follicle-stimulating hormone (FSH). Neoplasms that secrete prolactin, acromegaly (excessive secretion of growth hormone by the pituitary gland), and Cushing's syndrome may also result in amenorrhea.

Primary amenorrhea and delayed menarche may result from a number of other factors, including strenuous athletic activity and reduced body fat, infections, and stress. Heavier girls tend to begin menarche before lean ones, and physical maturation may be delayed in some adolescents involved in strenuous athletics. Sev-

eral factors may be interrelated and associated with delayed menarche, including minimal levels of critical body fat, delayed hypothalamic-pituitary or LH secretory patterns, and sleep-related disorders. In about 90% of delayed puberty cases, no cause is found.

Precocious puberty often is difficult to define because of the normal range of variation when puberty begins. Generally, puberty that begins before age 8 in girls is considered precocious. In approximately 80% to 90% of cases, no cause is apparent. The normal hypothalamic actions associated with puberty occur, and subtle cerebral abnormalities may be found. Precocious puberty is probably the result of a central nervous system (CNS) dysfunction.

Early development of secondary sexual characteristics with an increase in the size and activity of the ovaries is known as "true" precocious puberty; it is referred

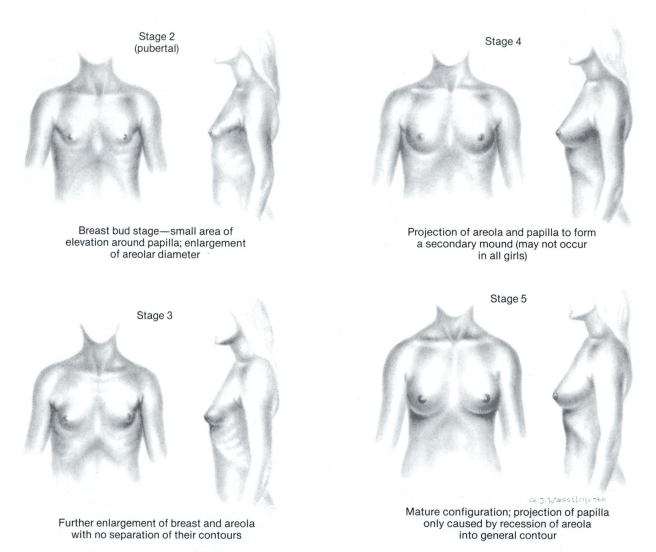

Stage 2 (pubertal)

Breast bud stage—small area of elevation around papilla; enlargement of areolar diameter

Stage 3

Further enlargement of breast and areola with no separation of their contours

Stage 4

Projection of areola and papilla to form a secondary mound (may not occur in all girls)

Stage 5

Mature configuration; projection of papilla only caused by recession of areola into general contour

FIGURE 13-3
Development of the breasts in girls—average age span, 11 to 13 years. Stage 1 (prepubertal—elevation of papilla only) is not shown. (Modified from Marshall WA, Tanner JM[76a]; and Daniel WA, Paulshock BZ.[28a])

to as "pseudopuberty" when there is no change in the hypothalamic-pituitary-gonadal subsystem of the endocrine system. A pathologic condition such as a tumor or cyst is the most common cause of excessive exogenous gonadal hormones, resulting in precocious pseudopuberty. The central nervous system may mature with prolonged exposure to exogenous gonadal hormones, resulting in true precocious puberty.

Menarche that occurs in very young children or even infants usually is associated with McCune-Albright syndrome, a fibrous dysplasia of the skeletal system. Congenital adrenal hyperplasia often is related to a deficiency of the 21-hydroxylase enzyme, which causes a deficiency in cortisol, aldosterone, and ultimately weak androgens. Premature thelarche often is associated with a familial tendency. It may be caused by the secretion of a small amount of estrogen by the ovaries.

Adolescents may develop gynecologic disorders typically viewed as adult problems, such as dysmenorrhea, premenstrual syndrome (PMS), endometriosis, dysfunctional uterine bleeding (DUB), and vaginal infections. Primary dysmenorrhea may occur in 50% of young women, beginning 6 to 12 months after menarche when ovulation is established.

The most common cause of secondary amenorrhea during the teen years is pregnancy. Secondary dysmenorrhea associated with a pathologic condition is more likely to develop about 2 years after menarche. Secondary amenorrhea may result from pelvic inflammatory disease (PID) or endometriosis. Vaginal infections and vulvar inflammation may result from a number of causes such as feminine hygiene chemical irritation, secondary candidiasis from acne treatments, or irritation from normal secretions and tight clothing.

Laparoscopic examinations have shown that endometriosis does occur in adolescents. Pregnancy is the most common cause of DUB in adolescents, although anatomic anomalies, foreign bodies (e.g., forgotten tampons), and chronic illness may also promote bleeding.

CLINICAL MANIFESTATIONS

Girls usually begin puberty about 2 years before their male peers. The first visible sign of puberty in girls is usually the appearance of breast buds (Figure 13-3). Hormonal effects during puberty generally result in shorter limb length for women than men. Women also have narrower shoulders and broader hips than men. Estrogen secretion causes a softer, smoother, more vascular skin texture in women. Hair becomes darker and coarser and grows in the pubic and axillary areas during adolescence (Figure 13-4). The sebaceous, eccrine, and

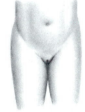
Stage 1 (preadolescent)
No distinction between hair on pubis and over the abdomen

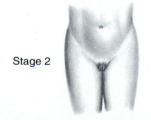
Stage 2
Sparse growth of long, straight, downy, and slightly pigmented hair extending along labia; between stages 2 and 3 begins to appear on pubis

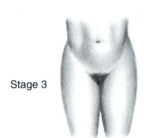
Stage 3
Hair darker, coarser, and curly and spread sparsely over entire pubis in the typical female triangle

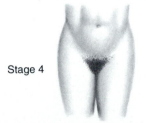
Stage 4
Pubic hair denser, curled, and adult in distribution but less abundant and restricted to the pubic area

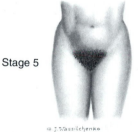
Stage 5
Hair adult in quantity, type, and pattern with spread to inner aspect of thighs

FIGURE 13-4
Growth of pubic hair in girls—average age span for stages 2 through 5, 11 to 14 years. (Modified from Marshall WA, Tanner JM[76a]; and Daniel WA, Paulshock BZ.[28a])

ADOLESCENCE: A TIME OF CHANGE

Adolescence is a time of psychosocial development as well as physical maturity. Self-concept risks, including factors related to the formation of a changed body image, and sex-role identity may emerge. Girls may develop poor posture and associated musculoskeletal problems from stooping or trying to appear shorter. Eating disorders are likely to surface during puberty. Hormonal shifts may compound cognitive and emotional changes, resulting in ineffective coping. Health risks, such as automobile accidents, drug abuse, or adolescent pregnancy, may be associated with adolescent behavior issues.

apocrine sweat glands become more active.

The development of secondary sex characteristics may be monitored or evaluated with maturation tools. The broadening of the pelvic girdle may be the first indication of puberty in girls. Physiologic leukorrhea occurs as the uterine and vaginal tissues expand and mature.

During puberty the heart size, blood volume, and blood pressure increase, while the pulse rate decreases.

Women usually have a higher pulse rate and lower blood pressure than men. Respiratory rates decrease during childhood and reach adult ranges in adolescence.

The gawky, long-legged appearance of early adolescence is caused by the rapid growth of the extremities, neck, and trunk. The hands and feet appear larger than other body parts. After the bone growth spurt, muscle develops and subcutaneous fat expands. Adipose tissue appears in the thighs, hips, buttocks, and breasts.

DIFFERENTIAL DIAGNOSIS

Atypical anatomic guidelines for puberty, including precocious and delayed characteristics, must be compared with physiologic factors such as amenorrhea and anovulation. The box on page 257 illustrates the diagnosis of delayed development.

If possible, primary amenorrhea from environmental factors should be differentiated from pathologic factors (e.g., gonadal dysgenesis, müllerian anomalies, hypothalamic-pituitary disorders).

DIAGNOSTIC STUDIES AND FINDINGS

Diagnostic test	Findings
Tanner staging system	Compares development of secondary sexual characteristics so that underlying pathologic condition can be determined
Thyroid function tests	To rule out asymptomatic hypothyroidism that could cause amenorrhea
Prolactin levels	To rule out hyperprolactinemia
Scanning procedures	To rule out pathologic condition (e.g., congenital defects, pituitary adenomas)
Pregnancy test	To rule out pregnancy as a cause of secondary amenorrhea
Progesterone challenge test	To determine if menses may occur
Chromosomal studies	To determine disorder and cause of inappropriate pubertal development

DIAGNOSTIC EVALUATION OF DELAYED DEVELOPMENT

Family history

History of delayed growth and maturation in parents and/or other relatives

Height and weight of siblings at comparable ages and their present measurements

Child's history

Prenatal—factors that could influence normal growth

Birth—height and weight (usually appropriate for gestational age)

Concurrent chronic diseases

Past illnesses such as head injuries and gastrointestinal, renal, or neurologic disorders

Dietary habits

Strength and stamina

Susceptibility to infection

Attainment of development milestones

School progress

Emotional problems or problems of social adjustment, especially those that may indicate past family instability (prolonged emotional upset has a significant influence on growth)

Previous growth pattern

Records available:

Decrease during any year or period (e.g., second year of life, just before puberty)

Remained relatively small throughout growth period with a growth curve parallel to or slightly below 3rd percentile

Records not available:

Determine when first noticed that the child was small compared with other children

Physical examination

Accurate measurements of height and weight (child stripped to underclothing)

Measurement of body proportions

Crown to pubis

Pubis to heel

Signs of sexual development using standard criteria

Breast budding in girls

Testicular enlargement (testicular volume greater than 2 ml) in boys

If present, normal sexual development can be expected to follow in 1 to 2 years

Bone age

Assessed from wrist x-ray films (always delayed)

Endocrine studies

Hormonal investigations essentially normal

Growth hormone (GH) response

Gonadotropin levels

Gonadotropin-releasing factor (GnRF) responses

Usually low for the child's chronologic age but consistent with bone age

Plasma testosterone and estrogen levels consistent with bone age

Urinary excretion of 17-ketosteroids consistent with bone age

Corresponding change in endocrine response consistent with normal pubertal changes occurs with maturation

(From Whaley and Wong.[107c])

MEDICAL MANAGEMENT

GENERAL MANAGEMENT

Reduce stressors that may be interfering with puberty such as stress, excessive exercise, or dietary extremes.

Treat underlying endocrine dysfunctions or pathologic conditions, such as chronic disease.

DRUG THERAPY

Treatment for acne, if needed.

Treatment as needed for infection, dysmenorrhea, etc.

Oral contraceptives and antiprostaglandins as appropriate for dysmenorrhea.

Medication to stimulate prolactin secretion if needed for amenorrhea.

Hormonal treatment if imbalance exists.

SURGERY

If congenital defect is present, surgical intervention may correct anomaly.

1 ASSESS*

ASSESSMENT	OBSERVATIONS
History	Age; previous growth patterns; family history of early or late puberty; chronic illnesses; previous scans and laboratory data (e.g., endocrine studies); life-style habits (e.g., diet, exercise, sleep patterns, emotional health)
Growth and development	Current Tanner scoring data of secondary sexual characteristics; bone age; body measurements
Psychosocial	Anxiety associated with knowledge deficit about growth and development

*Nursing care should be well documented in the patient's permanent health care record.

2 DIAGNOSE

NURSING DIAGNOSIS	SUBJECTIVE FINDINGS	OBJECTIVE FINDINGS
High risk for body image disturbance related to altered growth and development	States that her body does not look like that of her peers	Inappropriate Tanner scoring for age
	Expresses concern about early or late menarche; describes discomfort about changing body, especially in relation to growth of her peers	Scans or laboratory data indicate underlying pathologic condition; may observe normal range of development

NURSING DIAGNOSIS	SUBJECTIVE FINDINGS	OBJECTIVE FINDINGS
High risk for impaired skin integrity related to anomaly or infection	Patient describes itching, burning, or discharge, or parent states that child pulls, holds, or scratches her genital area	Vulvar or hymenal irregularity; signs of inflammation
Pain related to gynecologic condition, such as cyclic pain or infection	Describes pain during menses, or delineates symptoms of infection	Scans may indicate endometriosis; cultures may show infection
Knowledge deficit related to normal growth and development during puberty	Questions cause of normal anatomic or physiologic processes, such as increased vaginal secretions when sexually aroused	Vaginal discharge appears normal for developmental stage; Tanner scoring appropriate

3 PLAN

Patient goals
1. The patient will have normal growth and development within realistic parameters.
2. The patient will have a positive body image.
3. The patient will be free of infection or impaired skin integrity.
4. The patient will have no pain and will understand ways to decrease cyclic discomfort.
5. The patient and family will understand the normal changes that occur during childhood, puberty, and adolescence.

4 IMPLEMENT

NURSING DIAGNOSIS	NURSING INTERVENTIONS	RATIONALE
High risk for body image disturbance related to altered growth and development	Explain and assist patient and family with diagnostic procedures.	To provide support and information about tests.
	Encourage patient to describe her feelings about growth and body changes.	To promote acceptance of changing body image.
High risk for impaired skin integrity related to anomaly or infection	Describe potential causes and treatment of common gynecologic disorders.	To enhance learning and promote treatment choices.
Pain related to gynecologic condition, such as cyclic pain or infection	Encourage patient to ask questions about gynecologic discomfort.	To explore pain-relief measures and treatment for underlying condition.
Knowledge deficit related to normal growth and development during puberty	Help patient identify myths or dispel misinformation.	To clarify what is known about puberty and to identify areas where additional information is needed.

5   EVALUATE

PATIENT OUTCOME	DATA INDICATING THAT OUTCOME IS REACHED
Patient's growth and development are normal.	Tanner scoring is appropriate; scans and diagnostic tests show no abnormalities.
Patient has a positive body image.	Patient verbalizes acceptance of body changes and physical maturity.
Patient is free of infection, and there is no anomaly or skin breakdown.	Gynecologic structures and associated skin areas are intact, and there is no sign of inflammation.
Patient is free of cyclic pain.	Patient reports no discomfort with menses.
Patient and family understand changes associated with growth and development.	Patient and family can describe the normal range of development during childhood, puberty, and adolescence.

PATIENT TEACHING

1. Provide information about the cognitive, psychologic, and physical changes associated with childhood, puberty, and adolescence.
2. Present information about growth and development and common disorders, such as menstrual cycle conditions, and encourage the patient and family to ask questions.
3. If an underlying condition may exist, explain the appropriate diagnostic procedures and possible treatment choices.
4. Discuss ways to reduce the risk of infection and irritation, such as hygiene measures or treatment for vulvar irregularities.
5. Emphasize the importance of life-style habits such as good nutrition, adequate sleep, preventing accidents, and sex education.

Menopause and Postmenopause

Menopause is the cessation of menstruation. It is diagnosed after 1 year without menses. The term *climacteric* or *perimenopause* refers to the time surrounding menopause during which ovarian function decreases, resulting in decreased estrogen production. This is a normal life event, not a disease process, and women live many years after menopause. *Surgical menopause* occurs when the ovaries are removed. Premature or artificial menopause is the cessation of ovarian function as a result of radiation, surgery, immunologic disease, or bacterial or viral infection.

As the general population ages, more women are experiencing menopause. The average age for menopause is 51 to 52, although the age range is from 45 to 55. There are approximately 50 million women in the

United States over the age of 50 with a life expectancy of almost 80, indicating that women often live at least 30 years after menopause.

Some women (10%) have no symptoms of menopause other than cessation of menstruation; 70% to 80% are aware of other changes but have no problems. Approximately 10% experience changes severe enough to interfere with activities of daily living.

PHYSIOLOGY AND PATHOPHYSIOLOGY

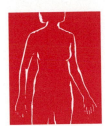 As ovarian function diminishes, a sequential loss in the function of estrogen-dependent tissues occurs. Ovulation and menstruation cease. There are changes in vaginal and vulvar tissue and other estrogen-dependent tissue such as the breasts. With aging, fewer follicles respond to gonadotropin stimulation, reducing the level of the estrogen estradiol. Although peripheral conversion of the estrogen estrone continues, it is a lower level estrogen, resulting in the symptoms associated with menopause.

Symptoms of perimenopause may vary greatly. Menstrual periods may stop abruptly but more commonly they become irregular, with decreased flow or hypermenorrhea. Cycles become anovulatory, and fertility decreases. These symptoms may last 2 to 3 years before menopause can be diagnosed appropriately.

The most common early symptom of menopause is vasomotor instability or "hot flashes" with sweats. The exact cause of hot flashes is unknown, although apparently they indicate hypothalamic autonomic instability resulting from the decline in estrogen. They occur most frequently at night.

The decrease in estrogen also causes changes in the reproductive structures. Atrophic tissue changes, including atrophic vaginal, vulvar, urethral, and general skin changes, may produce symptoms. As the myometrium thins, the size of the uterus decreases. Dyspareunia, pruritus, and urinary problems may occur in the postmenopausal years.

A variety of other symptoms have been related to menopause, although it is difficult to show causality. Anxiety, depression, tension, headaches, muscular aches and pains, palpitations, and changes in sexual functioning often occur during the climacteric.

Current research indicates that osteoporosis and heart disease increase after menopause, because estrogen has a protective effect in preventing these disorders. Issues of menopause must be concerned with both heart disease and osteoporosis because of the increased risk of each after menopause.

Complications of menopause include symptoms severe enough to interfere with normal activities. The increased risk of osteoporosis and heart disease is also noteworthy. Additional problems include dysfunctional uterine bleeding, endometrial cancer and hyperplasia, and issues related to estrogen replacement therapy.

Osteoporosis usually occurs after age 50 without any prior symptoms or warning. It can be painful and debilitating and can lead to death. Approximately 25 million Americans are affected by the disorder. Osteoporosis is a disease characterized by decreased bone mass, architectural deterioration of bone tissue, and increased risk for fracture. Risk factors for osteoporosis include fair hair and skin, thin build, Caucasian or Asian races, family history of the disease, early menopause, chronic illness, corticosteroid use, smoking, alcohol use, inadequate exercise, and calcium intake.

Prevention of osteoporosis focuses on stimulating bone formation and preventing resorption of bone. Although women are more at risk, probably because of their smaller bone size, men also develop osteoporosis. Treatment includes early education for the production of healthy bones, exercise, calcium supplements, and possibly, estrogen therapy.

DIFFERENTIAL DIAGNOSIS

Differential diagnosis includes consideration of the following:
Pregnancy
Dysfunctional uterine bleeding
Exercise-induced amenorrhea
Other hormonal factors including thyroid, adrenal tumor
Stress
Stenotic cervical os

ESTROGEN PRESCRIBING SCHEDULES

The most common protocols for the use of estrogen are described in the prescribing schedules chart (box on page 262). Doses will vary according to symptoms and side effects. There are a variety of estrogen preparations, each with different doses. In general it is recommended that the lowest possible dose for relief of symptoms be prescribed. Most protocols include the addition of a progestin for a specified period or at least discontinuing estrogen for a specified period during each month, after which cyclic bleeding is expected. The addition of the progestin serves as a protection against endometrial hyperplasia. Usual dosages and preparations include the following, though a variety of products is used.

VARIOUS ESTROGEN/ PROGESTOGEN PRESCRIBING SCHEDULES

Regimen 1

Estrogen—25 days
Progestogen—add at day 13

Regimen 2

Estrogen—every day
Progestogen—12-14 days on

Regimen 3

Estrogen—every day
Progestogen—every day

Conjugated estrogens, for example, Premarin, are available in oral tablets in 0.3, 0.625, 0.9, 1.25, and 2.5 mg doses.

Conjugated estrogen cream, 2 to 4 g daily for as short a time as needed to relieve symptoms of atrophic vaginitis.

Micronized estradiol, for example, Estrace, 1 to 2 mg daily orally.

Transdermal estradiol (Estraderm), 0.05 to 0.1 mg patch replaced 2 times per week.

Medroxyprogesterone (Provera), 5 to 10 mg, is added for at least 7, and more commonly, 10 to 14 days.

CONTRAINDICATIONS TO ERT:

Presence or history of estrogen-dependent tumor, breast, endometrial, or genital cancer, history of thromboembolism, acute myocardial infarction, undiagnosed vaginal bleeding, liver disease or abnormal liver function.

CAUTIONS TO ERT:

Women with fibroids, endometriosis, hypertension, diabetes.
Many women vary dosages or discontinue use, resulting in a variety of symptoms. If irregular bleeding should occur, an endometrial biopsy should be done.

IMPACT OF ESTROGENS ON HEART DISEASE

It appears that estrogen has a protective effect on the cardiovascular changes that lead to heart disease. Estrogen lowers cholesterol levels primarily by decreasing low-density lipoprotein (LDL) cholesterol and increasing high-density lipoprotein (HDL) levels. Estrogen also appears to have a direct physiologic effect on the walls of the blood vessels by mediating blood flow and opposing platelet aggregation. There is, however, some concern that the use of progestogens may interfere with some of the protective lipid effects of the estrogen. Therefore, for women who have had a hysterectomy and are not at risk for endometrial hyperplasia, the inclusion of progesterone with estrogen is not routinely used.

DIAGNOSTIC STUDIES AND FINDINGS

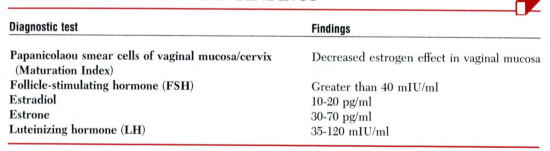

Diagnostic test	Findings
Papanicolaou smear cells of vaginal mucosa/cervix (Maturation Index)	Decreased estrogen effect in vaginal mucosa
Follicle-stimulating hormone (FSH)	Greater than 40 mIU/ml
Estradiol	10-20 pg/ml
Estrone	30-70 pg/ml
Luteinizing hormone (LH)	35-120 mIU/ml

MEDICAL MANAGEMENT

Management of menopause is usually provided by gynecologists, reproductive endocrinologists, internists, and family physicians.

Treatment depends on symptoms, risk profile for osteoporosis and heart disease, and contraindications for estrogens.

GENERAL MANAGEMENT

Extensive history including menarche, menstrual cycle, pregnancies, thyroid, medications, stress, psychosocial factors, systemic disease, risk factors for osteoporosis and heart disease.

Physical to include mammogram, guaiac, Pap smear.

Laboratory studies to include CBC, electrolytes, liver enzymes, thyroid, possibly glucose.

Counseling and teaching (50% of women have relief of some symptoms without additional intervention).

Treatment of hot flashes:

Estrogen and progesterone

Bellergal

Behavioral factors including self-awareness, adjusting the physical environment/ambient temperature, wearing layered clothing, and participating in support groups.

Lifestyle factors such as smoking cigarettes, drinking alcoholic beverages, and exercising.

Nonconventional remedies such as vitamin E, herbal remedies, and relaxation.

Treatment for prevention of osteoporosis:

Drugs used include:

Estrogen

Bisphosphonates

Calcitonin

Sodium fluoride

Growth hormone and growth factors

Parathyroid and other hormones

Nonpharmacologic approaches:

Calcium supplements

Weight-bearing exercise

DRUG THERAPY

Estrogen replacement therapy (ERT) is the most commonly prescribed drug for the treatment of menopausal symptoms. The general consensus is that the initial doses should be the lowest amount that will control symptoms. A woman who has not had her uterus removed should also take progesterone to produce endometrial sloughing. It is important to explain that with the cyclic administration of hormones, the woman will continue to have cyclic bleeding, and when hormones are stopped or missed she will have irregular bleeding and return of symptoms.

1 ASSESS*

ASSESSMENT	OBSERVATIONS
History	Complications associated with hormonal fluctuations, osteoporosis, and diseases that make hormonal treatment risky; previous breast or endometrial disease; vaginal bleeding; inactivity; alcohol consumption; dietary habits, especially intake of calcium; hepatic disease; chronic illnesses; skin color and racial ancestry; body build; thromboembolic disease; use of oral contraceptives.

*Nursing care should be well documented in the patient's permanent health care record.

2 DIAGNOSE

NURSING DIAGNOSIS	SUBJECTIVE FINDINGS	OBJECTIVE FINDINGS
Anxiety related to changes associated with menopause	Verbalizes anxiety related to menopausal symptoms.	Signs of anxiety, such as perspiration, elevated vital signs, or short attention span.
Potential for body image disturbance related to menopause	Expresses dissatisfaction with body; partner or family describes patient's change in outlook.	Poor eye contact; hides face or body areas.
High risk for impaired physical mobility related to the physiology of menopause and post-menopause	Complains that symptoms such as fatigue, hot flashes, and/or change in mobility prevent usual functioning.	Signs of fatigue, such as rings around eyes, or osteoporosis in spinal curvature.

3 PLAN

Patient goals

1. The patient will be free from anxiety and express knowledge about the usual changes associated with menopause.
2. The patient will have a positive body image.

3. The patient will have optimal physical mobility and independent functioning.

4 IMPLEMENT

NURSING DIAGNOSIS	NURSING INTERVENTIONS	RATIONALE
Anxiety related to changes associated with menopause	Explain physiologic process associated with menopause and postmenopause.	To provide information that will decrease anxiety and promote self-care.

NURSING DIAGNOSIS	NURSING INTERVENTIONS	RATIONALE
Potential for body image disturbance related to menopause	Encourage the patient to express feelings and ask questions concerning the effects of menopause, e.g., skin treatment, sexual function.	To provide information and options that may improve body image.
High risk for impaired physical mobility related to the physiology of menopause and postmenopause	Help patient and family assess life-style habits, such as diet, exercise, and rest, to increase mobility and decrease complications, such as osteoporosis.	To promote self-care and optimal wellness by decreasing risks associated with hormonal shifts and aging.

5 EVALUATION

PATIENT OUTCOME	DATA INDICATING THAT OUTCOME IS REACHED
Patient reports acceptance of menopause, without anxiety.	Anxiety regarding menopause is not evident in nonverbal behavior; patient and family describe accurate information concerning menopause.
Patient has a positive body image.	The patient's misconceptions are corrected and she expresses positive feelings about her body, sexuality, femininity, and age.
The patient's mobility and functioning are optimal.	The patient reports easy movements and relief of previous physical limitations associated with menopause or postmenopausal risks, such as osteoporosis.

PATIENT TEACHING

1. Assess the patient's knowledge and explain, as needed, the process of climacteric. Encourage the patient and family to ask questions.
2. Help the patient and family develop a wellness program that includes nutrition, rest, exercise, stress management, and risk prevention.
3. Reinforce correct information about menopause, sexuality, and body image, and correct any misconceptions.
4. Provide options for treating symptoms, such as hormonal therapy, vaginal lubrication with water-soluble solutions, and availability of counseling and support groups.
5. Provide educational materials that the patient and family may take home and refer to as needed.
6. Assess patient's general fitness, and identify signs of fatigue, immobility, or complications, e.g., tachycardia, syncope, osteoporosis associated with acute or chronic hormonal fluctuations or cessation.
7. Assess mobility, range of motion, and presence of kyphosis, and assess need for additional treatment or referral for osteoporosis.

CHAPTER 14

Health Promotion for Women

Health promotion is helping people change their life-styles to move toward a higher state of wellness. Inherent in this definition are *health* and *wellness*. Health involves a dynamic state of continuous balancing of a person's physical, emotional, social, intellectual, and spiritual components to produce happiness and a higher quality of life. This implies that the potential for change always exists and that a person's level of health is determined by the activities she engages in to prevent illness or promote wellness. Wellness is adopting attitudes and engaging in behaviors that enhance the quality of life and maximize personal potential. The responsibility for health and wellness lies with the individual and requires her participation in health-promoting behaviors.

Preventive medicine is a fairly new specialty that focuses on health promotion. Because of their expertise and their contact with individuals and groups in the community, and because they are members of a primarily female profession, nurses have a mandate and a unique opportunity in women's health care—to provide information and services that promote prevention, health care, and health maintenance for women.

Women are becoming more demanding consumers. They are more educated, knowledgeable, and sophisticated about their rights. Nurses must form partnerships with women to extend their abilities to care for themselves.

As we near the turn of the century, technology has developed to the point that most of those things that killed our forebearers have been eliminated as factors in the mortality of today's populations. In the early 1900s a woman could expect to live about 47 years. The life expectancy of women in the United States today is estimated to be about 78 years. Pneumonia, influenza, tuberculosis, and diseases of early infancy are no longer the major causes of death in women, as they were in the early 1900s. Today the five leading causes of death among women in the United States are cardiovascular disease, cancer, cerebrovascular disease, accidents and adverse effects, and chronic obstructive lung disease (noncancerous). In 1986, 76% of all deaths (women and men) in the United States were attributed to these conditions, which often are the result of individual decisions and life-styles.

The scientific community believes that technology has improved life expectancy as much as it can, and that the factors now responsible for the major causes of death among adults are due to life-style practices that could be changed, such as cigarette smoking, alcohol consumption, a high-fat diet, drug abuse, and lack of exercise. This chapter addresses some of the major health promotion issues for women.

ACCESS TO HEALTH CARE

Historically, women's health care focused on the female reproductive system. Women typically entered the health care system because they were pregnant, they wanted to become pregnant, or they wanted to avoid pregnancy. The change in women's roles has affected not only their health care needs, but also their perceptions of those needs. In addressing the needs of today's woman and the woman of the future, we must address her wholeness—her physical, emotional, social, intellectual, and spiritual being. Women's health must concern itself with the overall life experiences of women, not just their physical diseases or reproductive functioning—their "dis-eases" as well as their diseases.

Women are the primary users of the health care system. Much of that use is related to childbearing, but beyond that, women use more health care services than men. Even more significantly, they make 75% to 85% of the health care decisions for their entire family.

Factors that influence a woman's entry into the health care system include her socioeconomic status (can she afford the service), the availability and accessibility of health care providers, and the acceptability of the care to the woman. However, the most significant factor that influences a woman in seeking health care is education. Regardless of her socioeconomic status or the difficulty involved in obtaining care, if a woman has been educated as to the importance of specific health screening, care, or follow-up, she will often seek that care.

Some practitioners and health care groups recognize the influence of women on their practices and are developing "one-stop" centers to provide for all of a woman's needs in one place and at one time. The private sector has been doing this for several years, marketing aggressively to attract women to their centers. When the public sector incorporates this strategy, a positive change in women's overall health care will occur.

Often cultural differences affect whether, when, and where a woman seeks health care. To be effective with diverse populations, nurses must understand the customs and beliefs of individuals and groups in the area. They must be able to incorporate various beliefs into the traditional health care system and gain an understanding of how various beliefs affect the care of a woman and her family (Table 14-1).

WOMEN IN THE WORKPLACE

The impact of the workplace on women is becoming more evident each year—not just on their personal health, but also on the health and welfare of their families. There are inherent psychologic hazards associated with women working longer, more frequently, and in more responsible positions. If a woman is married, her husband often feels the stress of having to accommodate for the absence of his spouse and take on an unfamiliar caretaker role. Stress felt by both husband and wife has been related to the problems of juggling home, family, and careers, as well as to work-related concerns. Children present a whole myriad of concerns with both parents working outside the home.

Forty-three percent of the U.S. work force is made up of women. Even with a number of highly positioned, well-prepared women in the labor market, most working women are undereducated and underprepared for positions with an appropriate living wage. A majority have no health insurance. Women are often single parents and the sole support of the family. These, among other factors, contribute to an increase in the number of women living in poverty. Add to this the primary responsibility for providing care for children or during pregnancy or illness in the family, and the problems of women in the workplace begin to take on new dimensions. The lack of health care policies at the work site to encourage improved prenatal and child care or leave for family illness exacerbates problems for the

Table 14-1

CULTURAL GROUPS: HEALTH AND ILLNESS BELIEFS, PRACTICES, AND MORBIDITY PROBLEMS

Origin	Health beliefs	Health practices
ASIAN AMERICAN: China, Hawaii, Philippines, Korea, Japan, Southeast Asia (Laos, Cambodia, Vietnam)	Balance of yin and yang	Prevent imbalances of yin and yang and changes in climate
AFRICAN: West coast of Africa (as slaves), many African countries, West Indian islands, Dominican Republic, Haiti, Jamaica	Harmony with nature	Prevent disharmony; respect cleanliness and religion; avoid sick people
EUROPEAN: England, France, Germany, other European countries	Physical and emotional well-being; feeling OK	Respect proper nutrition, exercise, cleanliness, faith in God
NATIVE AMERICAN: 170 Native American tribes, western part of the United States, reservations, tribal homelands	Living in harmony with nature	Respect nature; avoid evil spirits
SPANISH AND CENTRAL AMERICAN: Spain, Cuba, Central and South America, Mexico, Puerto Rico	Reward for good behavior; balance of "hot" and "cold" humors	Wear amulets; use proper diet to maintain balance of "hot" and "cold"; pray

(From Potter and Perry.[89])

family of a working woman. The United States has no uniform policies on maternity leave, child care benefits, or time off for family illness.

Access to health care in the United States often is tied to the ability to pay for that care. Larger companies usually provide health care benefits, but most small businesses and individuals who hire only a few employees do not offer any health benefits. With health care as costly as it is, many women seek services from public health care sources. But gaining access to these public clinics can be difficult for a variety of reasons: (1) The operating hours of the clinics usually coincide with the woman's working hours; (2) usually only one type of service is offered at a specific time and place, fragmenting care; (3) waiting times can be long; (4) if the woman has children and cannot afford child care, she must take her children with her, often to more than one site; and (5) language barriers make it difficult to provide care, especially among the increasing number of immigrants in the United States.

At the worksite women may be exposed to additional health hazards, with no real understanding of how these affect her and her family's health. Attention to this concern is bringing more assistance to women who work. Legislation has been passed in many countries (e.g. Belgium, France, Great Britain, Italy, Japan, the United States, the former Soviet Union) to provide protection for women in the workplace. This legislation bans women from certain jobs and worksites that might expose them to teratogenic substances that could cause genetic anomalies in pregnant women. Besides protecting their potential to be mothers, other considerations for regulation include the size of the woman, the effort required for the job, the danger of the work, and the multiple responsibilities of working women. This protection has been a double-edged sword—serving to restrict women from many areas of employment whether fertility or responsibility was typical or not for the individual woman. The protective activities required are expensive for employers, often discouraging them from hiring women freely and without bias. This further narrows the job market for women. Many of the earlier restrictions on women in the workplace have been reversed because of the discrimination they imposed.

Illness beliefs	Illness practices	Traditional remedies	High morbidity incidence
Imbalance of yin and yang	Restore balance of yin and yang; use herbal remedies and acupuncture	*Huo li jian mei su* *Jen shen lu jung wan* Ginseng root Tiger balm White flower	Liver cancer Stomach cancer Coccidioidomycosis Hypertension Parasites
Disharmony	Use folk remedies and healers	Bangles Talisman *Asafoetida* Voodoo candles	Cancer of the esophagus Stomach cancer Coccidioidomycosis Hypertension Sickle cell anemia
Absence of well-being; feeling bad	Use home remedies, liniments, poultices, and medical care	Amulets Syrup of Black Draught Father John's Medicine Swamp root *Olbas*	Breast cancer Thalassemia
Disharmony with nature	Use medicine man and traditional herbal remedies	Masks Sweet grass Thunderbird Sand paintings	Accidents Heart disease Cirrhosis of the liver Diabetes mellitus Lung cancer
Punishment for wrong-doing; imbalance of hot and cold	Restore body's balance; use folk healers and remedies	Amulets: *Mano Negro* Special soaps Candles *Manzanilla* *Anis*	Diabetes mellitus Parasites Coccidioidomycosis

Work site health promotion programs have been developed in many areas. On-site health educators and/or health care providers assist both women and men by providing health care information, health screening, and help with setting health goals for the patients and their families. These programs usually are developed in the industries that also provide other health care benefits; such programs still do not reach those individuals not covered by health insurance plans. A majority of women and children do not have health care plans. Most health care for this population is crisis-based and not preventive.

SEXUAL ORIENTATION AND GENDER IDENTIFICATION AS BARRIERS TO HEALTH CARE*

Health care professionals working with the general population will encounter individuals who present themselves in a gender role, or sexual orientation, different from the role they were assigned at birth. Nurses must be understanding of the needs of the individual and must respond professionally. These individuals need health care no matter which gender or sex they identify with. Nurses must be able to interact in a professional manner, permitting the patient to reveal her/his sexual orientation or transgender nature without fear of condemnation or ridicule. Only then can a comprehensive assessment be conducted.

A lesbian may choose to avoid traditional health care providers and receive little if any preventive health screening. A supportive attitude from a health care provider will promote health care among this population of women. The health care provider needs to anticipate these patients and learn as much as possible about special needs, assessment, interviewing techniques to acknowledge alternative life-styles, and prejudices they usually face in health care institutions. Confidentiality is critical among lesbian patients.

*Data from Phyllis Randolph Frye. Proceedings from the First International Conference on Transgender Law and Employment Policy, Houston, Texas, 1992; and Rothblatt, MA: Second Report of the Health Law Project, Second International Conference on Transgender Law and Employment Policy: Transsexual and Transgender Health Law, August 1993.

Nurses need to become aware of their own personal attitudes that could prejudice care, learn more about this population of individuals, and be aware of community resources available for lesbians.

Transgendered patients are another population the nurse may encounter. These patients are individuals who have accepted an alternative gender and have taken on that role. Conservative estimates range from 100,000 to 1,000,000 transsexuals worldwide. They usually seek routine health care from health care providers they trust and with whom they have had positive interactions. However, transgendered patients may enter the hospital or health care facility for routine or preoperative care or in an emergency situation.

Understanding the terms *transgendered* and *transsexualism* is basic to providing appropriate care for these clients. Different definitions of transsexualism have lead to considerable confusion. The medical and legal professions define sex in the noun form as a categorization of people into males and females depending on whether they have penises or vaginas. The medical and legal professions view transsexualism as a desire to actually change one's genitals to the other sex's genitals. When a transgendered client seeks gender correction and uses the medical and legal communities' definition, transsexual medical and surgical treatment is categorized as cosmetic rather than medically necessary, thereby negating any medical insurance coverage for treatment.

Sociocultural experts categorize people into "sex groups" as male, female, and androgenous subtypes depending on their individual behaviors and personal identity beliefs. To this group of experts, transsexualism is a process of changing from one set of sex-typed behaviors and beliefs to another. The person's sex is an important part of self-expression. At a basic level, transsexualism is changing one's expression of sexual identity. This identity may be expressed through speech, apparel, body language, changes in secondary sex characteristics after hormone therapy, and various cosmetic surgeries, including alteration of genitals.

Transsexuals seek to make their outward appearance match their inner view of themselves. A transgendered patient who presents himself or herself is either a crossdresser or a transsexual (either preoperative or nonoperative). There are specific distinctions among these individuals that help determine their care. The female-to-male crossdresser wears clothing usually worn by someone of the male gender. He may or may not reveal his crossdressing, since women dressing in men's clothes is usually a socially allowed practice. The postoperative male-to-female is usually undetectable on superficial inspection, but she requires regular hormonal treatment similar to that given to most postmenopausal women.

The postoperative female-to-male is more rare, since the genital surgery has not been perfected and is very expensive. She also requires regular hormone therapy (see Transgendered Individuals, Chapter 12). The transsexual patient has legally changed his or her sexual classification.

The male-to-female crossdresser is either a man in men's outer clothing and women's underclothing or a man completely dressed in women's clothing, passing as a woman to some degree. When dressed as a woman, he is a SHE; when dressed as a man, he is a HE. This person usually is heterosexual and married, and often has children. In most cases the individual did not plan to reveal this secret—the health care provider comes to know of it through emergency room admission. The patient often is embarrassed and frightened that a homophobic or transphobic person will leak the secret to others, especially to the employer or family.

As health care professionals, nurses must be sensitive to the needs of these patients. If an individual presents herself as a woman, the nurse must be understanding and thoughtful enough to treat her as a woman, regardless of her genital organs. Nurses should assist the transsexual client with the distress he or she feels in making this sexual transition—not question the individual's sexual identity.

Transgendered individuals have absorbed social rejection outside the health care system. The patient will recover faster, with less stress and fewer complications, if treated with kindness and respect. The nurse must serve as the patient's advocate, be professional, and treat HIM or HER in the gender with which the person needs to identify. This population will not seek routine preventive health care in a hostile environment.

HEALTH RISK PREVENTION

Risks are hazards that can be limited or avoided to prevent harm. Certain actions can be taken or avoided to reduce the chance of health problems. For example, wearing seat belts decreases the probability of serious injuries during an automobile accident. Seat belts do not prevent 100% of injuries, but they do decrease the risk or likelihood of physical harm. Some risks, like a family history of breast cancer, may place a woman at risk for developing the same condition. While the risk of breast cancer cannot be reduced directly, steps can be taken, such as regular examinations and mammographies, to detect and treat the disorder early and to improve survival and quality of life. The reason some women at risk for breast cancer develop it while others do not remains unknown. Nevertheless, the risk of metastatic disease and death is controllable.

Risk prevention involves identifying potential problems, minimizing hazards, and treating conditions in a timely manner to prevent serious consequences. Environmental health hazards, such as noise pollution, second-hand smoke, and asbestos exposure, and biologic risks, such as water pollution or pesticides ingested in food, can affect everyone. Toxic substances may cause a number of different problems, such as memory loss, confusion, depression, tremors, vision problems, and a variety of other physiologic and psychologic conditions. One toxin may affect all of the body systems, or a combination of substances may cause unusual symptoms. All labels should be read before purchasing consumer goods. Irritating and toxic substances should be avoided. Several risks are more pertinent to women than to men. Examples of these hazards are highlighted in Table 14-2 and in the box on page 272.

Table 14-2

COMMON RISKS AND PREVENTIVE MEASURES

Risk	Preventive measure
Irritation or contact dermatitis (rash, redness, itching, blistering) from cleaners, soaps, bleaches, solvents and enzymes in detergents, home pesticides, and toxic house plants	Wear rubber gloves when using irritating chemicals; remove rings and jewelry during cleaning; use mild, superfatted soap with moisturizers or neutral pH; purchase nontoxic house plants (lists available in most hardware stores).
Rubber glove dermatitis	Use cornstarch powder inside gloves to decrease irritation from latex. Gloves are made from mercaptobenzothizole and tetraethylthiuram.
Irritation from cosmetics and sunscreens	Purchase "allergy-free" and "sensitive skin" cosmetics; avoid preservatives, such as eyeshadow with quaternium 15, face powder with imidazolidinyl urea, eyeliner and face powder from dialozolidinyl urea, lotion containing paraben, and eye solutions with thimerosal.
Irritation from hair products	Perform patch tests; permanent hair dyes use paraphenylenediamine; shampoos may contain formaldehyde, so rinse thoroughly.
Irritation from jewelry	Use surgical steel, stainless-steel, or 18 karat gold jewelry; avoid objects containing nickel.
Reactions to clothing and paper goods	New clothes should be washed to decrease formaldehyde resins and dye irritants; test paper goods, such as particle board, and avoid items that cause irritation; test new carpets or fabrics.
Irritation from fragrances	Perfumes, toilet paper, female hygiene products, and cosmetics may cause local or respiratory reactions; use products marked "fragrance free"; use white toilet paper; perform small perfume and cosmetic patch tests.
Nail bed damage and fungus	Avoid products containing paratoluene sulfonamide resin; periodically remove acrylic products and glue; routinely check condition of nails and nailbeds and remove any irritating product; treat fungus promptly with keratolytic antifungal agents, such as salicylic acid; avoid high doses of vitamin A and medications contaminated with arsenic or thallium; avoid prolonged water immersion.
Nonimmunologic contact urticaria; food allergies	Avoid flavors, products, and foods that cause "tingling" or hives, such as mouth and teeth products with cinnamon aldehyde, cinnamon, or menthol; seek medical treatment for any possible food allergy, since serious anaphylaxis can develop; new allergies can develop over time.

COMMON IRRITANTS AND TOXINS

Clinical mani festation	Type of irritant/toxin
Infertility	Lead from flaking paint or old plumbing; formaldehyde from poor ventilation in mobile home, or from other paper, fabric, or carpet product; arsenic from natural well water contamination, or from home-distilled whiskey or wine; boric acid and other pesticides; fungicide or methylmercury ingested from seafood or seed grain; dietary supplements, cigarettes, street drugs contaminated with arsenic or lead; toluene inhaled from glue or adhesives; other chemical toxins used in photography, painting, furniture repair, pottery, glass blowing, jewelry and metal work, sculpting, target shooting, and gardening.
Teratogenic (congenital or birth) defects	Most medications (prescription and over-the-counter); alcohol; tobacco; marijuana and other street drugs; insecticides; herbicides; food additives; contaminants; environmental and work chemicals, such as lead, arsenic, mercury, solvents, radiation.
Heart and circulatory problems	Chemicals including antimony (pewter, typesetting products), cadmium (art and hobby supplies), carbon disulfide (putty, rayon, rubber cement, markers), radiation (x-rays), and other factory chemicals.
Coughing and breathing problems	Inhaled substances such as tobacco smoke, marijuana, or cocaine; air pollution; irritants, such as animal danders and pollens; heat and cooling systems without adequate filtering or humidifying; gardening (pollen, bacteria, fungi, or pesticide inhalation); work that causes sawdust, sandstone, or ceramic powder inhalation.
Nausea and diarrhea	Food contamination (inadequate refrigeration or cooking); laxatives; antacids; high iron supplements; herbs (many different herbs may be toxic in large quantities); seafood; dairy products (lactase deficient); gluten products; acidic fluids from metallic containers causing copper, zinc, or cadmium ingestion; hobby or work with metals: arsenic, lead, mercury, antimony; opiate withdrawal.
Vertigo or dizziness	Lead; formaldehyde; hazardous wastes; fireplace that burns arsenic-treated wood; halogenated hydrocarbon solvents, such as waterless cleaners; contaminated food or water; solvents, glue, typewriter correction fluid; street drugs containing arsenic and lead; cigarettes and secondhand smoke containing cyanide and formaldehyde; animal flea-killing spray; hobby and paint products; and work with computer terminals.
Hair loss	Frequent use of antifungal and antidandruff shampoo; dietary supplements and health food that may contain thallium, arsenic, or selenium; high doses of vitamin A.
Headache	Processed and Chinese food containing monosodium glutamate (MSG); fishborne food poisoning; foods containing tyramine (figs, coffee, alcohol, yeast, cheese, etc.); chocolate (may promote migraines); food dyes and flavorings; licorice; oil of peppermint; well water with high nitrates; work and hobby chemicals; frequent use of computer or video terminals.

HEALTH PROMOTION

Health promotion activities are designed to support behavior conducive to health. Areas explored in this chapter are (1) smoking and health, (2) misuse of alcohol and drugs, (3) nutrition, (4) physical fitness and exercise, and (5) control of stress and violent behavior.

SMOKING AND WOMEN'S HEALTH

Women have "liberated" themselves in many ways over the past few decades. They have entered the high-stress world of the workplace and have assumed new roles and taken on new life-styles and habits. One of the habits most damaging to their health is cigarette smoking. This may have begun as a response to peer pressure, to role modeling from parents or mentors, as stress reduction, as weight reduction, or for many other reasons. Smoking seriously compromises a woman's health and has caused an increase in death and illness rates from cardiovascular disease, cancer, and chronic obstructive lung diseases (Table 14-3).

Eighty-three percent of all cases of lung cancer are caused by smoking; 75% of women who develop lung cancer smoke. The incidence of lung cancer among women has risen 200%—tripled—in 15 years. This parallels the increase in cigarette smoking among women. Lung cancer now surpasses breast cancer as the most common type of cancer among women. Other health risks associated with women who smoke are an increase in stillbirths and low-birthweight babies; reduced fertility; and an increased risk of heart attack, stroke, or embolism for women who smoke and take

Table 14-3

DEATH RATIO OF SMOKERS TO NONSMOKERS FOR MAJOR DISEASES

Disease	Smoker to nonsmoker ratio
Heart disease	approx. 2 to 1
Lung cancer	approx. 11 to 1
Stroke	approx. 3 to 1
Oral cancer	approx. 4 to 1
Ulcers	approx. 3 to 1
Bronchitis and other pulmonary diseases	approx. 6 to 1

The National Cancer Institute provides a manual for physicians, *How to Help Your Patients Stop Smoking.* Other information can be obtained from the National Cancer Institute at 1-800-4CANCER or the Office of Cancer Communications, Building 31, Room 10A18, Bethesda, MD 20892.

EFFECTS OF SMOKING ON THE BODY

Brain	Restricts oxygen flow; constriction of blood vessels in the brain can lead to stroke
Lungs	Increases the risk of lung cancer, emphysema, bronchitis, and pneumonia from contact with carcinogens in cigarette smoke
Heart and circulatory system	Increases the heart rate, elevates the blood pressure, constricts blood vessels, contributes to fatty deposits in the arteries, and reduces the level of oxygen in the blood
Digestive tract	Potentiates cancer in the tissues of the mouth, throat, esophagus, stomach, and intestines through carcinogens found in cigarette smoke; increases the risk of duodenal and stomach ulcers by increasing secretion of digestive acids
Bladder	Increases the incidence of bladder cancer through increased contact with carcinogens found in smoke (which are eliminated from the blood and stored in and disposed of by the bladder)
Female reproductive organs	Increases the risk of cervical cancer, miscarriage, premature birth, and infant morbidity and mortality

oral contraceptives (see the box above for the effects of smoking on the body). Women who smoke have two to six times the risk of a heart attack.

Tobacco use promotes both a physical and a psychologic dependence, accounting for the difficulty individuals have in quitting smoking. Chemically nicotine produces a stimulatory effect that leads to mild euphoria. It relieves anxiety, controls the appetite, heightens alertness, and improves mental performance. As tolerance to nicotine develops, the individual begins to smoke more to maintain the level of nicotine and prevent withdrawal symptoms. The latter effects probably have more to do with the continuance of smoking.

Women smokers are more hesitant than men to quit smoking. Fear of gaining weight is a major obstacle for women. This seems to be integrated with other social and behavioral factors—not only does smoking relax

women and help them concentrate, it helps them control anger and stress (which are socially unacceptable emotions). Besides, according to the latest marketing campaigns, smoking makes women more glamorous and sophisticated while helping them maintain their weight.

The only "easy" way to stop smoking is not to start. There are many incentives to quit smoking: numerous regulations prohibit smoking except in designated areas; scientific studies link diseases with smoking and passive smoke; and more employers offer incentives and various programs to help their employees quit. Even though cigarette dependence is powerful, people have been able to quit. And the smoker who quits gains significant benefits—health risks decrease dramatically over the next 5 to 10 years. The essential conditions for helping a person to quit smoking appear to be desire to quit and confidence in one's ability to quit. Authorities who study smokers and their dependence on nicotine support various methods of cessation. Most feel that smokers will make more than one attempt to stop before they finally quit. They suggest that even if one method does not work, another method might, and smokers should continue to try to quit.

Nicotine patches and nicotine gum do not appear to reduce the level of nicotine for the patient, but the tar and other carcinogenic materials received from smoking are eliminated.

MISUSE OF ALCOHOL AND DRUGS

Alcohol has been an integral part of our culture, used for religious rites, ceremonies, celebrations, or mourning. Considered a *man's disease*, alcohol dependency was regarded as a rare occurrence among women until the 1960s when, with the emergence of the women's movement, women's addictions were recognized. In the 1990s a greater percentage of women are drinking alcoholic beverages, and younger women are drinking heavily. More women are being admitted for treatment of alcohol consumption, and some experts estimate that currently there are almost as many women alcoholics as there are men with the disorder.

It is estimated that 70 to 90 million people, or about two thirds of all American adults, drink alcoholic beverages. One third of these adults are light drinkers; one third are moderate to heavy drinkers; and about 1 in 10 (9 million to 10 million people) has a problem with alcohol. At least 40% of all adults who abuse alcohol are women. Women undergoing the stress of life changes often seek refuge in alcohol or drugs. Problem drinking begins subtly, without the woman realizing it. The onset usually is slow and insidious.

A multitude of social problems have been related to alcohol. In 1990 the cost of alcohol abuse and dependence in the United States was estimated to be $136.3 billion. Industry alone loses about $43 billion each year because of alcoholism, in the form of medical expenses, insurance premiums, lost wages, a decrease in productivity, injuries, automobile accidents, crimes, fires, and the grievance process, among other things. Alcohol is blamed in 50% of all fatal traffic accidents, 53% of deadly falls, and 38% of drownings. Approximately 6,000 fires and burns each year are associated with alcohol use. Alcohol use has been implicated in 67% of homicides, 50% of rapes, and 20% to 36% of suicides.

Alcohol is classified as a drug, a potent central nervous system depressant. The depressant effect occurs primarily in the brain and spinal cord. Alcohol often is mistaken as a stimulant because of the initial stimulant effect that gives the drinker a sense of boldness or releases personal inhibitions and temporarily relieves tension.

The effects of chronic alcohol overuse on health include irreversible damage to the liver, stomach, spinal

---

ALCOHOL-RELATED HEALTH PROBLEMS

Liver	Chemical imbalance: altered protein production, blood sugar imbalance, fat accumulation in the liver tissue
	Inflammation: impaired circulation, scar tissue formation, alcohol-related hepatitis
	Cirrhosis: impaired circulation, kidney failure, death
Digestive tract	Oral cavity: when combined with smoking, alcohol use promotes cancer of the mouth, tongue, and throat
	Esophagus: irritation, impaired swallowing
	Stomach: irritation, gastritis, ulceration
	Pancreas: inflammation (pancreatitis)
	Digestion: impaired absorption
	Nausea: diarrhea, vomiting
Cardiovascular	Cardiomyopathy: shortness of breath, heart enlargement, dysrhythmias
	Dysrhythmias: cardiac insufficiency
	Coronary artery disease: angina pectoris, myocardial infarction
Malnutrition	Faulty dietary practices: empty calories, obesity
Cancer	Prevalence: mouth, larynx, esophagus, liver; alcohol's role as a carcinogenic agent is not clearly understood
Woman's reproductive system	Dysmenorrhea, infertility, miscarriage, fetal alcohol syndrome

(From Payne and Hahn, ed. 3.[86])

cord, and brain, as shown in the box on p. 274. Long-term abuse can result in cancer, stroke, cirrhosis and other liver diseases, malnutrition, nerve damage, destruction of brain cells, birth defects, infertility, and various mental problems. Problem drinking should be recognized and steps taken to assist the person before physical changes are irreversible. The problem drinker is[*]:

- Anyone who must drink in order to function or "cope" with life
- Anyone who, by her own definition or that of her family and friends, frequently drinks to a state of intoxication
- Anyone who goes to work intoxicated
- Anyone who is intoxicated and drives a car
- Anyone who sustains bodily injury requiring medical attention as a consequence of an intoxicated state
- Anyone who, under the influence of alcohol, does something she contends she would never do without alcohol

Women are more at risk for multiple addictions for several reasons. They usually hide their alcoholism, and physicians traditionally prescribe tranquilizers, pain medications, and other psychotropic drugs for relief of fatigue, depression, etc. that add to the effects and addictive potential of the alcohol being consumed. Two thirds of the 100 million prescriptions for tranquilizers, pain medications, and psychotropic drugs are for women. Women receive twice as many of these drugs as men. These medications can be dangerous, especially if overprescribed, used in conjunction with alcohol, or prescribed for older adults.

When alcohol or other drug abuse interferes with the individual's daily life, health, and job performance, action must be taken as soon as possible to reduce the irreversible effects of these drugs. The entire family of the alcoholic is affected, and treatment must be sought for them all. Of particular concern are findings that children of alcoholics are four times more likely to become alcoholics than are children of nonalcoholics.

Significant differences exist between men and women alcoholics: (1) Women can identify a specific triggering event that initiated their drinking; (2) women begin drinking at an older age, but the alcoholism progresses more rapidly among them than with men; (3) women receive more prescribed mood-altering drugs, which can contribute to multiple addictions, drug interactions, or cross-tolerance; (4) men tend to divorce their alcoholic wives, reducing support systems

(From U.S. Department of Health and Human Services: *Facts about alcohol and alcoholism*, Rockville, MD, 1980, National Institute on Alcohol Abuse and Alcoholism.)

THE TWELVE STEPS OF ALCOHOLICS ANONYMOUS

1. We admitted we were powerless over alcohol—that our lives had become unmanageable.
2. Came to believe that a Power greater than ourselves could restore us to sanity.
3. Made a decision to turn our will and our lives over to the care of God *as we understood Him*.
4. Made a searching and fearless moral inventory of ourselves.
5. Admitted to God, to ourselves, and to another human being the exact nature of our wrongs.
6. Were entirely ready to have God remove all these defects of character.
7. Humbly asked Him to remove our shortcomings.
8. Made a list of all persons we had harmed and became willing to make amends to them all.
9. Made direct amends to such people wherever possible except when to do so would injure them or others.
10. Continued to take personal inventory and when we were wrong promptly admitted it.
11. Sought through prayer and meditation to improve our conscious contact with God *as we understood Him*, praying only for knowledge of His will for us and the power to carry that out.
12. Having had a spiritual awakening as the result of these steps, we tried to carry this message to alcoholics and to practice these principles in all our affairs.

(From Anspaugh, Hamrick, Rosato.[6])

RESPONSIBLE DRINKING

Following are suggestions to help each person be a responsible drinker and host.

- Drink slowly; never more than one drink per hour.
- Eat while drinking, but stay away from salty food.
- When mixing drinks, measure the amount of alcohol; never just pour.
- Serve and choose nonalcoholic drinks as an alternative.
- The host should always serve the guests or hire a bartender. It is never wise to have an open bar or serve someone who is intoxicated.
- Stop using or serving alcohol 1 hour before a party is over.
- Don't drink and drive. Either have a nondrinker drive the car or call a cab.

(From Anspaugh, Hamrick, Rosato.[6])

during attempts to quit drinking; (5) women do not seem to receive as much as social support as men; and (6) it is more difficult for a woman who is unmarried, divorced, or a single parent to take advantage of expensive treatment programs.

Treatment for alcoholism must include managing the acute episodes of intoxication, correcting chronic health problems associated with the alcoholism, and altering the long-term behavior of the alcoholic so that destructive drinking patterns are not continued. A variety of approaches are used in treatment and rehabilitation of alcoholics and drug abusers. Many recovering alcoholics credit Alcoholics Anonymous (AA) with their sobriety. More than 19,000 AA groups in the United States provide the support a recovering alcoholic needs. They advocate use of the Twelve Step Program shown on page 275. The Twelve Step Program has been adapted for victims of many dependencies such as drug abuse and codependency.

Alcohol use will continue in our society. Irresponsible use has deadly consequences, but many people continue to act irresponsibly with alcohol. Preventive programs must be escalated to reduce the destruction to families and society. Treatment and rehabilitation programs must be available, accessible, and affordable.

NUTRITION

Western society has become more aware of the relationship between nutrition and health, and its role in wellness and fitness. As a society we believed that medical technology could solve our major health problems. Scientific solutions provided *cures* or *extinction* for many diseases formerly caused by nutritional deficiencies. And yet, even today, many diseases with nutritional implications continue to plague us, primarily as a result of dietary imbalances and excesses. It is estimated that 50% of American men and 60% of American women are overweight by midlife; 2% to 15% of children and adolescents are also overweight. Obesity is currently defined as being more than 30% overweight when compared to the individual's *ideal* weight using a normative weight table adjusted for height, sex, and general body structure (Figure 14-1).

An individual's health risks are greatly increased by being 20% to 30% overweight. Seven of the 10 leading causes of death in the United States are related to eating practices. Increased weight has been implicated in osteoarthritis, cancer, cardiovascular disease, gallbladder disease, hernias, hypercholesterolemia, hypertension, kidney disease, pulmonary diseases, maternity-onset diabetes, stroke, and pregnancy-induced hyper-

---

ESTIMATING YOUR BASAL METABOLIC RATE

Calculations for estimating BMR use different constants for men and women. The constant for men is 1 calorie per kilogram (2.2 lbs) per hour; for women, 0.9 calories per kilogram per hour. These constants are referred to as the BMR factor. The method for estimating the BMR for a 125-pound woman follows:

1. Convert body weight in pounds to kilograms (kg): 125 lbs ÷ 2.2 lbs = 56.8 kg.
2. Multiply weight in kilograms by the BMR factor: 56.8 × 0.9 cal/kg/h = 51.5 cal/h.
3. Multiply calories per hour by 24 (hours): 51.1 cal/h × 24 h = 1,227.3 cal/24 h.
4. The BMR is 1227.3 calories per day.

To determine the total calories expended, you need to estimate the number of calories used in muscular movement during a typical day. This is a rough approximation but should be within your range if you follow the guidelines below and select the category that fits you best.

1. Sedentary—student, desk job, sitting during most of your work and leisure time: **add 40% to 50% of the BMR.**
2. Light activity—teacher, assembly line worker, walk 2 miles regularly: **add 55% to 65% of the BMR.**
3. Moderate activity—waitress, aerobic exercise at 75% of maximum heart rate: **add 65% to 70% of the BMR.**
4. Heavy activity—construction worker, aerobic exercise above 75% of maximum heart rate: **add 75% to 100% of BMR.**

To calculate your range of daily total calorie expenditure if your activity level is in the *light* category:

1. Multiply BMR by the level of activity
   a. 1227.3 × 0.55 = 675
   b. 1227.3 × 0.65 = 797.7
2. Add BMR calories to the level of activity calories to get total calories
   a. 1227.3 + 675 = 1,902.3 cal/day
   b. 1227.3 + 797.7 = 2,025 cal/day

(From Estimating your basal metabolic rate [BMR]. In Anspaugh, Hamrick, and Rosato: *Wellness: concepts and applications*, St. Louis, 1991, Mosby–Year Book.)[6]

tension. Much of this has been related to overeating—eating too many calories for the person's activity level—and imbalance in the nutrients consumed. Not only does good nutrition promote better health and prevent disease, it is essential for providing energy and endurance. This fact promotes the practice of eating an adequate diet at regular intervals to improve performance. Other factors influencing body weight include intake of food, activity, size and body type, metabolism, and genetics. Weight gain occurs when energy input exceeds energy output. Calculations for estimating an individual's basal metabolic rate (BMR) are shown in the box on page 276. Once a woman knows her BMR, she has a better idea how many calories she needs to take in to maintain her ideal weight.

Life-style traits that make women more susceptible to nutrient imbalance include *eat and run*—picking up high-calorie, high-fat, and high-sodium frozen dinners or fast foods from the local fast-food restaurant; *skimpy eating*—not eating nutritionally balanced meals and cutting back on certain foods needed such as milk and red meat; *fasting*—reducing the number of meals to reduce caloric intake; *fad dieting*—using trendy and nutritionally unsound methods to lose weight; *inconsistent or excessive physical activity*—using physical activity to maintain weight rather than regulating intake, or using dieting to maintain weight rather than increasing activity to increase metabolism. Using food in times of stress is a negative coping skill used by many women. Likewise some of the dietary habits of women influence their level of stress (i.e., consumption of too much caffeine, too few or too many calories, too much sugar, or too few complex carbohydrates).

Women may lack adequate knowledge of proper nu-

METROPOLITAN LIFE INSURANCE COMPANY WEIGHT CHART

Does your weight fall within the range established by this table? Weight tables published in 1983 reflect the fact that today's adults are on the average somewhat heavier than in recent decades. Figures include 5 pounds of clothing for men, 3 pounds for women, and shoes with 1-inch heels for both.

	Men				Women		
Height	Small frame	Medium frame	Large frame	Height	Small frame	Medium frame	Large frame
5 ft 2 in	128-134	131-141	138-150	4 ft 10 in	102-111	109-121	118-131
5 ft 3 in	130-136	133-143	140-153	4 ft 11 in	103-113	111-123	120-134
5 ft 4 in	132-138	135-145	142-156	5 ft 0 in	104-115	113-126	122-137
5 ft 5 in	134-140	137-148	144-160	5 ft 1 in	106-118	115-129	125-140
5 ft 6 in	136-142	139-151	146-164	5 ft 2 in	108-121	118-132	128-143
5 ft 7 in	138-145	142-154	149-168	5 ft 3 in	111-124	121-135	131-147
5 ft 8 in	140-148	145-157	152-172	5 ft 4 in	114-127	124-138	134-151
5 ft 9 in	142-151	148-160	155-176	5 ft 5 in	117-130	127-141	137-155
5 ft 10 in	144-154	151-163	158-180	5 ft 6 in	120-133	130-144	140-159
5 ft 11 in	146-157	154-166	161-184	5 ft 7 in	123-136	133-147	143-163
6 ft 0 in	149-160	157-170	164-188	5 ft 8 in	126-139	136-150	146-167
6 ft 1 in	152-164	160-174	168-192	5 ft 9 in	129-142	139-153	149-170
6 ft 2 in	155-168	164-178	172-197	5 ft 10 in	132-145	142-156	152-173
6 ft 3 in	158-172	167-182	176-202	5 ft 11 in	135-148	145-159	155-176
6 ft 4 in	162-176	171-187	181-207	6 ft 0 in	138-151	148-162	158-179

"Miracle Foods" to Improve the Immune System and Prevent Cancer

- Cruciferous vegetables (broccoli, cabbage, cauliflower, and brussels sprouts) decrease the risk of cancer through compounds called indoles.
- Cold-water fish, such as salmon, are rich in omega-3 fatty acids, which protect against heart disease, cancer, and rheumatoid arthritis.

FIGURE 14-1
Metropolitan Life Insurance Company weight chart shows ideal weights for women and men by height.

trition and eating practices. Add to this the continuous messages women receive from society about being lean and fit, and the foundation is laid for frustration, noncompliance, eating disorders, and various forms of malnutrition. (See Chapter 10, Systemic Disorders Affecting Female Health, for information on eating disorders.) A common practice among women is choosing foods they eat according to their perception of its effect on their weight, not its effect on their health. A good example of this is the reduction of milk and bread in their diets. Thirty percent of women in the United States are dieting at any given time: 31% of women ages 19 to 39 diet at least once a month, and 16% consider themselves to be perpetual dieters.

One of the major dietary concerns for women is getting enough iron, zinc, and calcium. Women lose both iron and zinc with menstrual periods, increasing the amounts needed in the diet. Adequate amounts of iron are found in red meat, fortified cereals, and prune juice, but women fail to consume these foods in adequate amounts. Zinc is abundant in red meats but can also be consumed in grains, legumes, nuts, seeds, and milk and other dairy products. Calcium is required at all ages but especially during periods of growth. Pregnant women must consume additional amounts for the fetus as well. Maximum bone density is reached at about age 35. After that women begin losing small amounts of calcium from their bones. Major losses do not occur until the onset of menopause, with a decrease in estrogen levels, putting women at high risk for osteoporosis. Most women fail to consume the amount of calcium needed in their diets and should seriously consider supplementing it (see Chapter 13, Life Cycle Changes, and the patient teaching guide on osteoporosis). Additionally, as women age, their activity level usually declines, resulting in a reduction in muscle mass and metabolism. Less food is needed to maintain the same amount of weight. A decrease in the amount of food also presumes a decrease in the amount of vitamins and minerals consumed. Choosing foods of higher nutrient value becomes essential for older women. Producers of most food products are required by federal regulation to provide the consumer with a nutritional breakdown of their products. This requires that the consumer be astute in reading labels and understanding the nutritional content of foods.

Current guidelines for Americans' nutrition are reflected in the Food Guide Pyramid (Figure 14-2). The guidelines recommend that the largest proportion of our intake—nine servings per day—be in bread, cereals, rice, and pasta. The next largest category is fruits and vegetables (four servings of vegetables and three servings of fruits daily). Foods recommended next include three servings of dairy products and two of fish

and meat. Fats and sugars should be eaten sparingly.

These guidelines are dramatically different from earlier recommendations, and educational programs are needed to relay and explain this information to the public. The use of vitamin and mineral supplements is controversial; many experts maintain that a balanced diet supplies all the nutrients required. Others point to the fact that very few people eat the nine servings of grains, three servings of fruit, and four servings of vegetables daily, leaving them deficient.

As a culture Americans are preoccupied with weight and impressed with a lean, youthful body. This is exhibited in our media, our clothes, our role models. Lean is healthy—obesity is a health hazard. Obese individuals find themselves discriminated against socially and emotionally and categorized as lazy. This same culture has replaced muscle power with machine power amid the increased development of labor-saving machines, and life-styles have changed drastically.

Millions of dollars are spent each year on miraculous weight-loss products and/or programs. At no time has it been more essential that consumers understand the basics of nutrition: how nutrition affects their health, the changes in nutritional needs over the life cycle, and what individuals can do to maximize the benefits of their nutritional intake.

Nurses can serve as role models and resources, relaying the latest findings to women in the community. The women of the 1990s need some guidance in making sense out of the often contradictory messages they receive about nutrition and health, and how they might go about reaching optimum physical well-being.

General guidelines for nutritional support:

- Conduct an assessment of the individual's life-style, intake of food, physical activity, size and body type, metabolism, cultural practices, and genetics.
- Help the patient establish realistic goals for overall good health and weight loss.
- Develop a personalized diet and exercise plan with the patient.
- Teach the patient about nutrition, exercise, and the health risks of obesity.
- Teach stress management skills, and explore potential responses to stressors that aggravate overeating.
- Refer for medical management if appropriate.
- Refer to a support group if appropriate.
- Evaluate short-term and long-term changes.

PHYSICAL FITNESS AND EXERCISE

Women have progressed from a society in which they primarily performed manual labor—cooking, cleaning, gardening, sewing, washing, and such—to a less active, industrialized, computerized, fast-food society. Their bodies are being challenged by increasing levels

Fat and Health
Cultural values and individual viewpoints differ concerning ideal body weight. Heavy people may *not* have health problems, body image disturbances, or low-self esteem. However, poor nutritional habits and obesity *do* correlate with certain health risks. Eating a balanced diet, therefore is as essential to health promotion as avoiding drug abuse and minimizing exposure to toxins. Following these recommendations will help a woman to maintain a healthy life style.

Food Guide Pyramid
A Guide to Daily Food Choices

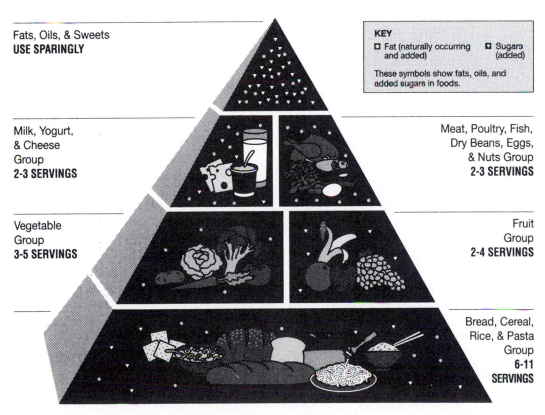

Fats, Oils, & Sweets
USE SPARINGLY

KEY
☐ Fat (naturally occurring and added)   ◩ Sugars (added)

These symbols show fats, oils, and added sugars in foods.

Milk, Yogurt, & Cheese Group
2-3 SERVINGS

Meat, Poultry, Fish, Dry Beans, Eggs, & Nuts Group
2-3 SERVINGS

Vegetable Group
3-5 SERVINGS

Fruit Group
2-4 SERVINGS

Bread, Cereal, Rice, & Pasta Group
6-11 SERVINGS

FIGURE 14-2
Food guide pyramid. (From U.S. Department of Agriculture and Health and Human Services.)

of inactivity. Lack of physical activity has been implicated in cardiovascular disease, diabetes, obesity, respiratory dysfunction, osteoporosis, and depression. The human body functions more efficiently when it remains physically active. Exercise maintains muscle tone, metabolism, circulation, cardiovascular fitness, and bone density. An important product of physical activity is mental well-being—an increase in self-esteem and relaxation, and improved self-confidence and alertness. Exercise promotes relaxation and provides a means to relieve the ailments that result from the stress of daily living, such as headaches, backaches, sleeplessness, fatigue, ulcers, and depression.

A fitness program should address flexibility, muscular strength and endurance, aerobic fitness, and body composition. A personal fitness plan should consider the individual's life-style, genetics, body structure, activities required daily, and leisure activities. Being "physically fit" means that a woman's body is healthy and functions efficiently to enable her to engage in rigorous tasks and leisure activities.

Cardiorespiratory endurance provides a foundation for overall fitness. It provides the energy needed to accomplish the activities of life. The body can process and support the delivery of adequate oxygen to muscle cells. This aerobic conditioning allows a person to work at a sustained level of intensity for a longer period. Additional structural and functional benefits result from cardiorespiratory (aerobic) fitness (see the box at right).

Aerobic exercise is the key to cardiorespiratory fitness, weight management and fat loss, and increased mental well-being. Essential components in the development of an effective cardiorespiratory and muscular fitness program are (1) the mode of activity, (2) the frequency of training, (3) the intensity of training, (4) the duration of training, and (5) resistance training. To be of benefit, aerobic exercise (using the large muscles of the body) must increase the breathing and heart rate continuously for 15 to 20 minutes at least three times a week. An aerobic activity should be stimulating but not exhausting or overly strenuous. When an activity becomes exhausting or overly strenuous, it also becomes anaerobic and the benefits to cardiorespiratory fitness are lost. Brisk walking, jogging, or swimming are three good examples of aerobic activities.

Stretching and range-of-motion activities improve and maintain flexibility while preventing injury and promoting back health, muscle health, and relaxation. Adding resistance to range-of-motion exercise promotes muscle strengthening and endurance. Weight training can be added to range-of-motion exercises to accomplish this.

Currently a great deal of emphasis is focused on body composition—the structure of the body in terms

---

STRUCTURAL AND FUNCTIONAL BENEFITS OF CARDIORESPIRATORY (AEROBIC) FITNESS

Aerobic fitness can help you:
- Complete your daily activities with enjoyment
- Strengthen your heart muscle and make it more efficient
- Increase your proportion of high-density lipoproteins
- Increase your capillary network in your body
- Improve collateral circulation
- Control your weight
- Stimulate bone growth
- Cope with stressors
- Ward off infections
- Improve the efficiency of your other body systems
- Bolster your self-esteem
- Achieve self-directed fitness goals
- Reduce negative dependency behaviors
- Sleep better
- Recover more quickly from common illnesses
- Meet other people with similar interests
- Receive lower insurance premiums

(From Payne and Hahn, ed. 3.[86])

---

of body fat, bone, and other elements. Body composition (measured as gross body weight) has been used to determine obesity and general wellness without a real understanding of why it is important to know a person's gross body weight. This measure gives the actual composition of the body in terms of lean body mass versus body fat. Muscle tissue is heavier than fat tissue. A woman may maintain her body weight over a span of years, but replace lean muscle tissue with fat tissue, with a resulting change in endurance, wellness, and risk for disease. Likewise, when a woman begins an exercise and diet program, muscle tissue (which weighs more) begins to replace fat tissue and the woman becomes discouraged if she doesn't see an immediate weight loss and doesn't understand the concept. Simple tape measurements (chest, waist, arm girth, and thigh girth) can help the woman follow the change in body composition.

Women of all ages must be taught the benefits of physical fitness, the physiologic and psychologic effects of food, exercise, genetics, life-style, stress, and environment on their well-being. They must understand what their personal health risks are and how to develop control over these factors. The woman with a family history of heart disease (genetic propensity) must realize how she can take control of other factors (e.g., obesity and smoking) to decrease her overall risks of heart disease. A sound program of physical fitness must be individualized to educate and motivate the participant. People who are beginning a new physical fitness program should be cautioned to have a good physical examination before starting if they have an existing medical condition that warrants it or if they are over 30 years of age and have not been physically active for the past 5 years.

Changing old habits requires a change in attitude and changes in life-style. For example, park farther away when going to work, school, or the grocery store. Take the stairs even if it is only a few flights a day. Walk a few blocks before dinner at least three evenings a week. Exercise with a video or start a lunchtime walking group at work; go dancing; have fun. Regardless of age or limitations, many activities can provide the cardiorespiratory conditioning needed for good health. Keep moving!

STRESS

One of the most elusive terms in our society is *stress*. It is used in many ways. Stress is cited both as the cause of illness and as the impetus for progress and achievement. It almost takes on a spiritual air of inspiration. Hans Selye, noted for research on stress, felt that stress is like relativity—a scientific concept that is too well known and too little understood. Usually stress has a negative connotation—stress from pressure or strain, being felt from something happening around or to someone. A person "under stress" may be ill, be under financial pressure, have a deadline to meet, or face one of many other conditions. Students feel stress from tests or impending deadlines. Parents feel stress from family needs or the demands of daily tasks. Anything that causes a person to experience stress is called a *stressor*. Stressors can be *internal* (a fever, response to hormonal changes such as in pregnancy or menopause, or an emotion) or *external* (changes in temperature, changes in a social or family role that originate outside the body).

Stress has been described as a nonspecific response of the body to any demand made on it—physiologic and/or psychologic. Physiologic reactions to stress are depicted in Figure 14-3. Selye developed a model to explain the human response to stress, the *general adaptation syndrome (GAS)*. The body strives to maintain a state of homeostasis. At times of illness, injury, or prolonged stress, the body's homeostatic control is compromised and inadequate. Serious illness or death can occur. The general adaptation syndrome is a complex set of neurologic and endocrine responses that speed up the body's processes (e.g., heart and respiratory rates) to prepare it for physical action or what is more

commonly known as the *fight or flight* reaction. This was probably very appropriate in primitive societies, when this reaction was often lifesaving, but it seems to work to the detriment of society today. Even though we no longer have the need to fight or flee, our bodies prepare us to do just that and produce a prolonged state of tension.

INDICATORS OF STRESS

Behavioral indicators
- Decreased productivity and quality of job performance
- Tendency to make mistakes or poor judgment
- Forgetfulness and blocking
- Diminished attention to detail
- Preoccupation, including daydreaming or "spacing out"
- Inability to concentrate on tasks
- Reduced creativity
- Increased use of alcohol or drugs
- Increased smoking
- Increased absenteeism and illness
- Lethargy
- Loss of interest
- Accident proneness

Physical indicators
- Elevated blood pressure
- Increased muscle tension (neck, shoulders, and back)
- Elevated pulse or increased respiration
- "Sweaty" palms
- Cold hands and feet
- Slumped posture
- Tension headache
- Upset stomach
- Higher pitched voice
- Change in appetite
- Urinary frequency
- Restlessness, including difficulty in falling asleep or frequent awakening

Emotional indicators
- Emotional outbursts and crying
- Irritability
- Depression
- Withdrawal
- Hostile and assaultive behavior
- Tendency to blame others
- Anxiousness
- Feeling of worthlessness
- Suspiciousness

(From Potter and Perry.[89])

Relaxation Techniques
- Visualization
- Deep breathing
- Meditation
- Biofeedback
- Progressive relaxation
- Music
- Humor
- Time management
- Exercise

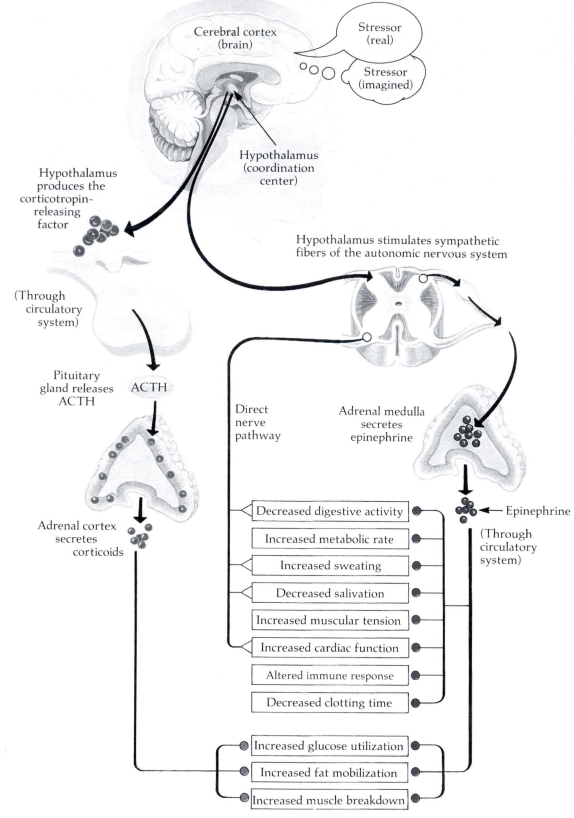

Cerebral cortex (brain)

Stressor (real)

Stressor (imagined)

Hypothalamus (coordination center)

Hypothalamus produces the corticotropin-releasing factor

Hypothalamus stimulates sympathetic fibers of the autonomic nervous system

(Through circulatory system)

Pituitary gland releases ACTH

ACTH

Direct nerve pathway

Adrenal medulla secretes epinephrine

Adrenal cortex secretes corticoids

Decreased digestive activity

Increased metabolic rate

Increased sweating

Decreased salivation

Increased muscular tension

Increased cardiac function

Altered immune response

Decreased clotting time

Epinephrine

(Through circulatory system)

Increased glucose utilization

Increased fat mobilization

Increased muscle breakdown

FIGURE 14-3
The stress response: physiologic reactions to a stressor.
(From Payne and Hahn.[86])

STRESS, NUTRITIONAL STATUS, AND IMMUNITY: AN INTERACTIVE EFFECT

Although the mechanism is not completely understood at this time, stress significantly affects nutritional status and thereby immunity. Several nutritional factors have implications for how our bodies respond to stress.

- **Energy:** Stress can increase the body's basic caloric needs by as much as 200%. The stress hormones increase body heat production. When this heat is released, it is not available for cell metabolism. The caloric inefficiency induced by stress accounts for the increased need for energy intake.
- **Protein:** Stress may increase the body's need for protein from 60% to as much as 500%. The integrity of the body's tissues, such as the skin and the tissue lining the mouth, lungs, and nose (called mucosal tissue), depends on adequate protein repair and maintenance of secretions of biochemicals that serve as protective agents. The formation of antibodies also requires protein.
- **Fats:** Dietary fatty acids influence the synthesis of a group of fatty acid derivatives called *prostaglandins*. Prostaglandins stimulate or depress other cellular and immune functions in relation to stress.
- **Vitamins:** Vitamin A functions to maintain healthy skin and mucous membranes. Individuals who are vitamin A deficient have fewer mucus-secreting cells and those they do have produce less mucus—thus the protection provided by the mucous lining is diminished. Vitamin C has been shown to enhance the engulfing or "eating" actions of the immune cells called *macrophages*. If vitamin C is deficient, macrophages are less mobile and less able to consume disease-causing organisms. Deficiencies of vitamins A, B_{12}, and folate can impair production of the cells that enable antibody responses. Large doses of vitamin E have been associated with suppression of B cells, which are vital to the immune response. Finally, metabolic requirements for thiamin, riboflavin, and niacin are increased in response to a stressful situation.
- **Minerals:** Deficiencies of zinc impair immune cell reproduction and responsiveness.

(From Anspaugh, Hamrick, and Rosato.[6])

Stress has been linked to various diseases and illnesses. These run the gamut from colds to cancer. One of the major concerns is the relationship of stress to heart disease, the leading cause of death in the United States (approximately 700,000 individuals die each year of heart disease). Cancer, ulcer, and migraine headaches are only a few of the other diseases linked to prolonged stress. The interactive effect of stress, nutritional status, and immunity is illustrated in the box above. The need to reduce stress-induced disease is obvious.

A little stress can heighten performance—too much can be debilitating. Each individual has the potential to manage the stressors of life. Effective stress management requires a change in attitude and life-style. Guidelines to help deal with stress are listed in the box at right. Stress management is not so much a way to cure illness as it is a means to improve the quality of life.

DEPRESSION AND SUICIDE

It is estimated that one out of five people in the United States will experience depression in his or her lifetime. Two thirds of these individuals are women. Depression is considered the most common emotional disorder in the United States, and more individuals seek counseling for depression than for any other emotional problem.

GUIDELINES FOR DEALING WITH STRESS

Some guidelines for dealing effectively with potentially harmful stress are:

- **Schedule time effectively:** Practice good time management techniques by using time wisely. This means taking time out for yourself every day and scheduling work when you are usually at peak ability.
- **Set priorities:** It is necessary to know what is important to you. Don't attempt to work on four or five projects simultaneously. Keep efforts focused on one or two major items.
- **Establish realistic goals:** Although it is good to aim high, goals must also be achievable. Don't establish impossible expectations and then become frustrated when they are not accomplished as quickly as you would like. Write down long-range goals and then establish bench marks as checks for keeping you on track and monitoring progress. Short-term goals help you see how you are moving toward your goal and provide rewards as you advance toward success.
- **See yourself as achieving the goals:** Visualize yourself as being successful. Go over in your mind what it will look and feel like to accomplish the goal.
- **Give yourself a break:** Take time every day to exercise and relax.

(From Anspaugh, Hamrick, and Rosato.[6])

Depression is a mental state of varying duration characterized by feelings of sadness, rejection, apathy, hopelessness, and/or withdrawal. Theories as to the cause of depression vary. Depression can have a physiologic or biochemical basis (endogenous), such as with a hormonal imbalance, or an external basis (exogenous), as in the loss of a loved one. The symptoms of depression for both types are similar: unexplained fatigue, the blues, insomnia, decreased or increased appetite, withdrawal from friends and family, decreased sex drive, hopelessness and, in extreme cases, inability to engage in the activities of daily living or a desire to die. Commonly a person who is depressed has low self-esteem and feels helpless.

Prolonged depression can lead to suicide. Suicide ranks eighth among the leading causes of death in the United States. Among adolescents and young adults ages 15 to 24, it is the third highest cause of death. Three times as many women as men attempt suicide, but more men succeed in killing themselves.

Any threat of suicide should be taken seriously—it is a cry for help. Listen to the person who talks about suicide; call for help if needed. Many cities have a crisis hotline or crisis intervention team. If nothing else is available, call 911 or the police. Stay with the person until someone arrives to help.

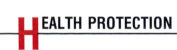

HEALTH PROTECTION

Health protection measures are designed to safeguard women from sexual harassment, rape, incest, domestic violence, and sexual abuse.

SEXUAL HARASSMENT

Sexual harassment can occur anywhere—at work, at play, or at school—and can come from a peer or a supervisor. Sexual harassment is "unwanted attention of a sexual nature that creates embarrassment or stress." According to guidelines set forth by the Equal Employment Opportunity Commission:

Unwelcome sexual advances, requests for sexual favors, and other physical conduct of a "sexual nature" constitute sexual harassment when any of three criteria are met: (1) submission to such conduct is made, either explicitly or implicitly, a term or condition of an individual's employment, OR (2) submission to or rejection of such conduct by an individual is used as a basis for employment, OR (3) such conduct has the purpose or effect of unreasonably interfering with an individual's work performance or creating an intimidating, hostile, or offensive working environment.

Sexual harassment may include unwanted physical contact, pressure from someone for dates, inferences or re-

marks of a sexual nature, or an offer of rewards for sexual favors. Some examples of sexually related conduct that may be considered unwelcome, even though it may not provoke verbal disapproval, include giving someone a kiss on the cheek; invitations for dinner or a date; massaging, touching, or brushing against a person's body; "leering" or "ogling"; commenting on the way clothing fits or looks; commenting on physical attributes; using demeaning or inappropriate terms in mixed groups; discussing sexual activities with others; calling a person by an undesired nickname or corruption of their name; standing closer than appropriate; making gestures or expressions that convey sexual connotations; giving gifts when inappropriate and/or unwanted. Recent court rulings have determined that the existence of harassment would be based on what the "reasonable woman" would consider sexual harassment.

Corporations, businesses, and schools have regulations governing sexual harassment. However, most women fail to report harassment for various reasons, including fear of losing their jobs or a reference; fear of ridicule or being labeled a troublemaker; embarrassment; and reluctance to reveal such personal acts in public, especially when they might be blamed for the other person's actions.

If sexual harassment occurs, documentation is imperative. The woman should determine what regulations are in place to protect individuals from sexual harassment and proceed as appropriate and according to policies in effect. Any incidents should be reported to the appropriate person or department. Each occurrence should be documented and witnessed, if possible. Sexual harassment is uncomfortable, unproductive, and illegal and can become dangerous. The employer has a legal responsibility to prevent, investigate, and respond to any report of sexual harassment and to provide appropriate education for employees regarding what it is and how acts of harassment will be handled. Sexual harassment is against the law.

RAPE

Rape, sexual assault, and incest are more frightening to women than are most other crimes. Rape appears to be on the increase. It is an act of violence, has nothing to do with passion or sex, and has a psychologically devastating effect on the victim. A list of guidelines for preventing rape appears in the box on p. 285.

In caring for the rape victim, areas of concern that the nurse should incorporate in a plan of care are screening and counseling for sexually transmitted diseases (STDs), human immunodeficiency virus (HIV), and pregnancy. Not only has the woman been personally and violently attacked, she has been exposed to deadly diseases and pregnancy. Follow-up is imperative for the victim.

RAPE PREVENTION GUIDELINES

- Never assume that you are an unlikely candidate for personal assault.
- Think carefully about your patterns of movement to and from class or work. Alter your routes frequently.
- Walk briskly with a sense of purpose. Try not to walk alone at night.
- Dress so that the clothes you wear do not unnecessarily restrict your movement or make you more vulnerable.
- Always be aware of your surroundings. Look over your shoulder occasionally. Know where you are so you won't get lost.
- If you think you are being followed, look for a safe retreat. This might be a store, a fire or police station, or a group of people.
- Be especially cautious of first dates, blind dates, or people you meet at a party or bar who push to be alone with you.
- Let trusted friends know where you are and when you plan to return.
- Keep your car in good working order. Think beforehand how you would handle the situation should your car break down.
- Trust your best instincts if you are assaulted. Each situation is different. Do what you can to protect your life.

(From Payne and Hahn, ed. 3.[86])

Many women who are raped do not report it to the police, and horror stories about the degrading treatment of rape victims do nothing to encourage reporting. A rape assault examination is conducted to collect evidence for prosecuting the rapist. This examination is thorough, and all evidence collected is sealed and given to the police for a trial. Rape counseling should be provided for both the victim and her family. Rape often has far-reaching effects on the victim, her spouse, and other members of her family. They should be referred to a local support group for continuing help. Help for the rape victim is outlined in the box below.

HELP FOR THE RAPE VICTIM

If you have been raped, you must seek help immediately.
- *Call the police to report the assault or go to the emergency room* of a local hospital immediately. Information and evidence collected will assist the police in apprehending and prosecuting the attacker. Specially trained nurses or women police officers are used in some hospitals to counsel rape victims and collect information and evidence in a caring and humane way.
- *Call the local Rape Crisis Center or Crisis Hotline* if you do not want to call the police. A special counselor usually can be reached at a 24-hour telephone number to assist rape victims in evaluating their options. They can escort the victim to the hospital, call the police, and provide counseling.
- *Maintain the evidence.* Do not bathe, douche, or change anything about you or the scene of the rape. A crime has been committed, and the evidence must be secure to make a definite identification and prosecution.
- *All injuries (including cuts, bruises, and scratches) need to be reported.* You may even think some are insignificant, but you need to report everything about the attack completely and accurately.
- *A thorough pelvic examination usually is performed.* Evidence is collected during the examination, injuries are assessed, and specimens for tests for STDs and pregnancy are collected. You may have to ask for the pregnancy and STD tests, as well as screening for AIDS.
- *Request that the police withhold your name from the media* as long as possible.

(From Helton.[51])

INCEST

Incest is the sexual abuse of a child by a family member. It is a hidden disorder, an insidious, destructive act that has long-term effects on the child and other members of the family as well. The rate of reported child abuse in families has risen dramatically in the past few years. Perhaps this is another spin-off of the women's movement—women feel empowered to reveal the unconscionable acts against them as children, or against their children if it is still occurring. Public awareness of the prevalence of incest increased during the 1970s, when the child protection lobby was incorporated. It connected child sexual abuse to the battered child syndrome and the women's movement (which recognized child sexual abuse as rape). Women's experiences are addressed in this section.

It has been estimated that 4.5% of adult women experienced an incestuous relationship with their fathers before the age of 18. One of three girls and one of seven boys are sexually abused before the age of 18. In comparing the incidence of incest to child abuse, theories are that one third of all child sexual abuse is committed by a family member. It is estimated that only one in every five cases is reported.

Symptoms or behaviors that might suggest the occurrence of incest are listed below. They pertain to children, adults, and fathers or father substitutes.*

SYMPTOMS OR BEHAVIORS IN AN *ADULT* THAT MIGHT SUGGEST INCEST

Nightmares

Recurrent pain, especially abdominal or genital, that cannot be explained medically

*Adapted from Bass and Davis[9b] and Helton.[51]

Sexual dysfunction or avoidance of intimacy

Compulsion either to become promiscuous or to avoid sex

Eating dysfunction

Lying, stealing, gambling

Change in behavior

Workaholism

Overly religious

Panic attacks

Overly safety-conscious

Hallucinations/flashbacks

SYMPTOMS OR BEHAVIORS IN *FATHERS OR FATHER SUBSTITUTES* THAT MIGHT SUGGEST INCEST

Open sexuality that seems inappropriate

Physical contact that seems inappropriate

Domineering, manipulative, oppressive, or coercive behavior

Alcohol or drug dependency

SYMPTOMS OR BEHAVIORS IN *CHILDREN* THAT MIGHT SUGGEST INCEST

Physical signs: Abdominal or pelvic pain and/or bleeding; vaginal or anal irritation or redness; pain, irritation, or redness around mouth

Change in behavior: Difficulty sleeping, nightmares, night terrors; grades fall off; lying, stealing, gambling; fear of being alone; inappropriate behavior between abuser and person abused when around others (especially daughters acting more like adults than children in relationships with the abusing father); role reversal with the mother

The damage to children who are victims of incest does not end when the abuse stops. It continues throughout

---

HOW THE HEALTH PROFESSIONAL CAN HELP A VICTIM OF INCEST

Learn everything you can about child sexual abuse, incest, and the adult survivor, so that you can help the person who has been abused and her family.

Support the survivor; don't doubt her story, and don't sympathize with the abuser.

Help the survivor determine how this has affected her and what she needs to do to heal.

Help the child (or adult) understand that she is not the person at fault; the abuser is.

Help the abused person know that what happened was awful and you understand how bad she feels. Let her know how bad you feel about what happened to her.

Give the person support over time. It will take time, and the abused person needs to know that you care and that you share her feelings of outrage and sadness.

Refer the person for counseling and to a support group.

If the person is suicidal, stay with her until she can get help.

Do not treat the person as a victim—she is a survivor, and it took a lot of courage and strength to survive.

The survivor will be changed as a result of the process of healing, and your relationship will likewise change.

the abused person's lifetime. But healing is possible, and nurses must learn more about incest and sexual abuse to be able to support these victims (see the box on page 286). The survivors of incest and/or child abuse need more than time. We are now finding that many children coped by repressing the memory of the abuse. However, throughout the years, the person had unexplainable reactions to being touched, to taking her clothes off in front of others (as in gym class), or to being alone with the abusing parent. As adults many of these individuals experience what has been described as posttraumatic stress syndrome—flashbacks, nightmares, and hallucinations remembering what happened in snatches. Some who have been unable to escape the reality of what happened to them have developed multiple personalities, have attempted (or succeeded at) suicide, or have ended up somewhere in between.

In *The Courage to Heal* (1992), Ellen Bass and Laura Davis proposed several stages of healing for victims of sexual abuse or incest. Briefly these are:

- The decision to heal—recognizing the effects of the abuse in your life and committing yourself to the arduous task of healing.
- The emergency stage—beginning to deal with the memories. This is very traumatic.
- Remembering—this brings back both memory and feeling of what happened.
- Believing it happened—accepting that the abuse actually happened and hurt you.
- Breaking the silence—and sharing the secret.
- Understanding that it wasn't your fault—placing the blame on the abuser, where it belongs.
- Making contact with the child within—getting in touch with your compassion and your anger, and beginning to express greater intimacy with others.
- Trusting yourself—learning to trust yourself again, your perceptions, feelings, and intuitions.
- Grieving and mourning—letting go of the pain and moving into the present.

MYTHS AND FACTS ABOUT ABUSE AND BATTERING

Myth	Fact
Battering occurs in a small percentage of the population.	Physical assault reportedly occurred in 28% of all American homes in 1976 (Strauss et al, 1980).
Battering occurs only in lower-class families.	Although lower-class families have a higher incidence of battering (Gelles, 1979), it also occurs in middle- and upper-income families. The incidence is not really known, because middle- and upper-income families tend to hide their battering.
Battered women like to be beaten and deliberately provoke the attack. They are masochistic.	Women are terrified of their assailants and go to great lengths to avoid a confrontation. In some cases the woman may provoke her husband to release tension that, if left unchecked, might lead to a more severe beating and possible death.
Batterers are uneducated men who are unable to cope with the world.	Many batterers are successful professionals, including politicians, ministers, physicians, and lawyers.
Men who batter their wives also beat their children.	One half of wife-batterers do not beat their children.
Battered women were battered children.	This myth holds true in only a few cases. Most battered women report that their husband was the first person to beat them.
Alcohol and drug abuse causes battering.	Gelles (1976) and Delgaty (1985) proposed that batterers use alcohol as an excuse to batter and shift the blame from themselves to the alcohol.
Once a battered wife, always a battered wife.	Many women who have battering relationships do not marry again. Those who stay in the relationships do so out of fear and financial dependence. Shelters have long waiting lists.
Batterers and battered women cannot change.	Counseling can effectively help resocialize both batterers and battered women.

(From Potter and Perry.[89])

- Anger, the backbone of healing—getting in touch with your rage and directing it to your abuser and those who didn't protect you.
- Disclosure and confrontation—directly confronting your abuser and/or family, which may be cathartic for many abused women.
- Forgiveness—for yourself; forgiving the abuser is not an essential part of the healing process.
- Spirituality—believing in a power greater than yourself, which can be an asset in the healing process.
- Resolution and moving on—progressing through these stages again and again, which allows you to reach a point of integration. You can't erase what happened to you, but you will make deep and lasting changes in your life. Having gained awareness, compassion, and power through healing, you will have the opportunity to work toward a better life.

DOMESTIC VIOLENCE AND SEXUAL ABUSE

Violence against women has been occurring for longer than can be documented, but physical abuse and battering are poorly understood. Some common misconceptions about violence against women in the United States are shown in the box on p. 287. Acts of violence against women are committed by men of all races, educational levels, professions, cultures, and socioeconomic classes. Characteristics of the victim and the abuser are outlined in the box below.

Battering is a crime punishable by law. Significantly, 90% of family homicides are preceded by family violence. Many women who commit suicide were battered (25% of white women, 50% of black women). Battering, abuse, and family violence all include repetitive episodes, demonstrable injuries, and evidence of deliberate, severe violence. Indicators of possible battering for women, men, and children are given in the box below.

The number of incidents of physical violence are staggering, and although most of these assaults are against women, men may also suffer abuse. Women are the vast majority of the victims, and health care providers must be aware of the clinical signs of abuse of women. These may include:

1. Drug or child abuse
2. Repeated injury to the head, face, neck, chest, abdomen, and upper extremities
3. A time delay between the injury and seeking treatment
4. Previous abuse

CHARACTERISTICS OF VICTIM AND ABUSER

Victim

Childhood influences

Many raised to be submissive, passive, and dependent
Likely to accept traditional female role in marriage
Accepts female sex-role stereotypes

Personality characteristics

Attributes beating to some personal inadequacy
Low self-esteem and feelings of worthlessness
Learned helplessness reduces problem-solving ability
Low tolerance for frustration
Easily upset, critical, aloof, and reserved
Severe stress reactions and psychophysiologic symptoms
Can't trust anyone
Some attempt suicide
Punishment justified if marriage fails
Unable to make "I" statements or maintain eye contact and denies and/or minimizes abuse

Life-style factors

Isolated from family and friends
Totally dependent on husband for financial and emotional support

Abuser

Childhood influences

Raised in family where men reign supreme
As a child may have used violence to problem solve
Accepts "macho" values

Personality characteristics

Feelings of inadequacy, inferiority, and insecurity
Emotionally immature and/or aggressive
Extremes in behavior and overreacting are typical
Low self-esteem with high degree of self-loathing
Intolerant of having masculinity threatened
Lacks respect for women
Poor impulse control
Excessive possessiveness and jealousy
Some use aggressive sexual attacks to punish and enhance own self-esteem
Alcohol or substance abuse may be present

Life-style factors

No particular profession, occupation, or socioeconomic group
Often has difficulties at work
Severely restricts wife's freedom and mobility

(From Bobak and Jensen.[13])

5. Chronic depression
6. Inappropriate use of sunglasses (assess with glasses removed for bruises around the eyes)
7. Broken bones
8. Serious bleeding injuries (nosebleed, lacerations)
9. Burns from a variety of sources
10. Vague or evasive answers in recounting the injuries

An appropriate method of assessing a battered women follows.
A cycle of violence has been described as including three phases*:

1. *The tension-building phase*—a period of increasing tension that leads to the battering; it usually includes anger, blaming, and arguing
2. *The acute battering incident*—the intense battering phase, which includes slapping, hitting, use of objects as weapons, sexual abuse, and verbal threats

*Adapted from Helton A: *A protocol of care for the battered woman*, White Plains, NY, 1987, March of Dimes Birth Defects Foundation.[51]

3. *The kindness and contrition, loving behavior phase, or calm stage*—the period of reconciliation and contrite behavior when the batterer promises never to do it again; he has taught the woman a lesson and will not have to beat her again. This stage may decrease or disappear.

Many factors enter into the decision of most women to remain with a batterer. Finances, lack of job skills, children to support, religion, fear of retaliation, and low self-esteem are among the most prevalent reported.

Pregnancy is a prime time for battering to begin or to escalate. The couple should be evaluated for risk factors, especially during prenatal visits and classes. The nurse should observe for poor communication and lack of support in interactions. The nurse also should provide education for preventing violence, and the options available if it occurs; screening and referral for signs of abuse; and care, counseling, and follow-up when

VIOLENCE AGAINST WOMEN IN THE UNITED STATES
- Each year 1 million to 6 million women are abused.
- A woman is beaten every 18 seconds.
- A rape or attempted rape occurs every 3½ to 6 minutes.
- Ten percent to 20% of all reported crimes are rapes.
- Eighty percent of rapes go unreported, and the victims do not seek health care.
- More than 100,000 cases of incest occur each year; many pregnancies result.

INDICATORS OF POSSIBLE BATTERING

(Not necessarily in order of prevalence)

IN WOMEN
- Change in appointment pattern; either increased appointments with somatic, vague complaints or frequently missed appointments
- Self-directed abuse, depression, attempted suicide
- Severe anxiety, insomnia, violent nightmares
- Alcohol or drug abuse

IN MEN
- Explosive temper
- Criticizing and denigrating partner, frequent "put-downs"
- Controlling of woman, attempts to control health care setting environment (may arrive unexpectedly)
- Breaks, throws objects when angry
- Makes all decisions on money and family

IN CHILDREN
- Child abuse, unexplained injuries, scars
- Somatic, emotional, and behavioral problems
- Violent behavior (particularly in boys)
- Sleep disturbances

- Complains of jealous, possessive male partner
- Frightened of partner's temper
- Defends partner's behavior ("rescues")
- Has been hit, slapped, kicked, shoved, or had objects thrown at her by partner
- (For some women) Abused as a child or saw mother abused

- Overprotective
- Jealous, suspicious
- Has hit, slapped, or pushed partner
- Alcohol or drug abuse
- Witnessed abuse as a child or was abused as child
- Defensive, particularly about inquiries regarding relationship with partner

- Difficulty in school, poor attention span
- Complains of headache, stomachaches
- Increased fears

(From Helton.[51])

PREPARATION

1. Always assess women for battering in a private place, away from her partner. Questioning a woman in front of her partner may place her in danger. Batterers frequently threaten the woman to maintain the secret of violence.
2. If children are present with the woman, ask staff members to watch the children to allow privacy when assessing the woman for battering.

PROCESS

1. Maintain eye contact when assessing a woman for battering. (In some cultures this may be inappropriate.) Battering is a health problem. Approach the topic as you would when assessing for other health risks. If a woman denies being battered or becomes upset at being questioned about it, explain that all your patients are screened for battering. Explain the concern health care providers have about the problem of violence against women.
2. Encourage but do not badger the woman to respond to the abuse assessment questions. A woman will choose when to share any history of violence with a health care provider. More time may be necessary for some battered women. Once the topic of battering has been opened, trust in the health care provider is necessary to encourage disclosure.
3. If you suspect or have evidence of battering, describe the cycle of violence and review the process of repetitive and escalating violence. Permit the patient to describe her situation; she may identify it as containing some or all of the elements of the cycle. Provide an environment that allows her to speak freely. *You may be the first person*, particularly the first *professional*, to acknowledge the problems she has experienced.
4. Provide all women patients (battered and nonbattered) with written referral information for community resources for battered women (police emergency, shelter, counseling, legal, etc.).

(From Helton AS: *A protocol of care for the battered woman*, White Plains, NY, 1987, March of Dimes Birth Defects Foundation.[51])

abuse is evident and the woman must leave the abusive situation.

Efforts aimed at preventing abuse and promoting health focus on several areas:

- Identifying the men at risk of becoming abusers
- Identifying the women and/or children at risk, or early in the abusive relationship
- Providing women with the information needed to recognize an abusive relationship before a commitment is made
- Assisting the victim in identifying her options and sources of support
- Giving women the support and information needed to reestablish a feeling of control and leave an abusive relationship
- If the woman is pregnant or has other children, protecting the unborn infant and other children
- Educating the legal authorities to assist the victim through the legal process

NURSING—HELPING WOMEN TAKE CHARGE

Nursing has a unique function in society—to provide care for patients while encouraging self-care. Working with patients to determine the course of their health care, nurses can help individuals reach their optimum level of wellness. Nurses do more than just provide health care services. They serve as patient advocates and change agents, helping the patient get through an illness, promoting positive changes in a person's life-style, and providing guidance and insight into maintaining those changes. As advocates for women, nurses must provide the information and support women need.

Understanding human behavior and what encourages an individual to seek change is a science that requires nursing to remain diligent and alert to new strategies and techniques. General guidelines for behavior change include:

- *Determine what needs to be changed* to assist the individual in reaching a higher level of wellness. This is where those assessment skills become so valuable. With the patient, assess her level of wellness and life-style to identify risk areas. She must be aware of the potential consequences of the health choices she makes.
- *Collect baseline data to determine the current level of risk* for the woman and how much effort is needed to make the needed behavior change. This may involve testing to determine blood levels of glucose in the case of a diabetic, maintaining a log if the concern is overeating or alcohol consumption, keeping a stress diary, or whatever seems to be relevant for the individual. Help the woman determine what kind of change she wants to make.
- *Determine what kind of motivation or commitment the individual has to make a change.* Help her be realistic and/or make the change in increments, a little at a time. Do not start a major change project until the person is ready. Build in success, not failure.
- *Set specific goals.* The woman needs a clear overall picture of what she wants to change and how

she can accomplish it.

- *Make a plan and analyze it.* Be realistic and decide specifically what habits need to be changed, what steps must be taken, and how long it may take to meet the objectives the woman sets.
- *Identify obstacles to the plan.* Plan strategies to overcome these obstacles as they may occur. Deal with anything that might interfere with meeting the objectives—lack of time, fear of harassment, weather conditions, comfort, or even lack of knowledge.
- *Evaluate success and plan rewards.* Record keeping and a supportive person can help an individual stay on target. The reward increases motivation and helps the person realize success. This would be an appropriate time to reevaluate the goals made. Are they still realistic? Do objectives previously made need to be changed?
- *Develop a support system to reinforce efforts* and keep up the motivation for change. Review the original plan. How have changes affected the individual? How far has she come? How will she maintain the change?

Actually seeing and feeling the effects of positive change encourage individuals to maintain a healthy lifestyle. It empowers women to strive for a higher level of wellness and puts them in charge of their health. Women must understand how they can play an active part in their health care and participate in the decision-making and treatment process. Women can begin taking charge of their own wellness by adopting a few basic habits to promote good health (see the preceding box).

PERIODIC HEALTH SCREENING TO PROMOTE WELLNESS

Wellness is a process that continually changes. Periodic health screening allows the individual and the health care provider to follow the woman's health status, identify risks and/or illnesses, make positive changes to minimize disability or disease, and optimize health. Specific tests and health screening procedures have been recommended for women throughout their lifetime by various health care groups, such as the American Cancer Society. Women need to know what these tests are, why they need them, and the appropriate schedule for them (see the box on p. 292).

THE FUTURE OF WOMEN'S HEALTH

Despite the ever-growing amount of information and the phenomenal technical advances in health care, we still have a long way to go to understand women's health. We do not know if any of the therapies for major diseases actually benefit women because they have never been tested on women. A lot has been written about the lack of research in women's health, and efforts to improve this are currently under way. Harvard University's long-standing Women's Health Study and the NIH Women's Health Initiative have joined forces to study the major diseases in postmenopausal women including cancer, heart disease, and osteoporosis. Other major studies are in progress as well, looking at disease and disability in women. Other studies are looking at hormone replacement therapy and heart disease; the influence of a low-fat diet on breast cancer, colon cancer, and heart disease; use of calcium and vitamin D in preventing osteoporosis; and the relationship of blood pressure and dietary habits with disease. We have a basic understanding of hormonal influences on the physical and emotional health of women, but only beginning knowledge on how we can assist women to control these influences. We have made great strides, but we still cannot adjust hormones at will and get the response desired.

These are some of the efforts in the physiologic basis of health, but what of the psychosocial aspects of disease? Why are 20% to 25% of women who are pregnant being battered? Why has incest survived the women's movement? Why do only 15% of women over the age of 50 take advantage of having a mammogram when they are at higher risk for breast cancer and this screening can identify a cancerous mass 3 years before it can be felt on exam? Why is heart disease the major killer of women when we know it is mainly a result of life-style practices? Why are the incidence and death from lung cancer and other lung diseases rising among women when we know that they are a direct result of smoking cigarettes, which is on the increase among women? Why is poverty so prevalent among women? Why are women and children going hungry and homeless in this technology-rich world?

We as health care providers must address these questions, and we must find methods to help individuals change their life-styles to move toward a higher state of wellness. Some answers can be found in empowerment of women: giving them the information and services that promote prevention, health care, and health maintenance, and teaching them how to make positive changes in their health practices. We see major efforts in health care and legislative reform, such as in legislation for family leave, but other legislative loopholes negate the benefits for some (only 60% of women are affected by this legislation).

Our job is clear—we must be advocates for those women who do not have the ability to care for themselves today and make sure that they are prepared for that task in the future. People in leadership positions must be enlightened to the benefits of providing for future generations by caring for today's women.

Women's Health in the United States
A new survey shows that more than one third of the 95 million adult women in the United States did not have any of the basic preventive services, such as a Pap smear, in the past year.

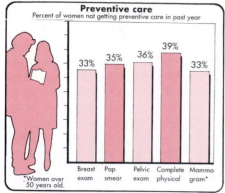

Preventive care
Percent of women not getting preventive care in past year

33% 35% 36% 39% 33%

Breast exam, Pap smear, Pelvic exam, Complete physical, Mammogram*

*Women over 50 years old.

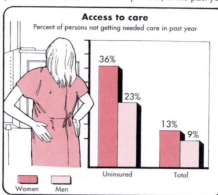

Access to care
Percent of persons not getting needed care in past year

36% 23% 13% 9%

Uninsured — Total

Women — Men

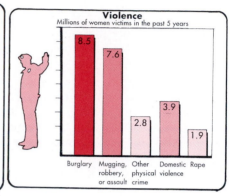

Violence
Millions of women victims in the past 5 years

8.5 7.6 2.8 3.9 1.9

Burglary, Mugging robbery or assault, Other physical crime, Domestic violence, Rape

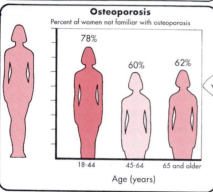

Osteoporosis
Percent of women not familiar with osteoporosis

78% 60% 62%

18-44 45-64 65 and older
Age (years)

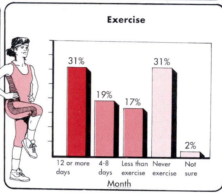

Exercise

31% 19% 17% 31% 2%

12 or more days, 4-8 days, Less than exercise, Never exercise, Not sure
Month

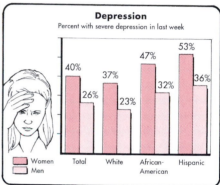

Depression
Percent with severe depression in last week

40% 26% 37% 23% 47% 32% 53% 36%

Total White African-American Hispanic

Women — Men

GUIDELINES FOR PERIODIC HEALTH SCREENING

- *Cholesterol testing*—every 5 years, beginning in early teen years; twice or more per year if extreme changes in weight or activity have occurred, if the woman has been ill or had previously tested high, or with any other life changes or chronic disease that requires cholesterol screening.
- *Hemaglobin and hematocrit*—every 5 to 10 years if not indicated earlier.
- *Blood glucose*—every 3 to 5 years after age 20, if within normal limits.
- *Blood pressure*—every year age 14 to 40; two or more times per year after age 40 or earlier if a woman has elevated or borderline blood pressure; takes oral contraceptives; has a history of heart disease; smokes; is overweight; has chronic diseases that require periodic blood pressure screening; takes steroids; or has kidney disease.
- *Pelvic examination*—every 1 to 3 years beginning at age 18 or when a woman or girl becomes sexually active; every year after age 40.
- *Pap smear*—begun at age 18 or when a woman or girl becomes sexually active; then every 1 to 3 years after two negative smear results; every year after age 40.
- *Breast self-examination*—monthly.
- *Endometrial tissue biopsy*—the American Cancer Society recommends one screening test if a woman is anovulatory, has a history of infertility, or has abnormal uterine bleeding; also if the woman is postmenopausal and is considering estrogen replacement therapy (ERT) or the use of tamoxifen.
- *Professional breast examination*—every 1 to 3 years ages 16 to 39; every year after age 40.
- *Mammogram*—one baseline test at age 35 if there is no family history of breast cancer before age 35; every 1 to 2 years after age 40; every year after age 50.
- *Digital-rectal examination/occult blood*—once a year after age 40.
- *Proctosigmoidoscopy*—every 3 to 4 years.
- *Bone scan*—baseline 1 year to 18 months after menopause.

CHAPTER 15

Patient Teaching Guides

The responsibility for health and wellness lies with the individual and requires that the individual who strives for optimal health participate in health-promoting behaviors. Today, women are more educated, knowledgeable, and sophisticated about their rights and responsibilities where health care is concerned. Nurses have a unique opportunity in women's health care because they can provide information and services that promote health awareness, health care, and health maintenance, and thus help women care for themselves.

Often women do not take advantage of opportunities for health-promoting activities because they do not understand the value of prevention. Patient teaching is the key to health promotion for women. Nurses can provide women with the information they need to participate in making decisions regarding their own health care.

This chapter provides handouts that can be photocopied and given to patients and their partners or families to take home and use as guidelines for self-care. Several of these guides facilitate early detection of breast disorders and sexually transmitted diseases by demonstrating procedures for self-examination and symptom detection. Other patient teaching guides explain specific disorders—their prevention, detection, and treatment. These include fibrocystic disease of the breast, breast cancer, sexually transmitted diseases, pelvic inflammatory disease, and urinary tract infections. Still others discuss conditions associated with body changes, such as premenstrual syndrome, menopause, and osteoporosis. Also, procedures such as hysterectomy and contraception are explained for the patient. Finally, guides discussing measures for preventing transmission of STDs are included.

These teaching guides are not intended to replace direct teaching. They are to be used by the nurse to reinforce patient teaching and to encourage the patient's participation and compliance in her own health care management.

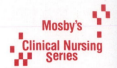
Breast Self-Examination

Performing breast self-examination once a month could save your life. Many breast cancers are discovered by patients who had regularly done self-examination and thus were able to distinguish a change from what is normal in their breasts. If you are still menstruating, examine your breasts right after your period ends. If you have reached menopause, pick a day of the month that is easy to remember.

How to perform breast self-examination

1. Undress and stand in front of a mirror with your arms at your sides (Figure 1). Look for any changes in the shape or size of your breasts or for anything unusual, such as discharge from the nipples or puckering or dimpling of the skin.
2. Raise your arms above and behind your head, and press your hands together (Figure 2). Look for the same things as in step 1.
3. Place the palms of your hands firmly on your hips (Figure 3); look again for any changes.
4. Raise your left arm over your head. Examine your left breast by firmly pressing the fingers of your right hand down and around in a circular motion until you have examined every part of the breast (Figure 4). Be sure to include the area between your breast and armpit and the armpit itself. You are feeling for any lump or mass under the skin. If you find a lump, notify your doctor.
5. Gently squeeze the nipple, and look for any discharge (Figure 5). Some discharge is normal, but report pinkish or reddish discharge to your doctor.
6. Repeat steps 4 and 5 on your right breast. (You may also perform steps 4 and 5 in the shower.)
7. Now, lie down on your back with a pillow under your right shoulder. Put your right arm under your head (Figure 6). This position flattens the breast and makes it easier to examine. Examine your right breast just as you did in steps 4 and 5. Repeat on your left breast.

Don't panic if you notice anything unusual. This doesn't necessarily mean you have cancer. Call your doctor, nurse, or clinic to schedule a professional breast examination. *Remember: breast self-examination is important, but it is not a substitute for a doctor's examination and regular mammograms for women over age 35.*

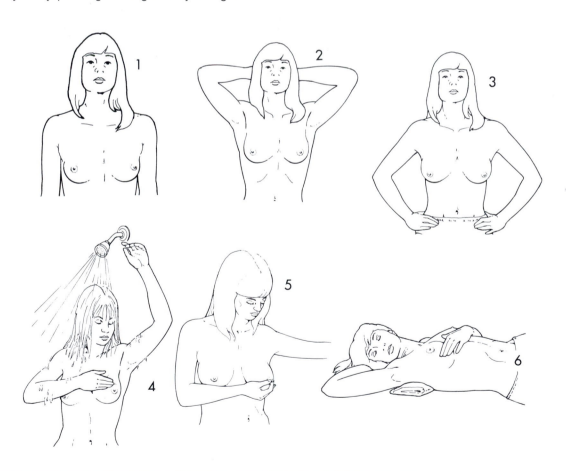

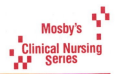

Mosby's
Clinical Nursing
Series

Fibrocystic Changes of the Breast

What are fibrocystic changes? Does this mean I have breast cancer?

Fibrocystic changes are the most common cause of breast lumps in women 30 to 50 years of age. These changes may also be referred to as fibrocystic disease, cystic disease, chronic cystic mastitis, or mammary dysplasia. This condition is not cancerous. At least 50% of women in their reproductive years have lumpy breasts as a result of this noncancerous condition.

How are breast changes diagnosed?

Usually fibrocystic changes can be diagnosed by physical examination or mammography, an x-ray of the breast. Fibrocystic changes may also be found with a biopsy, in which a small amount of tissue or fluid is removed from the breast and examined in the laboratory. Fortunately, only about 5% of women who require biopsies for a fibrocystic condition have the type of changes that would be considered a risk factor for cancer.

What causes fibrocystic changes?

Fibrocystic changes occur because of the way breast tissue responds to monthly changes in the levels of estrogen and progesterone, two female hormones produced by the ovaries during a woman's reproductive years. Each month during the menstrual cycle, breast tissue alternately swells and returns to normal. Hormonal stimulation of breast tissue causes the blood vessels to swell, the milk glands and ducts to enlarge, and the breasts to retain water. The breasts frequently feel swollen, painful, tender, and lumpy at this time. After menstruation, the swelling decreases and the breasts feel less tender and lumpy; that's why the best time to examine your breasts is right after your menstrual period ends.

How do fibrocystic changes feel? What should I look for?

Repeated hormone stimulation from monthly changes causes breast tissue to become firmer, and pockets of fluid, called cysts, may form in obstructed or enlarged milk ducts. The breast tissue may feel like an irregularly shaped area of thicker tissue with a lumpy or ridgelike surface. Fibrocystic tissue may also feel like tiny beads scattered throughout the breast.

Fibrocystic changes usually are found in both breasts, most often in the upper outer quadrant and the underside of the breast, where a ridge may sometimes be felt. In premenopausal women with a fibrocystic condition, lumpy areas in the breast may increase in size, and the woman may feel discomfort ranging from a feeling of fullness or heaviness to a dull ache, extreme sensitivity to touch, or a burning sensation. For some women the pain is so severe that it precludes exercise or even lying on the abdomen. The condition tends to subside after menopause (change of life).

How do I tell fibrocystic changes from a "lump" in my breast?

Confusion arises because not all women with lumps have fibrocystic changes. The breast is naturally a lumpy gland. The lumpy consistency arises from the milk glands and ducts and the fibrous tissue that separates and supports them. Practicing breast self-examination (BSE) regularly helps a woman distinguish between normal lumps and ones that must be evaluated by a physician.

How is a fibrocystic condition treated?

Treatment of a fibrocystic condition may require surgical removal (biopsy) of lumps that fail to disappear after brief observation, and attempts to remove fluid by a physician. For painful breasts a physician may recommend aspirin or other pain relievers. Also, applying warmth to the breasts (such as with a heating pad), wearing a good support bra, and avoiding caffeine in coffee, tea, chocolate, and soft drinks may help decrease water retention. *Patients with cystic breasts should not have caffeine.* Occasionally a physician may prescribe medications such as vitamin E, danazol, or tamoxifen to help relieve the symptoms.

What is a mammogram?

A mammogram is a low-dose x-ray examination that can detect lumps infinitely smaller than fingers can feel, and with minimal risk. Women between the ages of 35 and 39 who have no symptoms of breast cancer should have a mammogram as a baseline for comparison; women ages 40 to 49 should have a mammogram every 1 or 2 years; and women age 50 or over should have a mammogram yearly.

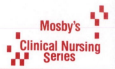

Discovery of Breast Cancer

I've found a lump in my breast. Does that mean I have cancer?

Every year thousands of women find a breast lump, and it's always an unsettling experience. However, most breast lumps aren't serious medical problems—they're simply noncancerous lumps. And thanks to breast self-examination and today's sophisticated technology, lumps that are cancerous often are diagnosed earlier, when they're smaller and can be treated more successfully. Although all lumps must be evaluated, most are noncancerous *(benign)* and give little cause for worry. Others are cancerous *(malignant)* and need prompt treatment.

What should I do first?

Have the lump evaluated as soon as possible. Mammography and other techniques can help determine whether the lump is benign or malignant. An evaluation also can indicate what type of treatment, if any, is most suitable for you. If you need treatment, your primary physician will recommend that you see a surgeon. There are several ways to decide what surgeon to see: (1) let your doctor refer you to one; (2) see a surgeon recommended by a friend you trust; (3) call the medical society in your area for a recommendation. Once you see a surgeon, talk with him or her about your options before you make a decision. It is a good idea (and often required by insurance companies) to obtain a second opinion. You'll find that more treatment options are available today than ever before.

What exactly is breast cancer?

The cells of malignant breast lumps grow uncontrollably and may invade other breast tissue or eventually spread *(metastasize)* beyond the breast. Often single, hard, and painless, these lumps usually don't change with the menstrual cycle. There are many different types of malignant lumps, but most develop in mammary ducts or glands. The size of the lump and how far it has spread determine the *stage* of breast cancer, which in turn influences the treatment approach.

How will my breast be tested?

A history and physical examination help your doctor begin to evaluate the lump and assess the likelihood that it is cancerous. A mammogram and ultrasound tests provide pictures of your breast that will reveal any abnormalities. In addition, a medical history provides medical information that helps in assessing your risk of cancer. You may be asked whether family members have had breast cancer. You may also be asked about your menstrual history and about the physical characteristics of the lump.

A physical examination helps determine the location, size, and general condition of the breast lump and lymph nodes. Using firm finger pressure, your doctor examines your breasts and underarm area, looking for lumps, dimpling or puckering of the skin, or fluid from the nipples.

Unless you've had a mammogram recently, your surgeon may request one. This breast x-ray, which may be a little uncomfortable, is the most helpful technique for spotting lumps too small to be felt. A pressure device slightly flattens your breast to provide a precise image. The x-ray is examined for lumps or clusters of tiny calcium deposits, which sometimes are associated with either cancer or benign conditions. Finally, an ultrasound scan may help distinguish solid lumps from fluid-filled cysts. "Echoes" from painless sound waves are converted into a visual image of the interior of your breast. Occasionally magnetic resonance imaging (MRI) is used for confirmation. All of these procedures help you and your surgeon decide whether a biopsy should be the next step.

What is a biopsy?

A *needle biopsy* is a simple procedure similar to taking blood. It takes only a few minutes and is easily performed in a doctor's office. Occasionally a local anesthetic is used to numb the breast area temporarily. After the breast has been cleansed with an antiseptic, the surgeon inserts a thin needle into the lump and extracts a few cells. If the lump is filled with fluid, the surgeon may be able to remove all the fluid, and no further treatment is likely. If the lump is solid, cells are removed and evaluated under a microscope to determine whether the lump is benign or malignant.

An *open biopsy* involves making a small incision in your breast and removing all or part of the lump for examination under a microscope.

The lump is malignant. Now what?

Hearing this diagnosis may be one of the most difficult things you ever experience. Whether you're told in person or over the phone, have someone with you or know whom you can call if you find out the lump is malignant. And remember, treatment will likely allow you to live a healthy life.

When you're ready, your surgeon will discuss treatment options with you, which you may, in turn, want to talk over with your family or a friend. You may also need other tests to help determine your best treatment options. You may take up to a few weeks to get a second opinion and talk with friends and women who have had breast cancer.

What are some of my treatment options?

Many more treatment options are available today than ever before for women with breast cancer. A *lumpectomy* is a fairly new procedure in which the breast is preserved but the lump and some normal tissue around it are removed. Axillary lymph nodes often are removed and examined for signs of cancer. *Radiation therapy,* a program of painless x-rays, usually follows a lumpectomy to eliminate any remaining cancer cells in your breast or lymph nodes. It typically is given in a few brief treatments every week for 5 or 6 weeks.

Another treatment option is a *modified radical mastectomy,* in which the breast and axillary lymph nodes are removed. Two variations of this technique are the *simple mastectomy,* in which the axillary lymph nodes are left intact, and the *radical mastectomy,* in which deep chest muscles and lymph nodes are removed. Most mastectomy patients can have breast reconstruction, either at the time of surgery or in the future.

How do I live with cancer?

- Take control of the options. Quiet or shy individuals may wish to appoint a spokesperson to insist upon certain conditions.
- There is a normal grief cycle that occurs with stress. For example, denial (or disbelief) occurs when cancer is first diagnosed.
- Ask for written material, so that confusing information can be re-read. Ask for a summary of treatment options, risks, and prognosis (potential outcome). Also, write down questions, and expect answers to these questions.
- Obtain the reasons behind various treatment and prevention plans. For instance, teeth may chip more easily, but these conditions can be corrected, or cosmetically repaired, especially if the teeth are kept in optimal condition.
- Be prepared for complications, and remember

that these conditions usually can be managed medically. For example, diabetes, high blood pressure, or thyroid disorders may surface for the first time, or become worse, during cancer treatment.

- Expect physical changes. Anticipate that hair loss will occur more than once.
- A cancer patient's quality of life can be excellent. For example, radiation therapy helps relieve pain. Pain killers, such as narcotics, can be taken without harmful side effects.
- Support groups are helpful for providing resources and psychologic help, and may assist family and friends.
- It is not wrong or harmful to discuss cancer with friends and family members, unless the topic of cancer becomes excessive or consuming.
- Keep a positive outlook and a good sense of humor! Laughter does seem to discourage illness and promote health!

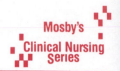

Mosby's
**Clinical Nursing
Series**

Premenstrual Syndrome

What is premenstrual syndrome?

Premenstrual syndrome, commonly known as PMS, is a collection of both physical and psychologic symptoms that usually occur 7 to 10 days before menstruation and disappear once the menstrual flow starts. It recurs at about the same time every month, and those who suffer from it tend to have the same symptoms each month. This predictable recurrence of symptoms is most significant in diagnosing the syndrome.

What causes PMS?

Doctors think the symptoms of PMS are related to changes in the levels of estrogen and progesterone, two hormones your ovaries produce during the menstrual cycle. These two hormones may interact with chemicals in your brain, producing this syndrome. It is also thought that prostaglandins cause the muscle or joint pain and headaches that often accompany PMS. Other theories suggest possible thyroid deficiency, a change in the body's ability to process carbohydrates, and a decrease in the opiate-like hormones naturally made by the body.

What are some of the most common symptoms of PMS?

Symptoms fall into two categories: emotional and physical. The most common emotional symptoms are depression, compulsive eating, assaultive behavior, panic attacks, food cravings, irritability, confusion, child abuse, alcoholic bouts, lethargy, anger, forgetfulness, self-abuse, tension, and increased sex drive.

The most common physical symptoms are migraine headaches, fainting, seizures, vertigo, asthma, rhinitis, sinusitis, breast engorgement and tenderness, cystitis, joint pain, backache, acne, sore throat, edema, herpes flare-ups, diarrhea, fatigue, nausea and vomiting, and swollen and painful varicose veins.

How common is PMS?

Any woman, from her first period until menopause, can suffer from PMS. It is estimated that 40% of all women have PMS in varying degrees at some time in their lives. Most develop PMS after a significant interruption of their hormonal cycles, such as occurs in pregnancy or through the use of oral contraceptives.

How can I find out if my problems are really caused by PMS?

The best thing you can do is chart your menstrual cycle and activities related to a possible premenstrual syndrome. Things you should keep track of on the chart are (1) symptoms (their type and severity); (2) medications (all prescription and over-the-counter drugs, both the kind and the time you take them); (3) foods (both unusual foods and unusual times you eat; include items you crave or eat more of than usual, such as salt, sugar, alcohol, or caffeine); and (4) especially stressful situations.

How is PMS treated?

Because PMS is a progesterone-deficiency illness, taking a synthetic progesterone may help, but by itself it will not control PMS. Treatment involves relieving the symptoms and, when possible, correcting the cause.

First, bloating and fluid retention may be relieved by reducing salt intake and using a diuretic drug to remove excess body water. Dietary changes may be made to increase protein and decrease sugars and alcohol; antianxiety drugs may be used to ease nervousness and lack of control. Seeing a therapist can help in modifying behavior and reducing stress; and adjusting your hormone levels may be helpful.

Can I do anything to prevent PMS?

You do have some control over your body's response to the menstrual cycle:

- Reduce your salt intake to prevent bloating.
- Do some form of moderate, enjoyable exercise four times a week.
- Cut back on caffeine and sugar.
- Keep your correct body weight. If you are 15 pounds or more over your desirable weight, consider a gradual weight-loss program.
- Reduce your stress level whenever possible. Don't schedule too many activities on the days you expect your symptoms to be severe.

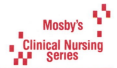
Mosby's
**Clinical Nursing
Series**

Before and After a Hysterectomy

I have been advised to have a hysterectomy to remove my uterus. Will my ovaries be removed, too?

Your first impression was right. A *hysterectomy* is an operation to remove the uterus. Sometimes the ovaries are taken out at the same time. Removal of the ovaries is called *oophorectomy*. It's important to know the difference between these two operations, because each has a different effect on your body. If you have only a hysterectomy, your periods will stop. But if you have your ovaries removed as well, the effects on your body will be greater. If your ovaries are removed, your body will no longer produce sufficient estrogen. This is called surgical menopause. It's just like natural menopause, except it happens more suddenly. And sometimes the effects are more severe, because of the sudden loss of estrogen.

What kind of reactions will my body have after an oophorectomy?

Most women (about 85%) feel some of the effects of the sudden, complete loss of estrogen immediately. At first you can probably expect hot flashes and night sweats. The hot flashes spread over the chest and neck area; the night sweats may wake you up from a sound sleep. This sleep disturbance may result in tiredness, depression, and nervousness. These may continue for several years. Some problems caused by estrogen loss may crop up later, but these can often be prevented by taking estrogen.

What's so important about estrogen?

Estrogen, a hormone made by your ovaries, prepares the uterus for either pregnancy or a menstrual period. It's needed, along with calcium, to keep bones strong; it also helps protect your vaginal and urinary tract tissues against thinning and drying.

What are the other health problems of surgical menopause besides hot flashes and night sweats?

One problem—changes in cholesterol levels—can slowly build up for years. After menopause it is very likely that cholesterol levels will increase more rapidly. Surgical menopause may also cause the lining of your vagina to become thin and dry, causing pain sometimes during or after sex. Over time, changes in the urinary system may cause bladder control problems, such as the need to urinate more frequently or some leakage of urine when coughing or sneezing.

Can anything be done to cure or prevent these problems?

Taking estrogen can help relieve or prevent many of these problems. It certainly relieves hot flashes and night sweats, helps prevent vaginal and urinary tract tissue from thinning and drying, and is the single best way to prevent osteoporosis. Replacing lost estrogen greatly lowers a woman's chances of breaking a bone or developing a humped back. Estrogen has no effect on rising cholesterol levels, but it does not affect them adversely.

I've heard that estrogen can cause cancer. Is this true?

Some studies have suggested a possible increased incidence of breast cancer in women taking *higher* doses of estrogen for prolonged periods of time, but most of these studies do not link breast cancer with taking the *usual* doses of estrogen *after* menopause. However, if anyone in your family has had breast cancer, let your doctor know before you start taking estrogen. Your doctor may very well recommend that you continue taking estrogen, even after any obvious symptoms have vanished. Taking estrogen continually lessens your chances of breaking a bone by as much as 50% to 60%. Taking estrogen along with calcium helps your bones stay strong. Almost half of the bone loss a woman suffers occurs in the first 7 years after surgical menopause. And if you have a hysterectomy at age 35 or 40, you can expect to live another 40 years or more without producing natural estrogen.

On the other hand, since taking any drug has some chance of side effects, estrogen may not be right for you. It's important to consult your physician about the best treatment for you to counter the effects of surgical menopause.

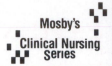
Vulvar Self-Examination

Cancer of the vulva is still a rare disease, but it is occurring more frequently. Women over age 50 are most susceptible to this cancer, but it can occur at any age. Examining your vulvar area once a month can help you discover the first symptoms of vulvar cancer, which can be cured if treated early. The vulvar area includes all the female external genital organs: the pubic mound, clitoris, urinary opening, vaginal opening, and anus (Figure 1).

How to perform vulvar self-examination

Use a flashlight and a hand mirror to make viewing easier. You may do the examination while sitting on the edge of the toilet seat, your bed, or the bathtub. Sit with your legs spread apart, and check the entire vulvar region (Figure 2).

Examine both sides of the labia (the opening folds of the vulva), and see if they are similar.

With your fingers, separate the inner lips of the vulva, and check the clitoris, the urinary opening, the vagina, and the skin between the vagina and anus (Figure 3).

Press down on all areas of the vulva, feeling for any lumps or masses (Figure 4).

Gently squeeze the vaginal opening between your thumb and forefinger. It should feel soft and moist (not tender or sore) (Figure 5).

If you notice any of the following, see your doctor:

Lumps, masses, or growths

Any change in skin color

Moles or birthmarks on the vulva that change color, bleed, or enlarge

Burning in the vulva during urination

Persistent itching

Soreness or tenderness that doesn't go away

Usually these signs don't indicate cancer, but check with your doctor to make sure.

What causes vulvar cancer, and what can I do to prevent it?

It is unclear what causes cancer in the vulvar area, but certain conditions are thought to lead to the disease. These include poor hygiene, certain types of sexually transmitted diseases, cancer of other reproductive organs, and a condition called dystrophy, in which the skin of the vulva may thin or thicken, and red or white patches and sores may appear. You can help prevent some of these problems by seeing your gynecologist at least once a year, reporting any changes you find during your vulvar self-examination, and practicing good hygiene. Good hygiene of the vulva includes the following:

Wiping from front to back after urination or a bowel movement

Avoiding scented and perfumed products such as tampons, sanitary pads, feminine hygiene products, and scented soaps

Using unscented, white toilet paper

Wearing all-cotton underwear

Avoiding tight clothing such as girdles, pantyhose, and form-fitting jeans

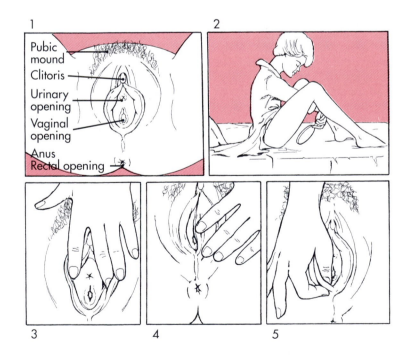

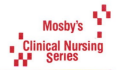

Signs and Symptoms of Sexually Transmitted Diseases

I've been told I may have a sexually transmitted disease. Does that mean I have AIDS?

No. There are over 50 known sexually transmitted diseases (STDs). AIDS (acquired immunodeficiency syndrome) is certainly the most talked about these days, but it's only one kind. Most STDs can be treated, others can be controlled, and all can be prevented. However, it's important to receive treatment for any STD, because left untreated, some STDs can cause serious health problems, including infertility, heart disease, brain damage, damage to unborn children, and even death.

Who is most at risk for getting a sexually transmitted disease?

Anyone who has sexual relations is potentially at risk, but particularly those who are not monogamous or have not been monogamous in the past. With the exception of AIDS and hepatitis B (which can be spread by sharing drug needles), if you don't have sex, you have virtually no risk of getting an STD. If you have sex with only one person who also has had no other sex partners, you have a low risk of infection. If you have sex with a few people you know well, your risk increases. The sex partners you choose determine the risk you face. If your partner has sex with others, your risk increases, and you lose control of that risk, because you have no control over your partner's choices. Finally, of course, if you have sex with many people, particularly people you don't know well, you are at highest risk of getting an STD.

What are the signs, symptoms, and treatment of the more common sexually transmitted diseases?

There are many different kinds of infections that can be transmitted during sexual activity. Never attempt to make a diagnosis on your own; the following list offers only a general description of a few of the most common sexually transmitted diseases.

Chlamydia—*Symptoms:* Pain on urination, vaginal discharge, or abdominal pain. Keep in mind, though, that often a woman doesn't have symptoms at first. Left untreated, chlamydia leads to serious infection, called pelvic inflammatory disease (PID); symptoms usually occur within 1 to 3 weeks after sex with an infected partner. *Treatment:* When diagnosed early, chlamydia can be cured easily with antibiotics.

Genital herpes—*Symptoms:* Early symptoms include burning or pain with urination, pain in the buttocks, legs, or genital area, vaginal discharge, or a feeling of pressure in the pelvic area. In a few days, small red bumps appear in the genital area; later the bumps develop into blisters, which open, crust, and then heal. Even after the sores disappear, the herpes virus remains in the body and can reactivate at any time, causing a new outbreak of blisters. The symptoms develop within 2 to 10 days after sex with an infected partner. *Treatment:* Herpes can't be cured, but it can be controlled. The drug acyclovir may speed healing and prevent recurrences. It also helps to keep the sores clean, dry, and free of irritation. Don't scratch them. Pregnant women who have had herpes should tell their doctors so precautions can be taken to protect the baby.

Gonorrhea—*Symptoms:* Often there are no signs. The person may experience pain or burning when urinating, or a woman may have a yellowish vaginal discharge. Advanced symptoms include bleeding between menstrual periods, swollen joints, fever, or pain in the pelvic area. Left untreated, gonorrhea leads to pelvic inflammatory disease (PID); symptoms usually occur within 2 to 10 days after sex with an infected partner. *Treatment:* Gonorrhea is a bacterial infection that can be quickly treated with antibiotics. Your partner should also be examined, and sexual activity should be avoided during treatment.

Genital warts (condylomata)—*Symptoms:* Genital warts are small bumpy warts that appear on or near the sex organs, usually 3 weeks to 3 months after sex with an infected partner. The warts sometimes develop inside the vagina, on the lips of the vagina, or around the anus, and they may grow into large masses. A mother may pass them on to her baby during childbirth. *Treatment:* Condylomata are most easily removed when they are small, so get treatment early. They're usually removed with chemicals such as podophyllin, but they may also be frozen off with liquid nitrogen or surgically removed. Repeat treatments often are necessary to remove all warts. A single wart can multiply.

Syphilis—*Symptoms:* The first symptom of syphilis, which usually occurs 1 to 12 weeks after sex with an infected partner, often is a painless sore on the genitals. The sore may occur inside the body and go unnoticed. The sore disappears within a few weeks, but the disease progresses. In the second stage, a skin rash appears, along with flu-like symptoms. These, too, eventually go away, but the disease doesn't. Left untreated, syphilis can lead to blindness, heart disease, brain damage, and even death. *Treatment:* Early antibiotic treatment is important. The symptoms of the infection may disappear, but the disease will remain in the body.

Human immunodeficiency virus (HIV) infection and AIDS—*Symptoms:* HIV infection and AIDS may produce no symptoms for months or years. As the immune system weakens, the symptoms include swollen lymph glands, fever, night sweats, severe fatigue, and weight loss. AIDS may be diagnosed when the person develops rare cancers and pneumonia. *Treatment:* If you have symptoms of HIV infection or are in a high-risk group or have sexual intercourse with someone in a high-risk group, see a doctor immediately. Although there is no cure for HIV infection or AIDS, treatments to fight the infection are available. For information, call the AIDS 24-hour hotline: 1-800-342-AIDS.

Vaginitis—*Symptoms:* Although vaginitis is considered mainly a woman's problem, it can be carried and spread by men. In fact, one form, trichomoniasis, often is considered a "ping pong" disease because sex partners don't know they have it and keep reinfecting each other. All forms of vaginitis share a common symptom of unusual discharge. Trichomoniasis produces a frothy yellow discharge with a persistent itching or burning and possibly an unpleasant odor. Yeast infection produces a discharge that looks like cottage cheese and possibly an intense itch. A *Gardnerella* infection causes a grayish-white, watery, strong-smelling discharge. *Treatment:* Both you and your partner should be treated with metronidazole for trichomoniasis to avoid reinfecting each other. *Gardnerella* infections are also treated with either metronidazole or ampicillin; yeast infections are treated with antifungal vaginal suppositories or creams, such as nystatin.

How can I reduce my chances of contracting a sexually transmitted disease?

Naturally, the best way to reduce your risk is by not having sex or by having sex with one mutually faithful, uninfected partner, or by using a condom during sex. **Remember, the more sexual partners you have, the greater your risk.** You can also reduce your risk by using condoms and spermicidals during sex; by urinating and washing after sex (but not douching; douching may actually force germs higher up into the body); by not having sex with someone who uses intravenous drugs or engages in anal sex; and by not engaging in oral, anal, or vaginal sex with an infected person. If you think you may have AIDS or an STD, seek treatment immediately.

How do I give myself a genital self-examination?

Start by examining the area that the pubic hair covers. It may help to position a mirror so that you can see your entire genital area. Even with a mirror, it may be difficult to see all areas. Experiment with positions that work best for you without making yourself uncomfortable. Start by spreading your pubic hair apart with your fingers. Carefully look for any bumps, sores, or blisters on the skin. Also look for warts. Genital warts may look like other warts; they may first appear as very small bumpy spots. Left untreated, they could develop a fleshy, cauliflower-like appearance.

Next, spread the outer vaginal lips apart and take a close look at the hood of your clitoris, which is at the top of the inner lips. Then gently pull the hood up to reveal your clitoris. Once again, look for bumps, blisters, sores, or warts.

Finally, examine both sides of your inner lips and the area around your urinary and vaginal openings for the same signs.

Besides these visual bumps and sores, what are other signs and symptoms of an STD?

Some STDs may cause a vaginal discharge that may be thicker, possibly yellow, and may also have an odor. Other symptoms or signs include a painful or burning sensation when urinating, pain in your pelvic area, bleeding between menstrual periods, or an itchy rash around the vagina.

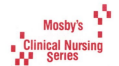
Pelvic Muscle Exercises

The pelvic floor is made up of muscles responsible for holding the body's lower organs, including the bladder. Because we walk upright, quite a bit of pressure is put on these organs as we walk, exercise, cough, or pick up something. When these muscles are weakened by childbirth or hormonal changes (such as those caused by menopause) or as a result of surgery or lower back injury, small amounts of urine may leak with physical activity. This condition is called stress incontinence, and it affects many women and some men.

Stress incontinence may be controlled without surgery in many cases. Exercising the pelvic muscles is a good way to strengthen them. Pelvic exercises (sometimes called Kegel exercises, after Dr. Arnold Kegel) are an excellent way to improve the fitness of the pelvic floor muscles.

Pelvic muscle exercises for women

First, it is important to locate and identify the correct muscles to exercise. The muscles you wish to exercise surround the urethra (the tube where urine leaves your body) and the vagina. You can find this muscle by practicing stopping your urine in midstream. Tighten (contract) the muscles to stop the urine; release the muscles to continue urination. Your nurse will help you locate the correct muscles. She may gently place a gloved finger in the vagina and ask you to contract the muscles around her finger, or she may use a special machine that helps you find and contract the correct muscles. The special machine uses sound or visual signals to help you understand how to contract and release the pelvic muscles. The nurse will also help you avoid tightening your abdominal or thigh muscles. Contracting these muscles will not help you strengthen the pelvic muscles.

It is helpful to practice Kegel exercises while urinating because correct muscle tightness will stop the flow of urine. During urination, tighten your muscles until the flow stops. The buttocks will be squeezed together. Hold back the flow for 3 to 5 seconds and then relax and start the flow of urine again. Repeat this stopping and starting of urinating flow 10 times, or until there is no more urine. Later you will be able to vary your muscle tightness from a rapid pace to a prolonged 10- to 30-second period.

As soon as you think you understand how to contract and release the pelvic muscles, here's how to proceed:
- Choose a time and place to exercise. You will need about 15 minutes to do your exercises.
- You will find the best position to do your exercises with practice. Some women prefer to sit or stand; others lie on the back with the head elevated on a pillow.
- Tighten the pelvic muscles as hard as you can.
- Hold the muscle tight for 10 seconds—you may find it helpful to count to 10—then relax the muscle for 10 seconds.
- Repeat this exercise 10 times.
- Ask your nurse or doctor how many times a day (repetitions) you need to perform the exercise (generally, it is best to begin with 10 repetitions and work up to 35 to 50 repetitions every other day). Remember that one repetition consists of 10 seconds of tightening and 10 seconds of relaxation.

You may wish to try a variation of this exercise.
- While sitting, standing, or lying with your head elevated, tighten and release the pelvic muscles in rapid succession. Repeat this 15 times.
- In the same position, tighten the pelvic muscles while you exhale. Hold the muscle for a count of 30. Repeat this exercise 10 times.

(From Gray.[39])

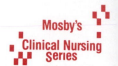

Mosby's
**Clinical Nursing
Series**

Contraception

How do I decide which kind of birth control is best for me?

No one type of birth control is right for everyone. You may want to talk with your partner and your healthcare provider to make the right choice. Some considerations to keep in mind are convenience (if you have to put a device in place every time you have sex, will you still be willing to use it?), willingness to handle your body, possible side effects and your willingness to tolerate those, and the degree of permanence you want from your birth control method. In any case, you'll want to choose a type of birth control that you can use safely and easily. Used correctly, any type of birth control works better than none. Incorrect use of a birth control method may end in unwanted pregnancy.

What is a condom and how do I use it?

A *male* condom is a thin covering that fits over the penis to catch sperm coming out of the penis during sex. Latex (rubber) condoms help protect you from AIDS and other sexually transmitted diseases (STDs). Condoms can be purchased in almost any drugstore or supermarket. In a year, 2 to 12 women out of every 100 become pregnant while using condoms. Condoms work best if you use them with a spermicide.

It's important to know how to put on a condom correctly, because it can't offer you any protection if it breaks. To minimize breakage, follow these steps: (1) put the condom on the head of the hard penis, leaving room in the tip to catch semen; (2) squeeze the air out of the tip of the condom and unroll it all the way down over the penis; (3) use only water-based lubricants, not oils (including petroleum jelly) or hand creams because they can cause condoms to break; (4) after sex, the wearer should hold the condom at the base of the penis and pull out of his partner carefully. Always keep a fresh supply of condoms on hand; never use the same condom twice.

Female condoms are relatively new devices that are similar to male condoms, except that the tube-like structure fits into the vagina rather than over the penis. The end opposite the tube fits over the opening of the vagina, or lips of the genital area.

What is a spermicide?

A spermicide is a gel, foam, cream, or tablet that kills sperm. It is inserted into the vagina, as close as possible to the cervix, a few minutes before having sex. Do this each time you repeat sex, leaving the spermicide in place afterward. Be sure to read the package insert for the spermicide. Some products require a waiting period before using and others must be inserted immediately before intercourse. Do not use tampons or douche for 6 to 8 hours. Spermicides can also help protect against some sexually transmitted diseases. They can be purchased at a drugstore or supermarket. In a 1-year period, 3 to 21 women out of every 100 become pregnant while using a spermicide.

Are sponges hard to use?

A sponge can be a little more convenient than a spermicide and condom. Sponges can also be used with them for even safer sex. Contraceptive sponges are small, round, specially made sponges filled with spermicide that fit into your vagina and over your cervix. It's a little more convenient, because you can have sex more than once while you have a sponge in place. To work, it must cover the cervix every time you have sex. The sponge should be put in your vagina (follow package instructions) 30 minutes to 18 hours before sex and kept in place for at least 6 hours after. Never keep the sponge in your body for longer than 24 hours. After you take out the sponge, throw it away. Sponges can be purchased at a drugstore or supermarket. In a 1-year period, 6 to 28 women out of every 100 become pregnant while using sponges.

What's the difference between a diaphragm and a cervical cap? Do they offer more protection than the sponge?

For both diaphragm users and cervical cap users, in a 1-year period, 6 to 18 women out of every 100 get pregnant. A diaphragm is a round, rubber cup that fits around the cervix to keep sperm out of the uterus and to hold spermicide in place. A cervical cap works the same way but is smaller and firmer. Both are used with gel or cream spermicide, and both must cover the cervix every time you have sex. Both must also be fitted by a doctor or health care provider. You should insert the diaphragm into your vagina a few minutes to 6 hours before sex; the cervical cap, 30 minutes to 40 hours before. Keep the diaphragm in place for at least 6 hours after sex; the cap, 8 hours after sex. Never keep the diaphragm in your body for longer than 24 hours;

the cervical cap must be removed within 48 hours. When using a diaphragm, remember to insert more spermicide into the vagina before each act of sexual intercourse, but leave the diaphragm in place. Do not remove the diaphragm for at least six hours after the last act of sexual intercourse. It's important to wash and carefully store the diaphragm or cervical cap after removal. Do **not** share a cervical cap or diaphragm, even among family members. They must be measured to fit you. If you have had a weight change or pregnancy, another fitting should be scheduled because you may need a new prescription.

What if I want stronger contraception protection than these other methods have offered, but I don't want anything permanent?

The pill, the implant (Norplant), and the intrauterine device (IUD) are all temporary contraceptive devices that offer stronger protection than the diaphragm, cap, spermicide, or condom. The birth control pill stops your body from sending out an egg each month and protects you 24 hours a day for as long as you take it every day at the same time. If you miss one pill, take it as soon as you remember. If you miss two, take both as soon as you remember, and use another type of birth control until you start the next package. In a year, only about 3 women out of every 100 become pregnant while taking birth control pills. Certain health risks are associated with the pill. Ask your health care provider about these risks before deciding whether they are right for you.

Norplant is a set of six small tubes filled with medication that stops your body from sending out an egg each month. It usually is placed under the skin of your upper arm. Norplant protects against pregnancy 24 hours a day for 5 years or until you have the tubes removed. The tubes are removed after 5 years. Ask for information about Norplant's side effects. In a 1-year period, almost no women have become pregnant while using Norplant.

An IUD is a small piece of plastic placed in your uterus to protect against pregnancy 24 hours a day for 1 to 6 years, depending on which type you use. The IUD is inserted into your uterus and through your cervix. You should feel for the strings on the IUD every month to make sure it is still in place. Call your doctor if the strings on your IUD are too long or too short or if you can't feel them. Ask about your possible risks with an IUD. In a 1-year pe-

riod, only about 3 women out of every 100 become pregnant while using an IUD.

What is natural family planning?

Natural family planning (NFP) is a way of telling which days of the month you can have sex without getting pregnant. To use NFP, you must learn how your body changes during your monthly cycle. A special trainer usually offers classes in NFP at hospitals, clinics, and churches. The procedure involves recording your temperature every day before you get out of bed and recording changes in the amount of mucus in your vagina. In a one-year period, 1 to 20 women out of every 100 become pregnant while using NFP. NFP works best if you follow all the steps taught in the program and have sex only on "safe" or "safer" days, meaning those in which you are least likely to conceive. (Remember: "Safer" days does not mean the same thing as "safer sex." Safer sex means always using a condom to help prevent disease.)

I'm ready for a permanent contraception solution. What's available?

Tubal ligation and vasectomy are two surgical solutions to contraception. Tubal ligation is a surgery that closes the tubes between your ovaries and uterus. It does not stop your monthly period; the egg simply cannot enter the uterus. Tubal ligation usually is permanent. It starts working right after surgery and lasts for the rest of your life. In a 1-year period, almost no women become pregnant after having a tubal ligation.

Vasectomy is a minor surgery that cuts the tubes between a man's testicles and penis. The penis can still get erect and release fluid (semen) during sex, but the semen no longer carries sperm. Vasectomy is also considered permanent; it usually starts working within 1 to 4 months after surgery. The man will need to have sperm count tests periodically after surgery and practice another type of birth control until his semen is free of sperm.

Over-the-counter (OTC) contraception, such as "male" and "female" condoms, spermicides, and vaginal sponges, usually come with excellent pictures and instructions. Read and follow these directions carefully. You should also receive package inserts with prescription birth control methods, such as oral contraceptives, cervical caps, and diaphragms. Materials are available for implants and IUDs. Don't hesitate to ask for more information from your nurse, physician, or pharmacist.

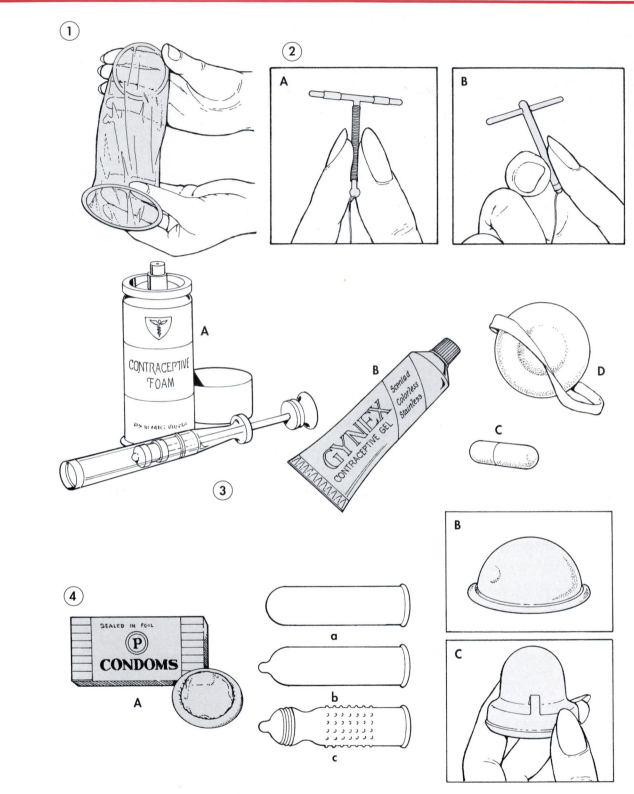

CONTRACEPTIVES. (1) Female condom. (2) IUDs. **A,** Copper-T 380A. **B,** Progestasert. (3) Vaginal spermicides. **A,** Foam with applicator. **B,** Contraceptive gel. **C,** Suppository. **D,** Sponge. (4) Mechanical barriers. **A,** Condoms (no prescription required). Types of condoms: **a,** Plain. **b,** Reservoir tip. **c,** Ribbed. **B,** Diaphragm. **C,** Cervical cap.

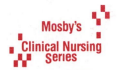

Safer Sex

What does it mean to practice "safer sex"?

The term "safer sex" refers to the practice of protecting yourself against sexually transmitted diseases (STDs), sometimes referred to as venereal disease (VD). There are at least 50 different kinds of these diseases, some of them even life-threatening. You can catch an STD by having sex with someone who is infected.

What if I have sex without actually having intercourse?

You can still get an STD without having vaginal intercourse or penetration. STDs are spread by having vaginal, oral, or anal sex with an infected person. STD-causing germs can pass from one person to another through body fluids such as semen, vaginal fluid, saliva, and blood; genital warts and herpes are STDs that are spread by direct contact with a wart or blister.

No one I date looks to me as if they could have an STD. They look really healthy.

You can't tell if a person has an STD just by appearance. In fact, some people with STDs have no signs at all and may not even know they are infected. Still, some signs to look for in your partner are a heavy discharge, rash, sore, or redness near your partner's sex organs. If you see any of these, don't have sex or be sure to use a condom.

How can I tell if I might have an STD?

You may have an STD if you experience burning or pain when urinating; sores, bumps, or blisters near the genitals or mouth; swelling around the genitals; fever, chills, night sweats, or swollen glands; or tiredness, vomiting, diarrhea, or sore muscles. In addition, you may have an unusual discharge or smell from the vagina; burning and itching around the vagina; pain in the lower abdomen; vaginal pain during sex; or vaginal bleeding between periods. *But don't forget; you may not have any warning signs at all.*

I think I have an STD! What should I do?

Get help right away. If you don't, you may pass the STD to your partner or, if you're pregnant, to your baby. In fact, without treatment an STD may make it impossible for you to have a baby at all. You may also develop brain damage, blindness, cancer, heart disease, or arthritis. In some cases you can even die. So go to a doctor or clinic right away.

If your health care provider determines that you do have an STD, tell your partner or partners to get tested, too. Take all of your medication; don't stop just because all your symptoms go away. Do not have sex until you have received full treatment. The disease could still be present in your body. Finally, keep all your appointments, and always use a condom and spermicide when you have sex.

What are the signs of STDs?

There are many different kinds of STDs, and some of them have similar symptoms. You should never attempt to make a diagnosis on your own. The nurse can give you a list with general descriptions of a few of the most common sexually transmitted diseases.

How can I reduce my chances of contracting an STD?

Remember, the more sexual partners you have, the greater your risk. Naturally, the best way to reduce your risk is by not having sex or by having sex with one mutually faithful, uninfected partner, or by using a latex condom and spermicide with nonoxynol 9 during sex. Some STDs may be avoided by placing spermicide in the vagina before having sex, because it kills sperm and some STD germs. It helps to urinate and wash after sex (but do not douche, because douching may actually force germs higher up into the body). Avoid having sex with someone who uses intravenous drugs or engages in anal sex. Don't engage in oral, anal, or vaginal sex with an infected person. If you think you may be at risk for AIDS or an STD, seek medical help immediately. Use a new condom each time you have sexual intercourse. *Recent research indicates that the prevention of HIV transmission and developing AIDS may be only 60% to 70% effective when using condoms as a barrier against this infection.*

What if the condom breaks? What should we do?

If a condom breaks, do not douche. Insert more spermicide into the vagina right away. Men should wash their genitals immediately. Go to a doctor or clinic for an STD examination as soon as possible.

PATIENT TEACHING GUIDE

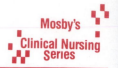

Urinary Tract Infections

How do people get urinary tract infections?

After the common cold, urinary tract infections (UTIs) are the most common infections to affect women and men. They usually are caused by bacteria, tiny microscopic agents that can invade just about any part of your urinary tract. Most come from the rectum, where bacteria occur naturally, and spread to the vagina and the urethra. They often travel into your system from outside the body, move up your urinary tract, multiply, and infect a specific organ. Women have more UTIs than men simply because of their anatomy. The urethra, which carries urine from the bladder outside the body, is shorter in women, allowing bacteria to travel easily from outside the body up into the urinary tract. Sexual intercourse and personal hygiene habits can help bacteria travel into the urethra. Infections also may occur because some women have a urinary tract with a low resistance to bacteria.

What is the best treatment for a UTI?

You can help your treatment be successful if you get an early diagnosis, understand the cause of your infection, and follow your entire treatment program to prevent the infection from returning. An early diagnosis gives you the best chance for successful treatment of your urinary tract infection and helps keep it from developing into a more serious problem. Most infections won't go away by themselves. You need medications and simple life-style changes, such as drinking plenty of water to flush bacteria from your body.

How will my doctor diagnose a UTI?

During your medical evaluation, your healthcare provider will ask about your medical history; be sure to describe all of your symptoms, any history of infections, what medication you are taking, if any, and whether you could be pregnant.

During your physical examination, your healthcare provider feels along the sides of your torso for tenderness and examines your genital area for redness and inflammation. Medical tests are extremely accurate in identifying the cause and location of your infection. One or several of the following tests may be recommended.

Urinalysis. Urine is examined for bacteria and inflammatory changes in cells.

Urine culture. Bacteria from your urine may grow on a culture plate.

Pyelogram. An intravenous drug is injected into your arm and an x-ray is taken of your urinary tract to identify anatomic problems.

Cystoscopy. A direct visual examination with a cystoscope reveals infection and anatomic problems.

Cystogram. X-rays of a fluid-filled bladder may spot anatomic abnormalities.

Are there different types of UTIs?

Yes, women can have several types of UTIs, including the following:

Cystitis. Cystitis is a bladder infection and the most common UTI in women. Symptoms may include an urgent or frequent need to urinate (called "urgency" or "frequency"), slight fever, pain, a burning feeling, or blood in the urine. Poor personal hygiene practices and sexual intercourse help spread bacteria to the urethra and bladder. Cystitis usually is treated with drugs.

Urethral syndrome. Urethral syndrome is an inflammation in the urethra, but the bacteria or other organisms that can cause it often are not detected by tests. You're likely to have pain in your lower stomach or back, urgency, or frequency. Long-term medications may be needed to eliminate the infection, which could have been triggered by intercourse or stress.

Pyelonephritis. Although less common, pyelonephritis, or kidney infection, can be the most serious UTI because it can damage your kidneys, which filter wastes for your entire body. Symptoms include pain in your upper back or side and a fever. This UTI may stem from bacteria, an obstruction, or a neurologic disorder that affects kidney or bladder function. Treatment depends on the cause.

How are UTIs treated?

For most infections, short-term antibiotics are all you need, but it may take several days to a week before you feel well. It's important to take all medication until it's gone. Long-term medications can take several months to cure an infection. In addition to adhering to your medication schedule, there are other steps you can take to help in both treatment and prevention of future UTIs:

- *Take your medication* for as long as it's prescribed so that you don't get a UTI again. You may want to write down when you need to take medications.

- *Drink enough fluids* (eight 8-ounce glasses of water or juice) every day to help flush out bacteria.
- *Practice good personal hygiene* by always "wiping" from front to back. Condoms, too, can help prevent UTIs caused by sexually transmitted diseases.
- *Empty your bladder frequently.* Women should always try to urinate after sex.
- *Avoid irritating foods,* especially spicy foods, caffeine, and alcohol.
- *Keep follow-up appointments.*

Is it possible I'll need surgery?

Most urinary tract infections do not require surgery, but surgery may be needed to relieve obstructions and to treat problems caused by scarring or long-term infections.

Preventing Urinary Tract Infections

A urinary tract infection (UTI) is any infection or inflammation located along the urinary tract. Most urinary tract infections occur in the bladder or urethra, the canal that carries the urine from the bladder to the urethral opening.

What causes urinary tract infections?

Urinary tract infections have a number of causes. Most are caused by bacteria from the bowel that invade the urinary tract. Because a woman's urethra is closer to the rectum than a man's is, women suffer many more urinary tract infections than men do. Other causes include overstretching of the bladder, urine left in the bladder (incomplete voiding), and lack of cleanliness when doing catheterization. Urethral inflammation can be caused by chemical irritants such as perfumed feminine hygiene products, sanitary napkins, spermicidal foams and jellies, and bubble baths.

What are the signs of a urinary tract infection?

Several signs indicate a urinary tract infection. You may have one or a combination of these symptoms:

1. A frequent and urgent need to urinate
2. Pain in the lower back and lower pelvic region
3. Cloudy, foul-smelling urine
4. Bloody urine
5. Chills or fever
6. Lack of appetite or lack of energy, or both
7. Sandlike material (sediment) in the urine

How to prevent a urinary tract infection or inflammation

The most important thing you can do to prevent a urinary tract infection is to practice good hygiene. Women should avoid wiping fecal matter into the urethral area. Wiping from front to back helps prevent germs and bacteria from entering the urethral opening. Showering or bathing daily also helps prevent the spread of germs, and drinking lots of fluids helps the bladder flush itself.

If you are catheterizing yourself, it is very important that you are careful to be very clean. It is very easy to insert germs along with the catheter into your urethra and bladder. Wash your hands frequently as you carry out the catheterization process. Wash the catheter in soapy water after each use and allow it to dry completely before using it again.

To prevent inflammation of the urinary tract, avoid perfumed feminine hygiene products, spermicidal jellies and foams, and bubble bath.

Seek treatment if you think you might have a urinary tract infection. Such infections can lead to bladder and kidney damage, kidney stones, and urine retention.

(From Gray.[39])

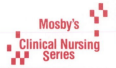

Menopause and Osteoporosis

What is menopause?

Menophause, the end of a woman's monthly menstrual periods, is a time of natural transition, usually reached by the age of 55. Most women go through menopause between the ages of 50 and 52, although it is perfectly normal to stop menstruating anytime between the ages of 45 and 55. A very small percentage of women go through premature menopause. A woman actually achieves menopause when she has gone 12 months without a period; however, the word "menopause" is often used to describe the entire period of change that comes before and after the actual date of menopause. This entire period, called the "climacteric," consists of three stages: perimenopause (the transition between fertility and the last menstrual period); menopause (when periods have actually ceased for a year); and postmenopause (the years after the end of menstruation).

What causes menopause?

By the time a woman reaches her late thirties or early forties, only a fraction of the original number of eggs in her ovaries remains. Less and less of the female hormone estrogen is produced from those eggs. After a while, estrogen dwindles to a level so low that it can no longer "tell" the body to menstruate.

What are the symptoms of menopause?

Some women experience only minor discomfort, whereas others need medical assistance to cope. In addition, some women feel the effects of menopause for a few years, others for the rest of their lives. Beginning in perimenopause, women may experience a variety of symptoms, such as menstrual irregularities, hot flashes, night sweats, vaginal inelasticity and dryness, weight gain, and skin changes. Menstrual changes, hot flashes, and night sweats usually are temporary responses to the waning of hormones, but estrogen deprivation also produces permanent changes in the body. For example, the skin may become drier, thinner, and itchy and may bruise more easily; hair on parts of the body may become dry and facial hair may increase; urinary tract tissues become thinner, resulting in greater frequency and urgency in urination or an inability to hold urine; the breasts may shrink, become softer, and begin to sag; the vaginal tissues may shrink and become thinner and drier; internal pelvic organs may shrink; and the risk of heart disease and osteoporosis increases.

What is estrogen replacement therapy?

Doctors prescribe estrogen replacement therapy (ERT) to correct some of the effects of deficiencies associated with menopause. This therapy is an especially effective treatment for hot flashes, night sweats, and vaginal dryness. If it is begun before menopause or soon after, the treatment can slow the often rapid loss of bone mass that occurs during the 5 to 7 years after the last period. It can also cut the incidence of heart disease in half. Not every woman needs additional estrogen when going through menopause, however. The decision whether to begin ERT depends on a woman's medical history, the severity of her symptoms, and her risk of bone loss. Each woman must weigh the risks against the benefits with her healthcare provider.

What other treatments are available for menopause?

The drug etidronate can lessen the frequency of crush fractures of the vertebrae that result from the loss of bone mass in osteoporosis, but prevention is best, which involves daily exercise and daily consumption before menopause of calcium equal to the amount in a quart of milk. Several drugs can relieve hot flashes and vaginal dryness as well, although some nonmedicinal measures can be taken to ease hot flashes and night sweats, such as dressing in removable layers of loose clothing made of natural fibers; using air conditioning or room fans when needed; sleeping with fewer blankets; avoiding caffeine, alcohol, and sugar; and eating a balanced, low-fat diet. Topical vaginal creams or gels can ease vaginal dryness.

I haven't had a period for about 10 months now. Does this mean I no longer have to bother with birth control?

Pregnancy in an older women can pose health risks for both mother and child. So all women who have menstruated even once within the prior 12 months should continue to use contraception until 1 year, maybe even 2, goes by with no menstrual period. In addition, the birth control method that a woman uses during her child-bearing years may not be appropriate during perimenopause. Because the risk of coronary and artery disease is increased in women over 40 years of age, some physicians do not recommend use of birth control pills for them, particularly if they smoke. An IUD may be an option for the older woman, but fewer kinds of IUDs are available today. And the irregularity of some women's menstrual cycles makes predicting their fertile time of the month difficult. Thus some women may come to rely on barrier methods of contraception such as condoms (used with a spermicide), diaphragms, and contraceptive sponges.

What is osteoporosis?

Osteoporosis is a condition caused by decreased density, or thinning, of the bone. It occurs when the skeletal "bank reserves" drop below your body's needs. Although the chemical composition of the existing bone is normal, the decreased bone mass results in weakness and brittleness of the bone, a key characteristic of the disease.

Why do so many women get osteoporosis?

About one fourth of the women in America have or will develop osteoporosis. If you are fair, thin-skinned, petite, Caucasian or Oriental, or have a family history of osteoporosis, you are at higher risk for developing this condition. You would be wise to exercise regularly and watch your daily intake of calcium.

The main cause of osteoporosis in women is the lack of the hormone estrogen, which their bodies stop producing at menopause. This loss of estrogen results in thinner, weaker bones. Hormone replacement may be an appropriate safeguard for many of these women.

A woman's bone reserves peak when she reaches 35 years of age. After that, her risk of osteoporosis is greater.

Who is at highest risk of developing osteoporosis?

You are at a greater risk for developing this condition if you have never been pregnant; you have experienced menopause; you have had your ovaries surgically removed; you breast-fed your child/children; you are allergic to milk and dairy products; you are inactive; your daily routine is stressful; you smoke; you consume large amounts of caffeine; or you drink alcoholic beverages.

What can I do to protect myself?

Be sure you're eating the recommended daily levels of dietary calcium and vitamin D (if you have a history of kidney stones, consult your doctor before increasing your calcium intake). Postmenopausal women and those whose ovaries have been surgically removed may need estrogen replacement to protect against bone loss.

Weight-bearing exercises such as walking and jogging are crucial to maintaining or building bone mass. Good nutrition is a basic tool in the prevention of osteoporosis. A lifelong, well-balanced diet that includes generous amounts of calcium-rich foods is the best protection against this condition and other bone disorders. Practically all foods contain calcium, but those highest in calcium include (in order of calcium content in an average serving): low-fat, plain yogurt; sardines; skim milk; low-fat milk; whole milk; Swiss cheese; cottage cheese; kale; cheddar cheese; ice cream; turnip greens; salmon (with bones); broccoli; and sunflower seeds.

Calcium needs increase with age. Before menopause a woman's minimum daily requirement is 800 mg; during menopause, 1,200 mg; and after menopause, 1,500 mg.

How is osteoporosis treated?

Medications may be prescribed that reduce the amount or slow the rate of bone loss. In addition, estrogen replacement therapy may be started in postmenopausal patients. Treatment is much the same as the prevention measures, with an emphasis on diet, exercise, and calcium supplements. Because the possibility of bone fractures is an ever-present danger for persons suffering from osteoporosis, observe these safety precautions to help prevent painful fractures:

- When possible, do not use drugs that alter the sense of balance.
- Use handrails when available and elevators instead of stairs or escalators when provided, to prevent falls.
- Wear comfortable clothing and soft shoes with cushioned insoles.
- Use extreme care when getting in and out of a bathtub. Equip your tub with railings or take showers.
- Do not lift heavy objects.
- Do not push or exert bodily force to move furniture or stubborn objects.
- Do not risk falling by climbing on chairs or stepladders to reach high places.
- Squat rather than stoop when picking things up from the floor.
- Ask for help when you need it rather than attempting tasks that could result in a painful injury.
- Develop a regular exercise program, such as swimming, walking, or supervised mild calisthenics.

Physical limitations, loss of independence, and the fear of being dependent on family members, friends, or neighbors are common concerns for victims of osteoporosis. Accepting the realities of the disease and adjusting to a restricted life-style can affect the personality as well. For this reason, it is vitally important to maintain a positive attitude. Learn to find joy in simplicity and moderation. Stay mentally alert. Surround yourself with supportive friends and pursue *wholeheartedly* every "permissible" activity!

CHAPTER 16

Pharmacologic Management of Women's Disorders

Antibiotics and Antiinfective Drugs

PENICILLINS

Penicillins are the most widely prescribed class of antibiotics. They inhibit the bacterial enzymes needed for cell wall synthesis. Penicillins are categorized by their structure and spectrum of activity. Penicillin G and related penicillins have a narrow spectrum of activity and are effective primarily against certain gram-positive bacteria. Aminopenicillins are effective against these organisms plus many gram-negative bacteria as well. Broad-spectrum penicillins are effective against an even wider range of organisms.

Indications: Treatment of mild to moderately severe infections caused by penicillin-sensitive microorganisms. For specific approved indications, refer to package literature.

Usual dosage: See the box on page 313 for dosages of major penicillins.

Precautions/contraindications: Do not use with a history of hypersensitivity to penicillins, cephalosporins, cephamycins, or penicillamine. Use during pregnancy should be limited to cases in which the drug is clearly indicated. Cautious use is required with nursing mothers; renal impairment; GI disease; infectious mononucleosis; or a history of asthma or allergies.

Side effects/adverse reactions: *CNS:* Seizures, hallucinations, confusion, hyperreflexia, dysphasia, encephalopathy. *GI:* Nausea, vomiting, bloating, flatulence, diarrhea, cramps, thirst, bitter taste. *Hematologic:* Eosinophilia, hemolytic anemia, thrombocytopenia, leukopenia, neutropenia, agranulocytosis. *Hepatic:* Cholestatic jaundice. *Hypersensitivity:* Rash, exfoliative dermatitis, erythema, contact dermatitis, hives, pruritus, wheezing, anaphylaxis, fever, blood dyscrasias, Stevens-Johnson syndrome, angioedema, serum sickness. *Renal:* Acute interstitial nephritis, electrolyte imbalance after IV administration. *Skin:* Pain, induration at injection site.

Pharmacokinetics: Penicillins are distributed throughout the body and cross the placenta. Most are excreted in the urine, largely unchanged, and also excreted in breast milk.

Interactions: Probenecid increases serum levels and prolongs the half-life of penicillins, an interaction used to therapeutic advantage whenever sustained therapeutic blood levels are desired, as in the treatment of acute pelvic inflammatory disease (PID) and gonorrhea. Natural penicillins may cause hyperkalemia if taken with other medications containing potassium or with potassium-sparing diuretics. Ampicillin may reduce the effectiveness of oral contraceptives.

Nursing considerations: Electrolyte imbalances may occur in patients receiving high doses of penicillins that contain sodium or potassium, as well in patients receiving any penicillins intravenously. Penicillins interfere with urine glucose tests that use cupric sulfate (e.g., Benedict's solution, Clinitest). Penicillins may cause a false-positive result on Coombs' test, interfering with hematologic studies and transfusion cross-matching.

PENICILLINS

Natural penicillins

Penicillin G benzathine (Bicillin) 2.4 million U IM—syphilis

Penicillin G potassium (Pfizerpen) 5-10 million U/day IM/IV—gynecologic infections

Penicillin G procaine (Wycillin) 4.8 million U IM—gonorrhea; 600,000 U/day IM—syphilis

Penicillin G sodium (generic) 4.8 million U IM—gonorrhea; 600,000 U/day IM—syphilis

Aminopenicillins

Amoxicillin (Amoxil, Larotid, Polymox) 250-500 mg q 8 h PO—gonorrhea, gynecologic infections, gonococcal urethritis

Amoxicillin/clavulanate (Augmentin) 250-500 mg/125 mg q 8 h PO—urinary tract infections

Ampicillin (Omnipen, Principen) 250-500 mg q 6 h PO—gynecologic infections, gonococcal urethritis; *or* 200 mg/kg/day IV/IM

Ampicillin/sulbactam (Unasyn) 1-2/0.5-1 g q 6 h IM/IV—gynecologic infections

Bacampicillin (Spectrobid) 1.6 g PO—gonorrhea; 400-800 mg q 12 h PO—urinary tract infections

Cyclacillin (Cyclapen) 250-500 mg q 6 h PO—urinary tract infections

Broad-spectrum penicillins

Amdinocillin (Coactin) 10 mg/kg q 4-6 h IM/IV—bacteremia, urinary tract infections

Azlocillin (Azlin) 100-300 mg/kg/day IV—urinary tract infections

Carbenicillin (Geocillin) 382-764 mg q 6 h PO—prostatitis, urinary tract infections; (Geopen, Pyopen) 200 mg/kg/day IM/IV—gynecologic infections, urinary tract infections; 4 g IM—gonorrhea

Mezlocillin (Mezlin) 100-125 mg/kg/day IM/IV—gynecologic infections, urinary tract infections

Piperacillin (Piperacil) 100-125 mg/kg/day IM—gynecologic infections, gonococcal urethritis, urinary tract infections; *or* 100-300 mg/kg/day IV

Ticarcillin (Ticar) 1 g q 6 h IM—gynecologic infections, urinary tract infections; *or* 150-300 mg/kg/day IV

Ticarcillin/clavulanate (Timentin) 3 g/100 mg q 4-8 h IV—urinary tract infections

(From Gray.[39])

CEPHALOSPORINS

Cephalosporins have mechanisms of action and pharmacologic properties similar to those of the penicillins. Like the penicillins, cephalosporins are classified by their antibacterial spectrum of activity as first-, second-, or third- generation drugs.

Indications: Treatment of upper and lower respiratory tract infections, skin and skin structure infections, and urinary tract infections. For specific approved indications, refer to package literature.

Usual dosage: Table 16-1 gives the dosage range for each type of cephalosporin.

Precautions/contraindications: Use during pregnancy should be limited to cases in which the drug is clearly needed. Cautious use is required with nursing mothers; a history of hypersensitivity to cephalosporins or penicillins; a history of GI disease or bleeding disorders; and impaired hepatic or renal function.

Side effects/adverse reactions: *CNS:* Dizziness, headaches, malaise, fatigue. High doses and renal impairment can cause seizures. *GI (common):* Nausea, vomiting, diarrhea, abdominal pain. *Hematologic (rare):* Mild and transient neutropenia, thrombocytopenia, anemia, lymphocytosis, agranulocytosis, aplastic anemia, pancytopenia, hemorrhage. *Hepatic:* Hepatic dysfunction. *Hypersensitivity:* Urticaria, pruritus, rash, fever, chills, reactions resembling serum sickness, eosinophilia, joint pain, edema, erythema, angioedema, Stevens-Johnson syndrome, erythema multiforme, exfoliative dermatitis, anaphylaxis. *Other:* IM injection causes pain, induration, and tenderness; IV infusion can cause phlebitis and thrombophlebitis.

Pharmacokinetics: Cephalosporins readily cross the placenta and are excreted in breast milk. Except for cefuroxime and cefpodoxime, food delays absorption. Cephalosporins are excreted primarily unchanged via the kidneys.

Interactions: A disulfiram-like reaction (nausea, vomiting) may occur if alcohol is ingested concurrently with or up to 72 hours after administration of cefamandole, cefonicid, cefotaxime, cefoperazone, cefotetan, or moxalactam. The antibacterial activity of aminoglycosides, penicillins, and chloramphenicol may be additive or synergistic with cephalosporins. Some cephalosporins increase prothrombin time, altering anticoagulant dosage requirements. Concurrent use with nephrotoxic drugs increases the risk of nephrotoxicity and should be avoided. Probenecid causes higher and prolonged serum levels.

Nursing considerations: Cephalosporins should be taken on an empty stomach, except for cefuroxime and cefpodoxime. Cephalosporins with a broad spectrum of activity may cause superinfection. Cephalosporins can interfere with a variety of tests, such as urine glucose tests that use cupric sulfate (e.g., Benedict's solution, Clinitest). Cephalosporins may cause a false-positive result on Coombs' test. Warn the patient not to drink alcohol for 72 hours after taking cefamandole, cefonicid, cefotetan, cefoperazone, cefotaxime, or moxalactam.

Table 16-1

CEPHALOSPORINS

Generic name	Trade names	Dosage range	Administration
First generation			
Cephalothin	Keflin	0.5-1 g q 4-6 h	IM, IV
Cefazolin	Ancef, Kefzol, Zolicef	0.5-1 g q 6-8 h	IM, IV
Cephapirin	Cefadyl	0.5-1 g q 4-6 h	IM, IV
Cephradine	Anspor, Velosef	500 mg q 12-24 h	Oral
		12.5-25 mg/kg/day q 6 h	IM, IV
Cephalexin	Keflet, Keflex, Keftab	250 mg-1 g q 6 h	Oral
Cefadroxil	Duricef, Ultracef	1-2 g/day q 12-24 h	Oral
Second generation			
Cefamandole	Mandol	0.5-1 g q 4-8 h	IM, IV
Defuroxime	Ceftin, Kefurox, Zinacef	250-500 mg bid	IM, IV
		0.75-1.5 g q 8 h	
Cefonicid	Monocid	1 g q 24 h	IM, IV
Cefoxitin	Mefoxin	1-2 g q 6-8 h	IM, IV
Cefaclor	Ceclor	250-500 mg q 8 h	Oral
Cefotetan	Cefotan	1-2 g q 12 h	IM, IV
Ceforanide	Precef	0.5-1 g q 12 h	IM, IV
Cefmetazole	Zefazone	2 g q 6-12 h	IV
Third generation			
Cefotaxime	Claforan	1-12 g/day q 6-12 h	IM, IV
Ceftriaxone	Rocephin	1-2 g once a day	IM, IV
Moxalactam	Moxam	2-4 g/day q 8-12 h	IM, IV
Cefoperazone	Cefobid	1-2 g q 12 h	IM, IV
Ceftizoxime	Cefizox	1-2 g q 8-12 h	IM, IV
Ceftazidime	Fortaz, Tazidime	0.25-2 g q 8-12 h	IM, IV
Cefixime	Suprax	400 mg/day	Oral

(From Grimes.[44])

SULFONAMIDES AND TRIMETHOPRIM

SULFONAMIDES

Sulfonamides are bacteriostatic drugs. They competitively antagonize paraaminobenzoic acid (PABA), which is necessary for folic acid synthesis. Sulfonamides are effective against microorganisms that must synthesize folic acid to replicate.

Indications: Broad spectrum of activity; most often used to treat urinary tract infections.

Usual dosage: Varies (see Table 16-2).

Precautions/contraindications: Do not use with hypersensitivity to sulfonamides; porphyria; or advanced renal or hepatic disease. Cautious use is required with severe allergies; bronchial asthma; blood dyscrasias; and G6PD deficiency.

Side effects/adverse reactions: *CNS:* Headaches, peripheral neuritis, tinnitus, psychosis. *GI:* Nausea, vomiting, diarrhea. *Hematologic:* Various blood disorders (e.g., acute hemolytic anemia, especially in patients with G6PD deficiency). *Hypersensitivity:* Fever, chills, arthralgia, photosensitivity, serum sickness, anaphylactic reaction, rash. *Renal:* Crystalluria, toxic nephrosis. *Other:* Hypoglycemia, diuresis, local reaction.

Pharmacokinetics: Sulfonamides are readily absorbed from the GI tract and eliminated mainly through the kidneys.

Interactions: Sulfonamides may displace highly protein-bound drugs (e.g., oral anticoagulants, anticonvulsants, and oral antidiabetic agents) from binding sites, increasing both the serum levels of those drugs and their therapeutic effects. The potential for toxic effects increases when sulfonamides are administered with hepatotoxic or bone marrow–suppressing drugs.

Table 16-2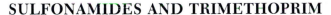

SULFONAMIDES AND TRIMETHOPRIM

Generic name	Trade names	Dosage range	Administration
Sulfadiazine	Microsulfon	2-4 g/day in 3-6 doses	Oral
Sulfacytine	Renoquid	250 mg q 6 h	Oral
Sulfisoxazole	Gantrisin	4-8 g/day in 4-6 doses	Oral
		100 mg/kg/day in 2-4 doses	SC, IM, IV
Sulfamethoxazole	Gantanol Urobak	1 g twice daily	Oral
Sulfamethizole	Proklar	0.5-1 g 3-4 times/day	Oral
Multiple sulfonamides*			
Trisulfapyrimidines	Triple Sulfa Neotrizine Terfonyl	2-4 g/day in 3-6 doses	Oral
Trimethoprim	Proloprim Trimpex	200 mg/day	Oral

Trimethoprim (TMP)/
  sulfamethoxazole (SMZ)
	Bactrim
	TMP-SMZ
	Comoxol
	Cotrim
	Sulfatrim
	Septra
		80 mg TMP/400 mg SMZ to 160 mg TMP/800
		  mg SMZ q 12 h
			IV, Oral

*Multiple sulfonamides provide the same therapeutic effect as the total sulfonamide content but reduce the risk of precipitation in the kidneys.
(From Grimes.[44])

Nursing considerations: Instruct the patient to take each dose on an empty stomach with a large glass of water and to increase her fluid intake to 2,000-3,000 ml (2 to 3 quarts) a day (to minimize the possibility of drug precipitation in the urine). If GI upset occurs, instruct the patient to take the drug with food. Caution the patient to avoid or minimize exposure to sunlight and to use a sunscreen when outside.

TRIMETHOPRIM

Trimethoprim blocks the conversion of folic acid into its active form, similar to the way the sulfonamides block folic acid synthesis.

Indications: Treatment of uncomplicated urinary tract infections.

Usual dosage: *Acute UTI:* 100 mg PO q 12 h, *or* 200 mg PO q 24 h for 10 days. *Recurrent UTI:* 100 mg PO daily at bedtime for 6 weeks to 6 months. Adjust dosage for renal impairment; do not use if creatinine clearance is below 15 ml/min.

Precautions/contraindications: Cautious use is required with renal or hepatic impairment or hypersensitivity to trimethoprim.

Side effects/adverse reactions: *GI:* GI disturbances may occur. *Hematologic:* Bone marrow depression, usually with prolonged administration. *Integumentary:*

Rash, pruritus, exfoliative dermatitis.

Pharmacokinetics: Trimethoprim is well absorbed after PO administration; primary elimination is through the kidneys.

Interactions: Administration with phenytoin increases the incidence of folate deficiency.

Nursing considerations: Monitor kidney function. Instruct the patient to increase her fluid intake to 2,000-3,000 ml (2 to 3 quarts) a day.

**SULFAMETHOXAZOLE/
TRIMETHOPRIM
(CO-TRIMOXAZOLE)**

Combining sulfmethoxazole and trimethoprim produces a dual block of folate synthesis, which provides a synergistic effect that increases activity and the antibacterial spectrum. The drug combination is used primarily to treat urinary tract infections and otitis media in children. See individual drugs for profile and nursing considerations.

Table 16-3 _____

ANTIBACTERIAL DRUGS FOR THE URINARY TRACT

Generic name	Trade names	Dosage range	Administration
Cinoxacin	Cinobac	1 g/day in 2-4 divided doses	Oral
Methenamine			
Hippurate	Hiprex, Urex	1 g 2 times/day	Oral
Mandelate	Mandameth	1 g 4 times/day	Oral
	Mandelamine		
Nalidixic acid		1 g 4 times/day	Oral
Nitrofurantoin	Furadantin	50-100 mg 4 times/day	Oral
	Furan		
	Macrodantin		
	Nitrofan		
Norfloxacin	Noroxin	400 mg q 12 h	Oral

(From Grimes.[44])

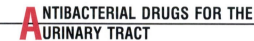

ANTIBACTERIAL DRUGS FOR THE URINARY TRACT

QUINOLONES

Cinoxacin

Cinoxacin is a synthetic organic acid related to nalidixic acid that inhibits the replication of bacterial DNA.

Indications: Treatment of urinary tract infections caused by susceptible organisms.

Usual dosage: 1 g PO daily in individual doses.

Precautions/contraindications: Toxicity may occur in patients with reduced renal function as a result of decreased renal elimination and increased serum drug levels.

Side effects/adverse reactions: *Most common:* GI or (GU) disturbances (nausea, vomiting, diarrhea, abdominal cramps, perineal burning).

Pharmacokinetics: Cinoxacin is completely absorbed after PO administration. It is partly metabolized in the liver, and the metabolites and remaining active drug are eliminated in the urine.

Interactions: Probenecid reduces renal elimination of cinoxacin, decreasing the urine concentration and increasing the systemic levels.

Nursing considerations: Caution the patient that cinoxacin may cause dizziness; it also may make her eyes more photosensitive.

Nalidixic Acid

Nalidixic acid has a drug profile similar to that of cinoxacin, but it may produce more GI side effects. See the preceding section on cinoxacin for a more detailed presentation.

Methenamine

Methenamine is a nonspecific bactericidal drug that is hydrolyzed to formaldehyde and ammonia in the bladder if the urine pH is kept at 5.5 or less. Methenamine is available as mandelate or hippurate salts; both forms contribute to acidification of the urine.

Indications: Prophylactic treatment of recurrent urinary tract infections and long-term prophylactic treatment of neurogenic bladder conditions.

Usual dosage: Varies (see Table 16-3).

Precautions/contraindications: Do not use with severe renal failure or dehydration. Also, do not administer to a patient with liver disease, since ammonia is one of methenamine's by-products.

Side effects/adverse reactions: Large doses can irritate the bladder. Other adverse effects include GI symptoms, stomatitis, and rash.

Pharmacokinetics: Methenamine and related salts are readily absorbed from the GI tract, with up to 25% subject to hepatic metabolism. The production of formaldehyde in the urine depends on an acid urinary pH and the duration of urine retention in the bladder.

Interactions: Drugs that raise the urinary pH (e.g., bicarbonate, acetazolamide) reduce the effectiveness of methenamine.

Nursing considerations: Acidification of the urine to a pH of 5.5 is required for the drug to be effective. This may be accomplished with ascorbic acid supplements or with foods high in ascorbic acid, such as cranberry juice or prunes.

Nitrofurantoin

Nitrofurantoin interferes with several bacterial enzyme systems.

Indications: Treatment of pyonephritis, pyelitis, and cystitis caused by susceptible organisms.

Usual dosage: *Adults and children ≥12:* 50-100 mg 4 times/day; for long-term suppression, 50-100 mg at bedtime.

Precautions/contraindications: Renal impairment, anuria, or oliguria reduces the effectiveness of nitrofurantoin and increases the risk of toxicity.

Side effects/adverse reactions: *CNS:* Peripheral neuropathy, headaches. *Hypersensitivity:* Rash, pruritus. *GI:* Anorexia, nausea, emesis. *Other:* Fever, pulmonary reactions (dyspnea, cough with fever and chills), hemolytic or megaloblastic anemia (rare).

Pharmacokinetics: Nitrofurantoin is rapidly and completely absorbed from the GI tract; absorption is enhanced if the drug is given with meals. Nitrofurantoin and its metabolites are excreted into the urine, where therapeutic levels are achieved.

Interactions: Probenecid reduces renal clearance, increasing serum levels to possibly toxic levels.

Nursing considerations: Administer with food or milk to enhance absorption and reduce GI upset. Monitor the patient for pulmonary changes, and instruct her to report any pulmonary symptoms to her nurse or physician.

ANTIFUNGAL DRUGS

Most fungal infections in women develop in the vagina. A fungal infection is common after a course of antibiotics if the natural vaginal flora have been destroyed. If the beneficial bacteria are eliminated, the pH of the vagina changes, enhancing the growth of pathogens.

Miconazole

Miconazole is a broad-spectrum fungicide that is effective against *Candida albicans* and many other fungi. Its mode of action is unclear, but it appears to inhibit the uptake of substances essential for cell reproduction and growth.

Indications: Topical treatment of vulvovaginal candidiasis.

Usual dosage: 1 applicatorful of vaginal cream at bedtime for 7 days, *or* 1 100-mg vaginal tablet at bedtime for 3 nights (both forms are inserted high into the vagina).

Precautions/contraindications: Do not use in children under age 2 or with pregnancy; nursing mothers; or a history of hypersensitivity to miconazole.

Side effects/adverse reactions: *GU:* Vulvovaginal burning and itching, pelvic cramps. *Integumentary:* Rash, urticaria, stinging, burning, contact dermatitis.

Nursing considerations: Advise the patient to wear a sanitary napkin to prevent staining of undergarments; to refrain from sexual intercourse to avoid spreading the infection; and to notify her physician if the condition does not improve within 4 weeks.

Nystatin

Nystatin is a nonsensitizing, nontoxic antifungal drug. It binds to the sterols in the fungal cell membrane, allowing leakage of intracellular components.

Indications: Treatment of topical infections, such as vulvovaginitis, caused by *Candida albicans*.

Usual dosage: 1 or 2 vaginal tablets daily for 14 days (inserted high into the vagina). The cream or ointment should be applied liberally to affected areas 2 times/day.

Precautions/contraindications: Do not use with pregnancy (category B); nursing mothers; or a history of hypersensitivity to nystatin.

Side effects/adverse reactions: *Integumentary:* Rash, urticaria, stinging, burning.

Pharmacokinetics: Symptomatic relief is rapid, often occurring within 24 to 72 hours of initial treatment.

Nursing considerations: Instruct the patient to do the following: cleanse the affected area thoroughly with soap and water and dry it well before applying the drug; wash her hands before and after each application, and wear plastic gloves when applying the drug to prevent further infection; wear a sanitary pad, since the drug may stain undergarments; stop using the drug and notify her physician if irritation occurs.

DRUGS FOR THE TREATMENT OF VAGINAL HERPES

Acyclovir

Acyclovir has been shown to reduce the frequency, duration, and severity of initial and recurrent herpes infections. However, it does not eliminate the infection. The drug should not be used to suppress recurrent disease in individuals with mild symptoms.

Indications: Treatment of herpes simplex virus, types 1 and 2, and varicella zoster (shingles) infections.

Usual dosage: *PO:* Initial genital herpes infection: 200 mg q 4 h while awake (total of 5 capsules/day) for 10 days. Chronic suppressive therapy for recurrent infection: 200 mg 3-5 times/day for up to 6 months. *Topical:* 5% ointment rubbed gently onto affected area q 3 h 6 times/day for 7 days.

Precautions/contraindications: Do not use with hypersensitivity to acyclovir. Safe use during pregnancy has not been established. Cautious use is required with nursing mothers and neurologic, renal, hepatic, or electrolyte abnormalities.

Side effects/adverse reactions: *GI:* Nausea, vomiting, diarrhea. *CNS:* Headaches, dizziness, fatigue. *Skin:* Rash.

Pharmacokinetics: Absorption of acyclovir is slow and incomplete after PO administration; elimination is via the kidneys.

Nursing considerations: Treatment may not reduce shedding of the virus. Caution the patient to refrain from sexual intercourse when visible herpes lesions are present to avoid infecting her partner.

DRUGS FOR THE TREATMENT OF ACUTE PELVIC INFLAMMATORY DISEASE

The treatment of choice for pelvic inflammatory disease (PID) has not been established, and no single drug is active against the entire spectrum of pathogens that cause this condition. Therefore treatment regimens involve a combination of different antimicrobial agents. The box at right gives examples of combination regimens with a broad spectrum of activity that are effective against most pathogens implicated in PID.

DRUG REGIMENS FOR PELVIC INFLAMMATORY DISEASE

Inpatient treatment

Regimen A
Cefoxitin, 2 g IV q 6 h, *or* cefotetan, 2 g IV q 12 h; **plus** doxycycline, 100 mg IV q 12 h.
Continue drugs IV for at least 48 hours after the patient improves. Then continue doxycycline, 100 mg PO 2 times/day for a total of 10-14 days of therapy.

Regimen B
Clindamycin, 900 mg IV q 8 h; **plus** clindamycin, 2 mg/kg IV or IM, followed by 1.5 mg/kg q 8 h in patients with normal renal function.
Continue drugs IV for at least 48 hours after patient improves. Then continue with doxycycline, 100 mg PO 2 times/day for a total of 10-14 days of therapy.
Alternatively: clindamycin, 450 mg PO 4 times/day for a total of 10-14 days of therapy.

Ambulatory treatment

Recommended regimen
Cefoxitin, 2 g IM with probenecid, 1 g PO; *or* ceftriaxone, 250 mg IM or equivalent cephalosporin. Followed by doxycycline, PO 2 times/day for 10-14 days.

Hormonal Therapy in Women

CONTRACEPTIVES

ORAL CONTRACEPTIVES

Oral contraceptives are highly effective in preventing pregnancy. Most preparations are combinations of a synthetic estrogen (ethinyl estradiol or mestranol) and a progestin (norethindrone, norethindrone acetate, ethynodiol diacetate, norgestrel, or levonorgestrel). Some preparations contain a progestin only. Combination products inhibit ovulation through a negative feedback effect in the hypothalamus. This alters the normal pattern of gonadotropin secretion by the anterior pituitary; both the follicular phase follicle-stimulating hormone (FSH) and the midcycle surge of gonadotropins are inhibited. The cervical mucus thickens (except with the most estrogenic preparations), creating an environment unfavorable to sperm penetration even if ovulation occurs. The progestin-only "minipills" cause the cervical mucus to thicken, making it relatively impen-

etrable to sperm. They may also increase tubal transport time and cause endometrial involution.

Indications: Prevention of pregnancy.

Usual dosage: Combination products are available in "low dose" (<50 μg of estrogen) and "higher dose" (≥50 μg of estrogen). Low-dose tablets may contain constant doses of estrogen and progestin (monophasic preparations) or variable doses (multiphasic preparations). Variable-dose combinations are either biphasic or triphasic, depending on the number of different dosage regimens in a cycle. The minipills contain a progestin only.

Combination oral contraceptives are taken for 21 days of the cycle, followed by 1 week without medication, during which withdrawal bleeding occurs. Most preparations are available in packets containing 21 active pills and 7 inert pills. Minipills are taken daily

Table 16-4

ORAL CONTRACEPTIVES

Progestin	Strength	Estrogen	Strength	Trade name
Products containing less than 50 µg of estrogen				
Norethindrone	0.5 mg	Ethinyl estradiol	35 µg	Brevicon Modicon
Norethindrone	0.4 mg	Ethinyl estradiol	35 µg	Ovcon
Norgestrel	0.3 mg	Ethinyl estradiol	30 µg	Lo/Ovral
Biphasic				
Norethindrone	0.5 mg (10 days) 1 mg (11 days)	Ethinyl estradiol	35 µg	Ortho-Novum 10/11
Triphasic				
Norethindrone	0.5 mg (7 days) 0.75 mg (7 days) 1 mg (7 days)	Ethinyl estradiol	35 µg	Ortho-Novum 7/7/7
Products containing 50 µg or more of estrogen				
Norethindrone	1 mg	Ethinyl estradiol	50 µg	Ovcon-50
Norgestrel	0.5 mg	Ethinyl estradiol	50 µg	Ovral
Products containing progestin only (minipills)				
Norethindrone	0.35 mg			Micronor
Norgestrel	0.075 mg			Ovrette

without a rest period. Table 16-4 lists examples of oral contraceptives.

Precautions/contraindications: Do not use with pregnancy; nursing mothers; breast or other estrogen-dependent neoplasms; or a history of or existing cardiovascular disorders. Cautious use is required with depression or a history of depression; preexisting hypertension; diabetes; gallbladder disease; or a history of migraine headaches.

Side effects/adverse reactions: *CV:* Thrombophlebitis, thrombosis, pulmonary embolism, MI; cigarette smoking increases the risk of cardiovascular side effects. *GI:* Nausea, vomiting, cholestatic jaundice. *Gynecologic:* Breakthrough bleeding, breast tenderness. *Dermatologic:* Melasma. *CNS:* Migraine headaches, depression. *Ophthalmologic:* Corneal changes. *Other:* Edema, rash, photosensitivity.

Pharmacokinetics: Estrogens are primarily metabolized in the liver and excreted in the urine. They can cross the placenta and are excreted in breast milk. Progestins are also metabolized in the liver and excreted in the urine, and a small amount is found in breast milk.

Interactions: Two types of drug interactions are possible: one in which the effectiveness of the oral contraceptive is reduced, and one in which the activity of the other drug is affected (see the box on page 320).

Nursing considerations: Assess the patient for pre-

vious cardiovascular and gallbladder disease. Pregnancy should be ruled out before starting oral contraceptives. The patient should use another means of contraception during the first week of the initial cycle. Tell the patient that she should have periodic tests, including a Pap smear, blood pressure check, mammogram, and pelvic examination. Stress that the risk of cardiovascular disease rises if the patient smokes while taking contraceptives.

DEPOT PREPARATIONS

Several long-lasting contraceptive depot preparations are available. These preparations usually contain a progestin only. The depot form of medroxyprogesterone acetate has received the most attention. Another preparation, the levonorgestrel implant (Norplant), is enclosed in Silastic capsules and implanted in the upper arm. It maintains contraceptive efficacy for 5 years.

Levonorgestrel implant (Norplant)

Indications: Prevention of pregnancy for 5 years.

Usual dosage: 6 capsules, implanted subdermally in the upper arm during the first 7 days of the onset of menses.

Precautions/contraindications: Do not use with hypersensitivity to levonorgestrel; pregnancy (category X); thrombophlebitis; undiagnosed genital bleeding; liver tumors; breast cancer; or liver disease. Cautious use is

ORAL CONTRACEPTIVE DRUG INTERACTIONS

Interacting drug	Effect
Aminocaproic acid	May increase clotting factors
Analgesics, antihistamines, antimigraine preparations	Reduce efficacy of oral contraceptive and increase incidence of breakthrough bleeding
Barbiturates, carbamazepine, chloramphenicol, griseofulvin	
Isoniazid, neomycin, nitrofurantoin	
Penicillin V, phenylbutazone, primidone, rifampin	
Sulfonamides, tetracyclines	
Broad-spectrum antibiotics	May cause failure of oral contraceptive
Troleandomycin	May cause jaundice

required with depression; psychosis; nursing mothers; fluid retention; and contact lens wear.

Side effects/adverse reactions: *CNS:* Dizziness, headaches, nervousness. *GU:* Amenorrhea, cervical erosion, breakthrough bleeding, dysmenorrhea, vaginal candidiasis, breast changes, vaginitis. *GI:* Nausea, abdominal discomfort. *Integumentary:* Alopecia, dermatitis, hirsutism, acne, hypertrichosis, infection, pain or itching at implant site. *Other:* Change in appetite, weight gain.

Pharmacokinetics: The dosage of progestin moving through the implant capsules into the bloodstream is initially about 85 µg/day, stabilizing at around 30 µg/day. Ovulation is inhibited, although the menstrual cycle is not usually disrupted. Progestin causes cervical mucus thickening, which discourages sperm mobility.

Interactions: Norplant's contraceptive effect is reduced when phenytoin or carbamazepine is taken concurrently.

Nursing considerations: Assess for menstrual irregularities. The implant should be removed if jaundice or thrombophlebitis develops. Inform the patient that physical examinations are necessary, and instruct her to see an ophthalmologist if vision problems occur.

POSTCOITAL CONTRACEPTION

When coitus has occurred and pregnancy is not desired, measures known as "morning after" contraception may prevent unwanted pregnancy and avoid abortion. Various estrogen regimens may be used for this purpose (see the box at right). The side effects of these regimens usually include breast tenderness, nausea, and vomiting.

POSTCOITAL CONTRACEPTIVE REGIMENS

Estrogen	Regimen
Ethinyl estradiol/norgestrel (as Ovral)	2 tablets q 12 h for 2 doses
Ethinyl estradiol	2.5 mg 2 times/day for 5 days
Conjugated estrogens	10 mg tid for 5 days
Estrone	5 mg tid for 5 days
Diethylstilbestrol (DES)	25 mg bid for 5 days

ABORTIFACIENTS

RU 486 (Mifepristone)

Although still not approved in the United States, RU 486 has received much attention. It is a progesterone receptor antagonist that can be used to induce abortions during early pregnancy. RU 486 also has potent antiglucocorticoid activity and has demonstrated usefulness in treating Cushing's syndrome. Because the federal Food and Drug Administration (FDA) has not approved its use, RU 486 is considered investigational and its use is strictly monitored.

Indications: Use as a safe and effective alternative to surgical abortion. Although RU 486 is not as efficacious as surgery, it eliminates the risk of complications from anesthesia and surgery. Patients may be treated as outpatients with close medical supervision until the abortion outcome is known. Because failed abortion and 55 days of amenorrhea may occur, the patient should be carefully evaluated before RU 486 is started.

Usual dosage: The optimum oral dosing regimen for

RU 486 has not been determined. Single doses of 600 mg and multidoses of 25-100 mg/day for 5-7 days, followed by a dose of prostaglandin, have been effective for inducing abortion.

Precautions/contraindications: Do not use with hypersensitivity to mifepristone. Cautious use is required with anemia. Pregnant women with more than 55 days of amenorrhea have a greater incidence of adverse effects and failed abortions.

Side effects/adverse reactions: *CNS:* Mild headaches (adequately controlled with mild analgesics). *GI:* Nausea and/or vomiting (controlled with antiemetics). *GU:* Mild to moderate uterine pain similar to that during heavy menses.

Pharmacokinetics: RU 486 reaches peak serum levels in about 3 hours after ingestion. It is highly protein bound and has an elimination half-life of 20-54 hours. Three metabolites of mifepristone have been identified. Less than 0.5% of the daily dose is excreted in the urine.

DRUGS FOR THE TREATMENT OF INFERTILITY

Clomiphene Citrate (Clomid)

Clomiphene is an oral nonsteroidal estrogen that induces ovulation in some women. Its exact mechanism of action is unknown, but it may prevent estrogen from binding with receptors in the hypothalamus.

Indications: Inducement of ovulation.

Usual dosage: *First course of therapy:* 50 mg/day PO for 5 days, started on day 5 of the menstrual cycle or at any time if the patient has no recent uterine bleeding. *Second course of therapy:* The first cycle is repeated until conception has occurred, or for 3 cycles. *No ovulation:* 100 mg/day for 5 days. Higher dosages increase the incidence of side effects.

Precautions/contraindications: Do not use in pregnancy or in cases of suspected pregnancy; neoplastic lesions; ovarian cysts; hepatic impairment; visual abnormalities; or thrombophlebitis.

Side effects/adverse reactions: *GI:* Gastrointestinal discomfort, nausea, vomiting, weight gain. *Ophthalmologic:* Visual disturbances (usually of short duration and reversible). *Reproductive:* Spontaneous abortion, multiple births. *Other:* Vasomotor symptoms similar to those manifested at menopause.

Pharmacokinetics: Clomiphene is absorbed from the GI tract and detoxified in the liver. The half-life is 5-7 days, and 50% of the drug is excreted in the feces after 5-7 days.

Nursing considerations: A medical history, pelvic examination, and liver function test should be done be-

fore treatment with clomiphene is started. The drug is administered after estrogen therapy has been discontinued. The patient and her partner should be well aware of the potential for multiple births. After administering the drug, monitor for manifestation of side effects. Subsequent treatment cycles should be started on day 5 of the cycle. Instruct the patient to take the drug at the same time each day to maintain the drug level; also, instruct her to report any visual abnormalities to her physician immediately. Evaluate the therapeutic response (fertility).

Menotropins

Indications: Used with human chorionic gonadotropin (HCG) in sequence to induce ovulation and subsequently pregnancy in infertile women with functional anovulation.

Usual dosage: *Induction of ovulation and pregnancy:* Initially, 75 IU of follicle-stimulating hormone (FSH) and luteinizing hormone (LH) IM daily for 9-12 days; followed by hCG (10,000 IU) 1 day after last dose of menotropins. Menotropins should not be given longer than 12 days. If ovulation occurs without pregnancy, this regimen may be repeated at least twice before increasing the dosage of FSH and LH to 150 IU. If ovulation again occurs without pregnancy, the higher dosage may be repeated at monthly intervals for 2 more courses.

Precautions/contraindications: Do not use with primary anovulation; thyroid and adrenal dysfunction; infertility caused by factors other than anovulation; abnormal bleeding of unknown origin; ovarian cysts; or ovarian enlargement.

Side effects/adverse reactions: Mild to moderate ovarian enlargement, abdominal distention and pain, ovarian hyperstimulation syndrome, fever, nausea, vomiting, diarrhea, release of multiple ova, follicular cysts, weight gain.

Pharmacokinetics: The exact fate of menotropins after injection is unknown. Approximately 8% of the dose is excreted unchanged in the urine.

Nursing considerations: Before treatment, rule out pregnancy, primary ovarian failure, neoplastic lesions, and husband's infertility. Measuring urinary excretion of estrogen serves as an index of follicular maturation.

DRUGS FOR THE TREATMENT OF ENDOMETRIOSIS

Danazol

Danazol is a synthetic androgenic steroid. It inhibits ovarian steroidogenesis by inhibiting gonadotropin secretion, resulting in amenorrhea. It probably also acts directly on the ovaries. Danazol inhibits the progress and pain of endometriosis by causing atrophy and involution of both normal and ectopic endometrial tissue.

Indications: Palliative treatment of endometriosis.

Usual dosage: 400 mg 2 times/day for 3-6 months. Started during menstruation or if pregnancy test is negative. Therapy may be extended for up to 9 months, and the regimen may be repeated if symptoms recur.

Precautions/contraindications: Do not use with pregnancy; nursing mothers; undiagnosed abnormal bleeding; impaired renal, cardiac, or hepatic function; or porphyria. Cautious use is required with migraine headaches.

Side effects/adverse reactions: *Androgenic (virilization):* Acneform lesions, oily skin, voice change, clitoral enlargement. *CNS:* Dizziness, headaches, sleep disorders. *Eye:* Visual disturbances. *GU:* Decreased libido. *Hypersensitivity:* Skin rashes. *Hypoestrogenic:* Menopausal symptoms, vaginitis. *Musculoskeletal:* Muscle spasms. *Other:* Elevated blood pressure, decreased levels of HDL cholesterol, and increased levels of other lipoproteins.

Pharmacokinetics: Peak plasma levels are attained in 1-2 hours. The plasma half-life is 4½ hours. Danazol is metabolized to water-soluble metabolites and excreted primarily in the urine.

Nursing considerations: Pregnancy should be ruled out before treatment is started. Baseline and periodic liver function tests should be performed. Advise the patient of the virilization effects of the drug. Treatment should be started during menstruation. Monitor cardiovascular functions, and monitor the patient for edema. Monitor the patient closely if migraines and epilepsy are preexisting conditions for worsening.

Interactions: The effects of oral antidiabetic drugs and oxyphenbutazone are increased. Prothrombin time is increased with anticoagulants. Edema occurs with use of ACTH or adrenal steroids. The effects of insulin are decreased.

DRUGS FOR THE TREATMENT OF MENOPAUSE

Estrogen

Most of the symptoms of menopause associated with low estrogen levels (vaginal and urethral atrophy) and vasomotor reactions (hot flashes, sweating, increased pulse rate) can be ameliorated or reversed with an estrogen preparation. Conjugated estrogens are most commonly prescribed. Other natural and synthetic oral preparations are also effective. The newest type of drug delivery system for estrogen preparations is a transdermal patch, which releases estradiol at a constant rate. A progestin, usually medroxyprogesterone acetate, is

added to the regimen if the uterus is still in situ. This has been found to reduce the incidence of endometrial hyperplasia and carcinoma. An intake of 500-1,000 mg/day of elemental calcium is also recommended to retard the onset of osteoporosis.

Therapeutic regimens

When the uterus is in situ, a cyclic regimen is used to avoid uninterrupted stimulation of the uterus. Estrogen is taken for 25 days, with 5 or 6 days off, or a transdermal patch is applied twice weekly. If a progestin is prescribed, it is added to the regimen the last 10-13 days of the cycle.

For women whose uterus has been removed, estrogen is prescribed either continuously or cyclically (25 days on and 5-6 days off). A progestin is not usually included in the regimen. However, some experts believe that adding progestin may protect a woman against breast cancer.

Indications: To relieve vasomotor and other symptoms that accompany the onset of menopause and to retard the progression of osteoporosis.

Usual dosage: See the box on page 323 for various estrogen preparations and their usual dosages.

Precautions/contraindications: Do not use with hypersensitivity to estrogen; breast cancer; or pregnancy. Cautious use is required with hypertension; gallbladder disease; diabetes mellitus; heart failure; and hepatic or renal impairment.

Side effects/adverse reactions: *CNS:* Headaches, dizziness, depression, libido changes. *CV:* Thromboembolic disorders, hypertension. *GI:* Nausea, vomiting, diarrhea, bloating, cholestatic jaundice. *GU:* Mastodynia, spotting, changes in menstrual flow and cycle. *Metabolic:* Reduced carbohydrate tolerance, fluid retention. *Other:* Leg cramps.

Nursing considerations: Tablets can be taken with the food or liquid of the patient's choice. A cyclic regimen is recommended for patients with the uterus in situ. Annual mammograms and Pap smears are recommended. Reinforce the dosing schedule with the patient.

Progestin (medroxyprogesterone acetate)

Medroxyprogesterone acetate is a synthetic derivative of progesterone with a prolonged, variable duration of action. It also possesses androgenic and antiestrogenic activity. Progestin induces and maintains the endometrium, preventing uterine bleeding; inhibits production of pituitary gonadotropin, preventing ovulation; and produces thick cervical mucus that resists the passage of sperm.

Indications: Used with estrogen replacement for menopausal symptoms and to treat secondary amenorrhea; also used as a contraceptive and for palliative treatment of inoperable, recurrent, metastatic endometrial or renal carcinoma.

Usual dosage: *Secondary amenorrhea:* 5-10 mg/day for 5-10 days beginning anytime if endometrium is adequately estrogen primed. *Abnormal bleeding due to hormonal imbalance:* 5-10 mg/day for 5-10 days beginning on assumed or calculated day 16 or day 21 of menstrual cycle. *Carcinoma:* 400-1,000 mg/week until disease stabilizes, then 400 mg/month.

Precautions/contraindications: Do not use with pregnancy.

Side effects/adverse reactions: *CNS:* Cerebral thrombosis or hemorrhage, headaches, depression. *CV:* Hypertension, pulmonary embolism. *GI:* Nausea, vomiting, cholestatic jaundice. *Reproductive:* Breakthrough bleeding, cervical erosion, dysmenorrhea. *Other:* Weight changes, breast tenderness.

Pharmacokinetics: Duration of action is 24 hours. Medroxyprogesterone acetate is metabolized in the liver and excreted in the urine and feces.

Nursing considerations: IM injection may be painful. Repeated IM injections may cause infertility and amenorrhea for 18 months.

ESTROGENS

Chlorotrianisene (TACE) 12-25 mg/day PO—atrophic vaginitis, prostate cancer

Conjugated estrogens (Premarin) 0.3-1.25 mg/day PO—atrophic vaginitis

1.25-2.5 mg/day topical

1.25-2.5 mg tid PO—prostate cancer

Dienestrol (DV, Ortho Dienestrol) Cyclic topical application (see manufacturer's instructions)—atrophic vaginitis

Diethylstilbestrol (DES) 1-3 mg/day PO—prostate cancer

Diethylstilbestrol diphosphate (Stilphostrol) 50-200 mg tid PO—prostate cancer; IV (see manufacturer's instructions)

Esterified estrogens (Estratab, Menest) 0.3-1.25 mg/day PO—atrophic vaginitis; 1.25-2.5 mg tid PO—prostate cancer

Estradiol (Estrace) Cyclic topical application (see manufacturer's instructions)—atrophic vaginitis; 1-2 mg tid—prostate cancer

Estradiol transdermal (Estraderm) 1 patch 2 times/wk topical—atrophic vaginitis

Estradiol valerate (Delestrogen) 10-20 mg q 4 wk IM—atrophic vaginitis; 30 mg q 1-2 wk IM—prostate cancer

Estrone (Estroject, Estrone-A) 0.1-0.5 mg 2 or 3 times/wk IM—atrophic vaginitis; 2-4 mg 2 or 3 times/wk IM—prostate cancer

Estropipate (Ogen) 0.75-6 mg/day PO—atrophic vaginitis

Ethinyl estradiol (Estinyl) 0.15-3 mg/day PO—prostate cancer

Polyestradiol (Estradurin) 40 mg q 2-4 wk IM—prostate cancer

(From Gray.[39])

APPENDIX A

Standard Laboratory Values: Pregnant and Nonpregnant Women

Laboratory value	Nonpregnant	Pregnant
Hematologic values		
Complete blood count (CBC)		
Hemoglobin, g/dl	12-16*	10-14*
Hematocrit, PCV, %	37-47	32-42
Red cell volume, ml	1,600	1,900
Plasma volume, ml	2,400	3,700
Red blood cell count, million/mm^3	4-5.5	4-5.5
White blood cells, total per mm^3	4,500-10,000	5,000-15,000
Polymorphonuclear cells, %	54-62	60-85
Lymphocytes, %	38-46	15-40
Erythrocyte sedimentation rate, mm/h	≤	30-90
MCHC, g/dl packed RBCs (mean corpuscular hemoglobin concentration)	30-36	No change
MCH/(mean corpuscular hemoglobin per picogram [less than a nanogram])	29-32	No change
MCV/μm^3 (mean corpuscular volume per cubic micrometer)	82-96	No change
Blood coagulation and fibrinolytic activity†		
Factors VII, VIII, IX, X		Increase in pregnancy, return to normal in early puerperium; factor VIII increases during and immediately after birth
Factors XI, XIII		Decrease in pregnancy
Prothrombin time (PT)	12-14 sec	Slight decrease in pregnancy
Partial thromboplastin time (PTT)	60-70 sec	Slight decrease in pregnancy and again decreases during second and third stages of labor (indicates clotting at placental site)
Bleeding time	1-3 min (Duke) 2-4 min (Ivy)	No appreciable change
Coagulation time	6-10 min (Lee/White)	No appreciable change

*At sea level. Permanent residents of higher levels (e.g., Denver) require higher levels of hemoglobin.
†Pregnancy represents a hypercoagulable state.
‡For the woman about 20 years of age; 10 years of age: 103/70; 30 years of age: 123/82; 40 years of age: 126/84.
(From Bobak/Jensen, ed. 5.[13])

324

Laboratory value	Nonpregnant	Pregnant
Platelets	150,000 to 350,000/mm^3	No significant change until 3-5 days after birth, then marked increase (may predispose woman to thrombosis) and gradual return to normal
Fibrinolytic activity		Decrease in pregnancy, then abrupt return to normal (protection against thromboembolism)
Fibrinogen	250 mg/dl	400 mg/dl
Mineral/vitamin concentrations		
Vitamin B$_{12}$, folic acid, ascorbic acid	Normal	Moderate decrease
Serum proteins		
Total, g/dl	6.7-8.3	5.5-7.5
Albumin, g/dl	3.5-5.5	3.0-5.0
Globulin, total, g/dl	2.3-3.5	3.0-4.0
Blood sugar		
Fasting, mg/dl	70-80	65
2-hour postprandial, mg/dl	60-110	<140 after a 100 g carbohydrate meal is considered normal
Cardiovascular determinations		
Blood pressure, mm Hg	120/80†	114/65 during midtrimester, then return to usual value by end of third trimester
Pulse, rate/min	70	80
Stroke volume, ml	65	75
Cardiac output, L/min	4.5	6
Circulation time (arm-tongue), sec	15-16	12-14
Blood volume, ml		
Whole blood	4,000	5,600
Plasma	2,400	3,700
Red blood cells	1,600	1,900
Chest x-ray studies		
Transverse diameter of heart	—	1-2 cm increase
Left border of heart	—	Straightened
Cardiac volume	—	70 ml increase
Hepatic values		
Bilirubin total	Not more than 1 mg/dl	Unchanged
Serum cholesterol	110-300 mg/dl	↑ 60% from 16-32 weeks of pregnancy; remains at this level until after birth
Serum alkaline phosphatase	2-4.5 U (Bodansky)	↑ from week 12 of pregnancy to 6 weeks after birth
Serum globulin albumin	1.5-3 g/dl	↑ slight
	4.5-5.3 g/dl	↓ 3 g by late pregnancy
Renal values		
Bladder capacity	1,300 ml	1,500 ml
Renal plasma flow (RPF), ml/min	490-700	Increase by 25%, to 612-875
Glomerular filtration rate (GFR), ml/min	105-132	Increase by 50%, to 160-198
Nonprotein nitrogen (NPN), mg/dl	25-40	Decreases
Blood urea nitrogen (BUN), mg/dl	20-25	Decreases
Serum creatinine, mg/kg/24 h	20-22	Decreases
Serum uric acid, mg/kg/24 h	257-750	Decreases
Urine glucose	Negative	Present in 20% of pregnant women
Intravenous pyelogram (IVP)	Normal	Slight-to-moderate hydroureter and hydronephrosis; right kidney larger than left kidney

Pregnancy Tests and Laboratory Results Influenced by Pregnancy

An illness or pregnancy-related complication may mirror the symptoms of a normal pregnancy. These conditions need to be ruled out when diagnosing pregnancy:

Appendicitis
Hydatidiform or partial mole
Ectopic pregnancy
Missed abortion
Pseudocyesis
Chorioepithelioma
Choriocarcinoma
Gastrointestinal disorders

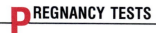 **P**REGNANCY TESTS

All pregnancy tests detect human chorionic gonadotropin (hCG), a hormone found only in pregnant women. The hCG hormone usually can be detected by 7 days after fertilization (4 to 6 days after implantation), or approximately 20 days from the first day of the patient's last menses. The hCG hormone is produced by the placenta; the level of hCG peaks in 8 to 12 weeks.

TYPES OF PREGNANCY TESTS

Latex agglutination inhibition (LAI): read within 2 min.

Hemagglutination inhibition (HAI): more sensitive, read within 1 to 2 hours

Radioreceptor assay: requires 1 hour and expensive equipment

Radioimmunoassay: measures beta subunits of hCG (specific antibodies); test results within 1-48 hours

Enzyme immunoassays and enzyme-linked immunosorbent assay (ELISA): colorimetric indicator of beta-hCG; can be read in about 5 minutes

Over-the-counter (OTC) pregnancy tests have a false-positive rate of about 5% and a false-negative rate of about 20% to 25%; first voiding of the morning has the highest level of hCG.

hCG (serum and urine)	Serum: Nonpregnant woman: <0.01 IU/ml
Pregnant (weeks)	
1	0.01-0.04 IU/ml
2	0.03-0.10 IU/ml
4	0.10-1 IU/ml
5-12	10-100 IU/ml
Pregnant 1-12 weeks	Urine: 6,000-500,000 IU/24 h
	Nonpregnant woman: negative or none
Nonpregnant, dead fetus, incomplete abortion	Decreased hCG level
Hydatidiform mole, erythroblastosis fetalis, choriocarcinoma, chorioepithelioma	Elevated hCG level
Anticonvulsants, phenothiazines, antiparkinsonism drugs, hypnotics	Elevated hCG level
Other Tests	
Glucose tolerance test (GTT)	Glycosuria, with normoglycemia, is common in pregnancy
Insulin clearance test	Clearance increased with hypermetabolic states and with pregnancy
Thyrotrophin-releasing hormone (TRH) stimulation test	Exaggerated results with oral contraceptives or pregnancy

Conditions Requiring Immediate Intervention

Several different conditions require prompt health care intervention for women. Treatment typically begins in a clinic, doctor's office, or emergency setting and is followed by hospitalization, if needed.

VASOVAGAL SYNCOPE

During procedures, a vasovagal response may occur. A loss of consciousness may follow from a drop in blood pressure and lowered heart rate. A decrease in peripheral resistance, cardiac output, and venous return results.

Typical Interventions

The woman should be placed in a position to maximize respiratory function and blood flow. Vasovagal response may be minimized if a procedure is suspended, and if comfort and perfusion measures are performed, such as a cool cloth to the forehead, or a *reverse Trendelenburg* position. The health care team may need to be notified, and the emergency (crash) cart obtained. Medications, such as atropine sulfate and epinephrine, should be ready for administration. The following parameters should be monitored: airway, breathing, and circulation; signs of shock, such as decreased or increased blood pressure; pulse.

SUPINE HYPOTENSION

Weight from abdominal contents may compress the vena cava and aorta, resulting in a drop in blood pressure. This phenomenon is known to occur during pregnancy when a woman is supine, but it may also occur in the nonpregnant woman, especially when lying in a lithotomy position.

Typical Interventions

The woman's position should be changed from a supine or lithotomy position to a *side-lying position*. Supine hypotension should resolve if compression of the large abdominal vessels is reduced. If the symptoms persist or other signs of shock develop, the health care team should be notified and an emergency cart obtained. The following parameters should be monitored: vital signs, especially blood pressure (hypotension) and respiratory rate (breathlessness), should be assessed; skin condition, especially signs of diaphoresis (clammy skin) or pallor.

TOXIC SHOCK SYNDROME (TSS)

Toxic shock syndrome, a bacterial infection, may lead to septic shock and the release of exotoxins. There is a high mortality rate if underlying disease or pathology exists, or if treatment is delayed or inadequate.

Typical Interventions

Fluid volume regulation is performed to restore intravascular volume. Usually 3 to 5 liters of saline, Ringer's lactate, or buffered ($NaHCO_3$) IV lactate solution is given for severe shock. *Blood plasma expanders* are given after the initial resolution of fluid balance is restored. Whole blood is used if massive hemorrhage occurs and if the hematocrit (Hct) is less than 30%. Packed red blood cells (PRBCs) are used if pulmonary capillary wedge pressure (PCWP) or right atrial pressure is elevated, or if underlying disease or pathology prohibits sudden volume expansion. For elevated PCWP (e.g., cardiogenic shock), diuretics may be needed. Central venous pressure (CVP) and other parameters are usually monitored in an intensive care setting.

DISSEMINATED INTRAVASCULAR COAGULATION (DIC)

Thrombosis or hemorrhage may result in disseminated intravascular coagulation (DIC) syndrome. This bleeding disorder occurs when fibrinogen transforms into fibrin clot (diffuse intravascular fibrin formation). Clots then form in the capillaries, leading to the depletion of clotting factors more rapidly than they can be replaced. Capillaries become dilated with stagnant blood. Metabolic waste from anaerobic metabolism leads to acidosis. Further hemorrhaging may result from increased fibrinolysis, low levels of antithrombin III, and depletion of clotting factors.

Typical Interventions

Heparin therapy is given to break the DIC cycle. Antibiotics are used, if infection exists or is suspected. *Blood products*, such as saline-washed PRBCs, platelets, clotting factors, or fresh-frozen plasma, are given to replace O_2 carrying capacity and deficient clotting factors. A *semi-Fowler's position*, *oxygen therapy*, a *warm environment*, and *vasopressors* (e.g., dopamine) are used to improve gas exchange and arterial hypotension. *Antiarrhythmic* (e.g., lidocaine) and *cardiotonic* (e.g., dopatrex) medications are given as needed.

The following parameters should be closely monitored: pulses and vital signs for abnormalities (tachypnea, dysrhythmias or gallop, hypotension, dyspnea); tissue perfusion for signs of cyanosis or pallor; bleeding, petechiae, ecchymosis; intake and output, renal function tests to detect decreased renal function; routine lab; clotting tests; blood gases, sensory, motor, and mental status.

DYSFUNCTIONAL UTERINE BLEEDING

Occasionally, dysfunctional uterine bleeding (DUB) results in uncontrolled hemorrhaging. Heavy menses (menorrhagia or hypermenorrhea) may result from underlying pathology, such as endometriosis, polyps, cysts, myoma, or malignancies. Mid-cycle hemorrhage is less common, but does occur.

Typical Interventions

Preoperative care is given, such as keeping the patient NPO or without oral intake, completing laboratory studies, and answering questions about surgery and postoperative care. Emergency surgery, including

D&C, removal of tumors by hysteroscopy, resectoscopy with cautery procedures, and abdominal or vaginal hysterectomy with partial or total salpingo-oophorectomy, may be required. First aid principles should be followed to detect hypovolemic shock or the development of DIC. The following parameters should be monitored for signs of abnormalities: vital signs; tissue perfusion; diaphoresis; routine blood counts; signs of DIC; signs of shock.

OVARIAN CYSTS

Ovarian cysts, although usually clinically insignificant, may cause severe pain from torsion (twisting) or uncontrolled hemorrhage. Surgery may be needed to rule out appendicitis, cancer, or ectopic pregnancy.

Typical Interventions

Preoperative care is given, if a *laparotomy* is required. Cyst removal is not usually a surgical emergency, unless the cysts are associated with torsion, hemorrhage, or rupture. Preoperative assessment includes ultrasonography to distinguish neoplastic cysts from functional cysts, abdominal x-rays to identify calcified structures, barium enema to rule out colonic disease, and a pregnancy test to distinguish between potential lutein cysts and pregnancy. The following parameters should be monitored: vital signs and physical symptoms of hemorrhage or shock; routine lab studies to prepare for surgery; diagnostic tests to determine cause of pain or hemorrhage.

CONCEPTION COMPLICATIONS

Ectopic (outside the uterus) pregnancy is the implantation of the trophoblast in areas that cannot sustain gestational growth. If implantation occurs within the uterine (fallopian) tubes, rupture will occur if there is no intervention. *Gestational trophoblastic neoplasms* include hydatidiform mole and invasive mole.

Typical Interventions

Preoperative care is given because emergency *laparotomy* is needed to remove an ectopic pregnancy and repair structures. Amniography and ultrasonography are used for early diagnosis of trophoblastic neoplasms that may decrease the risk of metastasis, especially with choriocarcinoma. Hydatidiform mole is removed with D&C techniques, if fertility is desired, followed by actinomycin-D treatment. *Hysterectomy* followed by chemotherapy and radiation therapy may be indicated. The following parameters should be closely monitored: vital signs and physical symptoms of hemorrhage or shock; routine lab studies to prepare for surgery; diagnostic tests to determine cause of pain or hemorrhage; observation of hCG levels to evaluate postevacuation success, if a neoplasm was present.

References

1. Akesson EJ, Loeb JA, Wilson-Pauwels L: *Thompson's core textbook of anatomy*, ed 2, Philadelphia, 1990, JB Lippincott.
2. American Cancer Society: *Cancer facts and figures—1993*, Atlanta, 1993, The Society.
3. American Heart Association: *1990 Stroke facts*, Dallas, 1990, The Association.
4. American Joint Committee on Cancer: *Manual for staging of cancer*, Philadelphia, 1992, JB Lippincott.
5. Andolina VF, Lille S, Willison KM: *Mammographic imaging*, Philadelphia, 1992, JB Lippincott.
5a. Andreoli T et al., editors: *Cecil's essentials of medicine*, Philadelphia, 1986, WB Saunders.
6. Anspaugh, Hamrick, and Rosato: *Wellness: concepts and applications*, St. Louis, 1991, Mosby–Year Book.
7. Asken S: *Liposuction surgery and autologous fat transplantation*, Norwalk, Conn., 1988, Appleton & Lange.
8. Baird SB, McCorkle R, Grant M: *Cancer nursing: a comprehensive textbook*, Philadelphia, 1991, WB Saunders.
8a. Baron EJ, Finegold SM: *Bailey and Scott's diagnostic microbiology*, ed 8, St. Louis, 1990, Mosby.
9. Barnett R: *The American health food book*, New York, 1991, Dutton.
9a. Belcher AE: *Cancer nursing*, St. Louis, 1992, Mosby.
9b. Bass E, Davis L: *The courage to heal*, New York, 1992, Harper–Collins.
10. Benjamin RB: *Atlas of office surgery*, vol 1, Philadelphia, 1989, Lea & Febiger.
11. Bevis R: *Caring for women: obstetric and gynaecological nursing*, ed 4, London, 1991, Bailliere Tindall.
12. Blanchard R, Steiner BW: *Clinical management of gender identity disorders in children and adults*, Washington, DC, 1990, American Psychiatric Press.
13. Bobak IM, Jensen MD: *Maternity and gynecologic care: the nurse and the family*, ed 5, St. Louis, 1993, Mosby.
14. Boskin W, Graf G, Kreisworth V: *Health dynamics: attitudes and behaviors*, St. Paul, 1990, West Publishing.
15. Bostwick J: *Breast reconstruction following surgery*, Atlanta, 1989, The American Cancer Society.
16. Bowers AC, Thompson JM: *Clinical manual of health assessment*, ed 4, St. Louis, 1992, Mosby.
17. Brandt BB, Harney J: An overview of interstitial brachytherapy and hyperthermia, *Oncol Nurs Forum* 16(6):833-841, 1989.
18. Brundage D: *Renal disorders*, St. Louis, 1992, Mosby.
19. Byyny RL, Speroff, L: *A clinical guide for the care of older women*, Baltimore, 1990, Williams & Wilkins.
20. Canobbio M: *Cardiovascular disorders*, St. Louis, 1990, Mosby.
21. Centers for Disease Control: *Sexually transmitted diseases: treatment guidelines*, Atlanta, 1990, US Department of Health and Human Services.
22. Cerrato, P: Helping food addicts kick the habit, *RN* 50:75-78, August 1987.
23. Chipps E, Clanin N, Campbell V: *Neurologic disorders*, St. Louis, 1992, Mosby.
24. Cohen S, Kenner CA, Hollingsworth AO: *Maternal, neonatal, and women's health nursing*, Springhouse, Pa., 1991, Springhouse Corp.
25. Cook MJ: Perimenopause: an opportunity for health promotion, *JOGNN* 22(3):223-228, May/June 1993.
26. Corbett JV: *Laboratory tests and diagnostic procedures with nursing diagnosis*, Norwalk, Conn., 1992, Appleton & Lange.
27. Crafts RC: *Textbook of human anatomy*, ed 3, New York, 1985, Churchill Livingstone.
28. *Current clinical strategies: gynecology and obstetrics*, Newport Beach, R.I., 1992, CCS Publishing.
28a. Daniel WA, Paulshock BZ: *Patient care*, 13 May 1979, pp 122-124.
29. DiSaia PJ, Creasman WT: *Clinical gynecologic oncology*, ed 3, St. Louis, 1989, Mosby.
30. Doress PB, Siegal DL: The midlife and older women book project in cooperation with the women's health book collective, *Ourselves, growing older*, New York, 1987, Simon & Schuster.
31. Droegemueller W et al.: *Comprehensive gynecology*, St. Louis, 1987, Mosby.
32. Everly GS, Feldman RHL: *Occupational health promotion*, Baltimore, 1985, Chevron Publishing.
33. Felig P et al.: *Endocrinology and metabolism*, ed 2, New York, 1987, McGraw-Hill.
34. Fogel CI, Woods NF: *Health care of women: a nursing perspective*, St. Louis, 1981, Mosby.
35. Foley D, Nechas E, Wallis L: *Women's encyclopedia of health and emotional healing*, Emmaus, Pa., 1993, Rodale Press.

35a. Frederickson HL, Wilkins-Haug L: *OB/GYN secrets*, St. Louis, 1991, Mosby.

35b. Frye PR: *Proceedings from the first international conference on transgender law and employment policy*, Houston, 1992.

36. Fudenberg H et al.: *Basic and clinical immunology*, ed 3, Los Altos, Calif., 1980, Lange Medical Publications.

36a. Gallagher SH, Leis HP Jr, Snyderman RK et al.: *The breast*, St. Louis, 1978, Mosby.

37. Glass RH: *Office gynecology*, ed 4, Baltimore, 1993, Williams & Wilkins.

38. Gomel V, Munro MG, Rowe TC: *Gynecology: a practical approach*, Baltimore, 1990, Williams & Wilkins.

39. Gray M: *Genitourinary disorders*, St. Louis, 1992, Mosby.

40. Gray H, Clemente C: *Anatomy of the human body*, ed 3, Philadelphia, 1985, Lea & Febiger.

41. Grazer FM: *Atlas of suction assisted lipectomy in body contouring*, New York, 1992, Churchill Livingstone.

42. Griffith HW: *Instructions for patients: medical tests and diagnostic procedures*, Philadelphia, 1989, Lea & Febiger.

43. Griffith-Kenney J: *Contemporary women's health: a nursing advocacy approach*, Redding, Mass., 1986, Addison-Wesley.

44. Grimes D: *Infectious diseases*, St. Louis, 1991, Mosby.

45. Gross PA et al.: *Managing your health*, New York, 1991, Consumer Reports Books.

46. Gusbert SB et al.: *Female genital cancer*, New York, 1988, Churchill Livingstone.

47. Haagensen CD: *Diseases of the breast*, Philadelphia, 1986, WB Saunders.

48. Harris JR et al.: *Breast diseases*, Philadelphia, 1991, JB Lippincott.

49. Hatcher RA: *Contraceptive technology: 1990-1992*, ed 15, New York, 1992, Irvington Publishers.

50. Heart disease: women at risk, *Consumer Reports*, 58(5):300-302, May 1992.

51. Helton AS: *Protocol of care for the battered woman*, White Plains, N.Y., 1987, March of Dimes.

52. Herman C et al.: Effects of coping style and relaxation on cancer therapy side effects and emotional responses, *Oncol Nurs Forum* 13(5):308-315, 1990.

53. Heywang-Kobrunner S: *Contrast-enhanced MRI of the breast*, Basel, N.Y., 1990, HD Medical Information Publishers.

54. Hirshmann JR, Hunter CH: *Overcoming overeating*, New York, 1989, Fawcett Columbine.

55. Holleb AI et al.: *American Cancer Society textbook of clinical oncology*, Atlanta, 1991, The Society.

56. Holmes KK et al.: *Sexually transmitted diseases*, ed 2, New York, 1990, McGraw-Hill.

57. Homer MJ, Sickles EA: *Mammographic interpretation: A practical approach*, New York, 1991, McGraw-Hill.

58. Hughes LE, Mansel RE, Webster DJT: *Benign disorders and diseases of the breast: concepts and clinical management*, London, 1989, Bailliere Tindall.

59. Hunter College Women's Studies Collective: *Women's realties, women's choices*, New York, 1983, Oxford University Press.

60. Hurley JS, Schlaadt RG: *The wellness life-style*, Guilford, Conn., 1992, Dushkin Publishing.

61. Iazzeho D: What's happening with women and body image? *The network news*, p 1, May/June 1992, National Women's Health Network.

62. Ingalls AJ, Salerno MC: *Maternal and child health nursing*, ed 7, St. Louis, 1991, Mosby.

63. Isaacs JH: *Textbook of breast disease*, St. Louis, 1992, Mosby.

64. Jacobs DS et al.: *Laboratory test handbook*, ed 2, Baltimore, 1990, Williams & Wilkins.

65. Jones JM et al.: *Women's health management: guidelines for nurse practitioners*, Reston, Va., 1984, Reston Publishing.

65a. Katz WA, editor: *Diagnosis and management of rheumatic disorders*, Philadelphia, 1988, JB Lippincott.

66. Kee JL: *Laboratory and diagnostic tests with nursing implications*, ed 3, Norwalk, Conn., 1991, Appleton & Lange.

67. Kenen RH: Protecting women in the workplace: what the US could learn from the European community, *The Network News* 17(4): 5-8, July/Aug 1992.

68. Kinne DW: *The surgical management of primary breast cancer*, Atlanta, 1991, The American Cancer Society.

69. Lascelles PT, Donaldson D: *Diagnostic function tests in chemical pathology*, Boston, 1989, Kluwer Academic Publishers.

70. Lauver D: Psychosocial variables, race, and intention to seek care for breast cancer symptoms, *Nurs Res* 41(4):236-241, 1992.

71. Lauver D: Addressing infrequent cancer screening among women, *Nurs Outlook* 40(5):207-212, 1992.

72. Lewis TLT, Chamberlain GVP: *Gynaecology by ten teachers*, ed 15, London, 1990, Hodder & Stoughton.

73. Loprieno N: Guidelines for safety evaluation of cosmetics ingredients, *Food Chem Toxicol* 30(9): 809-815, Sept 1992.

74. Lynch HT: The family history and cancer control: hereditary breast cancer, *Arch Surg* 125(2):151-152, 1990.

75. Malasanos L, Barkauskas V, Stoltenberg-Allen K: *Health assessment*, ed 4, St. Louis, 1990, Mosby.

76. Mansel RE: *Recent developments in the study of benign breast disease*, Park Ridge, N.J., 1992, Parthenon Publishing.

76a. Marshall WA, Tanner JM: *Arch Dis Child*, 44:291, 1969.

77. Martin LL: *Health care of women*, Philadelphia, 1978, JB Lippincott.

78. McNally JC et al.: *Guidelines for oncology nursing practice*, Philadelphia, 1991, WB Saunders.

79. Mickley JR et al.: Spiritual well-being, religiousness and hope among women with breast cancer, *Image* 24(4):267-272, 1992.

80. Miller GT Jr: *Living in the environment*, ed 7, Belmont, 1992, Wadsworth Publishing.

81. Mitchell GW Jr, Bassett LW: *The female breast and its disorders*, Baltimore, 1990, Williams & Wilkins.

81a. Mourad LA: *Orthopedic disorders*, St. Louis, 1991, Mosby.

82. Mudge-Grout CL: *Immunologic disorders*, St. Louis, 1992, Mosby.

83. Ornstein R, Sobel D: *Healthy pleasures*, Redding, Mass., 1989, Addison-Wesley.

84. Otto SE: *Oncology nursing*, St. Louis, 1991, Mosby.

85. Parker CW: *Clinical immunology*, Philadelphia, 1980, WB Saunders.

86. Payne WA, Hahn DB: *Understanding your health*, ed 3, St. Louis, 1992, Mosby.

87. Perry AG, Potter PA: *Clinical nursing skills and techniques: basic, intermediate, and advanced*, ed 2, St. Louis, 1990, Mosby.

88. Phipps WJ et al.: *Medical-surgical nursing: concepts and clinical practice*, ed 4, St. Louis, 1991, Mosby.

89. Potter PA, Perry AG: *Basic nursing: theory and practice*, ed 2, St. Louis, 1991, Mosby.

90. *Proceedings from the first international conference on transgender law and employment policy*, Houston, 1992, Phillis Randolph Frye.

91. Public Health Service: *Promoting health/preventing disease: year 2000 health objectives for the nations*, draft for public review and comment, USGPO, Washington, DC, 1989, US Dept of Health & Human Services.

92. Raff B, Friesner A: *Quick reference to maternity nursing*, Rockville, Md., 1989, Aspen Publishers.

93. Rocker I: *Pelvic pain in women: diagnosis and management*, New York, 1990, Springer-Verlag.

93a. Rothblatt MA; *Second report of the health law project, second international conference on transgender law and employment policy: transsexual and transgender health law*, August 1993.

94. Sandmaier M: *The healthy heart handbook for women*, National Institutes of Health, Bethesda, Md., 1987, US Department of Health and Human Services.

95. Seeley RR, Stephens TD, Tate P: *Anatomy and physiology*, ed 2, St. Louis, 1992, Mosby.

96. Seidel HM et al.: *Mosby's guide to physical examination*, ed 2, St. Louis, 1991, Mosby.

97. Sitruk-Ware R, Bardin CW: *Contraception: newer pharmacological agents, devices, and delivery systems*, New York, 1992, Marcel Dekker.

98. Smith DB: Sexual rehabilitation of the cancer patient, *Cancer Nurs* 12(1):10-15, 1989.

99. Sonstegard LJ, Kowalski KM, Jennings B: *Women's health: ambulatory care*, vol 1, New York, 1982, Grune & Stratton.

100. Speroff L, Glass RH, Kase NG: *Clinical gynecologic endocrinology and infertility*, Baltimore, 1983, Williams & Wilkins.

100a. Spiessl B, Beahrs OH, Hermanek P et al., editors: *TNM atlas*, ed 3, New York, 1990, Springer-Verlag.

100b. Stark DD, Bradley WG Jr: *Magnetic resonance imaging*, ed 2, vol 2, St. Louis, 1992, Mosby.

101. Stenchever MA: *Office gynecology*, St. Louis, 1992, Mosby.

102. Stine GJ: *The biology of sexually transmitted diseases*, Dubuque, Iowa, 1992, WC Brown Publishers.

103. Thibodeau GA, Anthony CP: *Structure and function of the body*, St. Louis, 1988, Mosby.

104. Thompson JM et al.: *Mosby's clinical nursing*, ed 3, St. Louis, 1993, Mosby.

105. Turner LW et al.: *Health concepts and strategies*, ed 2, St. Paul, 1992, West Publishing.

106. Upton AC et al.: *Staying healthy in a risky environment: the New York University Medical Center family guide*, New York, 1993, Simon & Schuster.

107. Vickers MJ: Understanding obesity in women, *JOGNN* 22(1):17-23, Jan/Feb 1993.

107a. Willson JR, Carrington ER: *Obstetrics and gynecology*, ed 9, St. Louis, 1991, Mosby.

107b. Whitney C, Daroff R: An approach to migraine, *J Neurosci Nursing*, 20:5, 1988.

107c. Whaley LP, Wong DL: *Nursing care of infants and children*, ed 4, St. Louis, 1991, Mosby.

108. Wistreich GA: *The sexually transmitted diseases: a current approach*, Dubuque, Iowa, 1992, WC Brown Publishers.

109. Wolfe SM, Jones R: *Women's health alert*, Redding, Mass., 1991, Addison-Wesley.

110. Women's Health Collective, *The all new our bodies, ourselves*, New York, 1984, Simon & Schuster.

Index

DUE DATE

MAR 1 9 1996			
JUL 1 5 1996			
NOV 2 8 1997			
APR			
DEC 1 8 2007			
			Printed in USA

RESOURCES TO ASSIST WOMEN IN THEIR HEALTH CARE

AIDS Network Hotline (National)
800-342-AIDS (2437)
800-344-SIDA (7432) for Spanish
800-AIDS-TTY for the hearing impaired

Alcohol Hotline
800-ALCOHOL (252-6465)

American Association of Retired Persons (AARP)
3200 East Carson Street
Lakewood, CA 90712
310-496-5233

American Cancer Association's Hotline
800-562-2623

American Cancer Society Helpline
800-227-2345

American Fertility Society
1209 Montgomery Highway
Birmingham, AL 32516
205-978-5000

Ask-a-Nurse
800-321-6877 or 800-535-1111

Association of Voluntary Sterilization, Inc. (AVS)
79 Madison Avenue
New York, NY 10016
212-351-2500

Cancer Information Service
800-4-CANCER (422-6237)

Cocaine Hotline
800-COCAINE (262-2463)

Consumer Information Center
18th and F Streets, NW
Washington, DC 20405
202-501-1794

Consumer Product Safety Commission Hotline
800-638-CPSC (2772)

Department of Health and Human Services (HHS)
Hubert H. Humphrey Building
200 Independence Avenue, SW
Washington, DC 20201
202-619-0257

DES Action USA
1615 Broadway, Room 510
Oakland, CA 94612
510-465-4011

Endometriosis Association
8585 North 76th Place
Milwaukee, WI 53223
414-355-2200 or 800-992-3636

Herpes-REACH
PO Box 649, Station P
Toronto, ON M5S 2Y4
Canada
Information 416-340-3959
Support group 416-449-0876

Medic-Alert Foundation International
2323 Colorado Avenue
Turlock, CA 95381-1009
209-668-3333

National Abortion Federation Consumer Hotline
800-772-9100

National Anorexic Aid Society, Inc.
1925 East Dublin-Granville Road
Columbus, OH 43229
614-436-1112

National Center for Health Information
Office of Disease Prevention and Health
  Promotion (ODPHP)
PO Box 1133
Washington, DC 20013-1133
800-336-4797 or 301-565-4167

National Council on Family Relations
3989 Central Avenue, NE, Suite 550
Minneapolis, MN 55421
612-781-9331

National Foundation March of Dimes
1275 Mamaroneck Avenue
White Plains, NY 10605
914-428-7100
800-326-2229